A HISTORY OF ITALIAN FERTILITY

This book is the third in a series on the decline of European fertility published for the Office of Population Research, Princeton University.

A History of Italian Fertility

During the Last Two Centuries

BY MASSIMO LIVI-BACCI

PRINCETON UNIVERSITY PRESS
PRINCETON, NEW JERSEY

Published by Princeton University Press, Princeton, New Jersey
In the United Kingdom: Princeton University Press, Guildford, Surrey

Library of Congress Cataloging in Publication Data will
be found on the last printed page of this book

Publication of this book has been aided by the Office of Population
Research and the Whitney Darrow Publication Reserve Fund of
Princeton University Press

This book has been composed in Linotype Times Roman

Printed in the United States of America
by Princeton University Press, Princeton, New Jersey

Foreword

About ten years ago Massimo Livi-Bacci committed part of his time and energy to collaboration in an ambitious demographic research project centered at the Office of Population Research in Princeton. The purpose of this project is to document and analyze the extensive reduction in human fertility that has been experienced in the past century or so in virtually every large geographic subdivision of every country in Europe. Although the occurrence of a decline has been practically universal, the time of its initiation and the pace at which it developed has been quite varied—birth rates were falling as early as the end of the eighteenth century in parts of France, and as late as the mid-twentieth century in Albania.

The conditions under which women begin to bear fewer children is a subject of great interest today; one of the most readily accepted ideas at the World Population Conference in Bucharest in 1974 is the belief in a virtually automatic reduction in fertility.

It is hoped that the books that emerge from this project will be valuable in two ways: in providing the quantitative history of a profound social change in each country (the decline in fertility itself), and as a contribution to better general knowledge of the circumstances under which women begin to bear fewer children. This project was originally supported by the Rockefeller Foundation and the National Science Foundation. In recent years, the National Institute of Child Health and Human Development has provided the bulk of the support, including Professor Livi-Bacci's research on Italian fertility.

Professor Livi-Bacci was the author of the first book to be published in the series presenting the results of the European Fertility Project—*A Century of Portuguese Fertility*, published in 1971. He has also written several articles on trends in fertility in Spain since the late eighteenth century. In this book he presents a detailed account and careful analysis of the varied experience in Italy. He includes, as background for the modern experience of falling birth rates since the unification of Italy in 1861, an examination of old records from fifteenth-century Florence and eighteenth-century cities in the south of Italy. (These records show that the number of surviving children per family was *positively* associated with income in these populations—a relation, the author speculates, that was reversed during the modern transition to low fertility, but may be restored when the practice of birth control becomes virtually universal.) The greater part of the book, however, is devoted to a presentation and analysis of the history of fertility since 1861, since which date, population records have included periodic censuses and virtually complete registration of births and deaths. The presentation includes maps, figures, and tables showing the evolution of fertility in considerable geographic detail for the century after unification.

The author has also examined the occasional Italian records that provide evidence on the number of children born to couples in different social and economic categories, as well as the more generally available evidence on geographic differences. He finds that some groups—Italian Jews, for one example, and titled families, for another—had reduced their fertility even before the nineteenth century. Certain categories of government employees for whom fertility information is fortuitously preserved had lower fertility by the mid-nineteenth century than the general population.

It is true that fertility is lower than in the past in all very highly modernized societies. As Professor Livi-Bacci once remarked, city apartment dwellers who have telephones, automobiles, and television sets do not have eight children. However, the existence of a simple relation between readily identified features of development and reduced fertility is challenged by the experience of sustained high fertility in countries that have enjoyed substantial social and economic progress (such as Mexico and the Central Asian Republics of the Soviet Union), and the reduction of fertility in areas that remain rural, not generally literate, and subject to high mortality (such as Bulgaria in the 1920s). The unparalleled detail and completeness of European demographic statistics provide the opportunity to examine the circumstances under which fertility declined in a large number of geographic areas (more than 700 provinces) with diverse cultures and economic conditions—and diverse dates at which the trend in question was initiated. The project includes separate studies of a number of countries, some conducted by demographers on the staff at the Office of Population Research, and some (as in this instance) by cooperating experts at universities or research centers in Europe or America.

His colleagues on the European Fertility Project and at the Office of Population Research will in years to come recall with pleasure and gratitude Professor Livi-Bacci's contribution to their ideas, during many hours of discussion and debate, and the permanent availability of his solid scholarship in the two books he has contributed to the project.

ANSLEY J. COALE
Director, Office of Population Research
Princeton University

Preface

This book on Italian fertility presents the results of research carried out during the last ten years. In 1965, I wrote an article in which the first data were presented and the first hypothesis was advanced on the fertility decline in Italy during the last century. In the following years, my research on the subject was abandoned and then resumed several times in a reflection of the strength of other competing interests and obligations. During the summers of 1965 and 1967, which were spent in Princeton at the Office of Population Research, I had the opportunity to discuss some of my plans as well as my first findings with colleagues in the European Fertility Project. It was only in 1973 that I started the actual writing of the book; it was completed in 1974 at Princeton during part of a sabbatical supported by the Population Council.

A particular debt of gratitude is owed to two persons. One is Ansley J. Coale, director of the project, with whom I have discussed practically every part of this book. The other is my father, the late Livio Livi, a demographer and social scientist who, through discussions and in other mysterious ways, passed on to me much of his vast knowledge of the Italian population.

My grateful thanks go also to my friends and colleagues of the Office of Population Research in Princeton and of the Dipartimento Statistico in Florence. Etienne van de Walle, Jane Menken, and Allan Hill in Princeton and Carlo Corsini and Antonio Santini in Florence helped me in various ways and at various stages of my work; all deserve my gratitude.

I had the courage to write this book in English, in spite of my limited command of the language. Patricia Taylor did her best to ensure conformity of my manuscript to the laws of the English language, although I am told that the Latin structure that pervaded the original text is still evident here and there. She also edited the text and the tables; in short, she transformed a poor manuscript into what I hope to be now an acceptable book. Ann Ryder patiently typed the more than one hundred tables that appear in the manuscript as well as the text itself; Richard Boscarino did the illustrations; and statistical checking was performed by Kirsten Yocom.

Finally, I have also the pleasure of acknowledging the financial help of the National Institute of Child Health and Human Development, which has supported the overall work of the European Fertility Project and my specific research on Italy.

Massimo Livi-Bacci

Florence
November 1975

Contents

List of Tables

CHAPTER 1

CHAPTER 2

CHAPTER 3

LIST OF TABLES

CHAPTER 4

CHAPTER 5

CHAPTER 6

CHAPTER 7

APPENDIX A

APPENDIX B

List of Maps and Figures

A HISTORY OF ITALIAN FERTILITY

Introduction

This book deals with demographic change in Italy during the last two centuries, or, more precisely, with a particular aspect of demographic change: the decline of fertility.

Approximately 150 million Italian children were born between the beginning of the nineteenth century and 1961, the year that marked the centennial of Italian independence and unification. During this time span the demographic behavior of the Italian population, as of all European populations, radically changed. Women, once inexorably destined for marriage, frequent childbirth, and early onset of old age, have been freed from the tyranny of biological events. At the same time, death has become relatively less frequent and the life span has doubled; frequent mortality crises (from typhus, cholera, smallpox, or famine) have disappeared, with the tragic exception of war. Mobility has increased and people have emigrated from the country by the million. Internal migration has profoundly changed the pattern of settlement, depopulating the mountain and rural areas and inflating the urban ones.

With a few variants, this summary of the main aspects of demographic change could fit the description of the history of any European country during the nineteenth and the twentieth centuries. The Italian population, therefore, is not a special case and fits very well in the general pattern of demographic change within European populations. So does the change of fertility, of course with its own peculiarities.

The birth rate of Italy started declining at the end of the nineteenth century, about a century later than that of France, a few decades later than that of other western European countries, and a few decades earlier than that of other Mediterranean populations. The timing of the decline is in agreement with the place and role of Italy in Europe and with her double soul, Continental and Mediterranean at the same time.

At the other end of the time scale, the same situation is reproduced. Low fertility, compatible with the pace and structure of modern times, was not reached until after World War II, a couple of decades later than in the other western countries, but well in advance of Spain and Portugal, where the transition to low levels of fertility had not yet come to an end. What is true of fertility, is true of many other indicators of social and economic development: the level of Italian education, income, and industrialization is behind that of western Europe and ahead of that of the Mediterranean countries. The last of the European countries and the first of the Mediterranean ones, as a popular and abused expression used to say.

The detailed analysis of Italian fertility presented in this book does not modify the terms of the generalization concerning the place of Italy in the European demographic scene. But generalizations on the basis of superficial analogy and parallelism are extremely dangerous and often of little heuristic value in the social sciences. They do not help very much in determining casual factors and in assessing relationships between the various phenomena. Indeed, when the analysis uncovers the hidden aspects and patterns of change, the detailed features of territorial and class differences, and the varying correlates of the phenomena under study, then generalizations appear to be what they are: summaries, more or less correct, of past events rather than laws or models. This is also the lot of the theory of the demographic transition: a summary of demographic change over a given historical period and geographical area rather than the essence and the core of an articulate system of functional relationships empirically tested and proved. Even as a summary, the theory of the demographic transition has to allow for too many exceptions (why did the fertility decline start earlier in rural France than in industrial England?) to be convincing.

In the social sciences (and demography is no exception), the process of knowledge goes through steps and stages often in a dialectical sequence. Constants, regularities, and laws are too often the consequence of our inability, for lack of documentation or insufficiency of research, to know the facts with precision. For example, the hypothesis that fertility behavior was more or less uniform in predecline times, as a consequence of the lack of fertility control, has melted like snow under the sun in the light of a deeper and more methodical historical research, which has made evident an unsuspected variety of situations. New historical analysis helps in testing, and generally in destroying, generalizations (or theories) formulated at a lower level of knowledge. Then, of course, the need for a new systematic presentation of facts for new generalizations arises. The new theories may be similar, different, or complementary to the old ones, but they will never be identical because they are formulated at a higher level of knowledge. This book, along with the other monographs on European countries in the Princeton Fertility Project, tends precisely to fulfill this task. The aim is to test, dismantle, and possibly rebuild with more refined elements the accepted generalizations as to the modes, patterns, and factors of the secular process of fertility decline. But many difficulties stand in the way.

First, there are several problems concerning the sources and the methods. We have to establish the facts: we have to analyze fertility change as precisely as possible and with detail. When possible, we have exploited the available statistical material with a uniform methodology that will ensure comparability with the results of the other studies conducted on other European countries. Of uniformity, however, we have not made a myth, and we have used a variety of measures and data every time this was helpful in establishing facts and testing hypotheses.

Second, there was the problem of choosing the historical limits of the investigation. The temptation was to start the analysis with 1861. This is the year of Italian unification and of the first national census; and, in practice, it marks the beginning of the national statistical system. At that time, fertility had not yet started to decline, at least at the national level, so that the process could be followed from the start with uniform data and uniform methodology. But, there were other, equally valid reasons to start at an earlier date: (1) the existence of a substantial body of statistical material and of a respectable volume of research for the first part of the nineteenth century: (2) the belief that the demographic history of modern Italy, and particularly the history of differential demographic change of the territorial areas, cannot be well understood without a precise knowledge of the character of the states before unification; and (3) the hypothesis, readily confirmed by our findings, that fertility decline, although starting at the national level in the 1890s, had already occurred in geographically and socially delimited areas well before unification.

To start systematically from the time of the Napoleonic hegemony over Europe and Italy (although we will frequently intrude into earlier historical periods) seems a just compromise; indeed, the Napoleonic times spread long lasting seeds of social change on a soil already made fertile by the age of Enlightenment and by reformism.

The third set of problems relates to the necessary links between demographic analysis and the analysis of the social, economic, and cultural changes in Italian society. We have dealt with this problem in a very empirical and unsystematic way, in part under the constraint of the lack of quantitative material, and in part as a consequence of the unsatisfactory state—theoretical and methodological—of the relationships between demography and the other social sciences. Although we have done our best to establish the links between demographic and social change, there is still ample ground for further research.

A fourth set of problems was posed by the need—deeply felt by the author—to link the results of demographic analysis with the pace and patterns of the cultural modifications in the Italian society. Unfortunately, we have done little more than acknowledge a need for a higher level of knowledge in this field. Fertility changes are the consequence of deliberate and conscious decisions taken at the individual level by couples. They imply complex modifications in the systems of preferences and values attached by individuals to the children and to the family. These preferences and values are part of a more general system involving the relations between individuals and between individuals and society. In this respect, we do not know very much about our contemporaries, but we know far less about our ancestors. The history of social psychology and the "histoire des mentalités" have a long way to go, and demographers have still to devise ways of taking advantage of their findings.

With the ambitions and limitations explained in these pages, this book is composed of seven substantive chapters. Chapter 1 examines the situation of the states from Napoleonic times to 1860. With the limitations of the material, we have tried to outline trends and differentials. Chapter 2 deals with the analysis, carried out with uniform methodology, of fertility and nuptiality trends of the regional populations from 1861 to 1961. Chapter 3 examines urban-rural differentials in fertility and nuptiality, and Chapter 4 is devoted to a detailed geographical analysis of fertility at the provincial level and, in some cases, for several hundred smaller administrative units. Chapter 5 consists of a multivariate analysis of the relations between fertility and a few indicators of the demographic, social, and economic characteristics of the provinces, from 1881 to 1961. In Chapter 6 we have studied differential fertility, trying to reconcile the different patterns of differential behavior before, during, and after the secular decline of fertility. Chapter 7 discusses several demographic, biological, and social factors that, although relevant to fertility, did not fit into the structure of the analysis in the preceding chapters. These factors are the role of breastfeeding and of other biological characteristics in determining the predecline levels of fertility as well as the territorial differentials; and the role of family structure, of emigration, and of the demographic policy of fascism in determining the differential pace of change in the various areas and sectors of the population. The main findings and conclusions of the book are reappraised in the final chapter, while the technicalities concerning the quality and the comparability of the data, as well as the reconstruction of comparable regional and provincial series, are contained in Appendixes A, B, and C.

Chapter 1: From Napoleonic Times to National Unification

1.1 *Hypotheses and Facts*

The modern demographic history of the Italian state cannot begin before 1861, which was both the date of national unification and the year of the first national census. In the ensuing years, a methodical and continuous collection of vital statistics also started in the several thousand comuni that form the smallest administrative units of the country.

Before 1861, however, there is much of demographic interest: some of the events before 1861 have a direct bearing on Italy's demographic circumstances in the latter part of the nineteenth century. Although fertility only began to fall in Italy as a whole at the end of the nineteenth century, in some areas (notably Toscana, Piemonte, and Liguria) the decline started well before the end of the century and, in some instances, in the decade following unification. Moreover there is as yet no definite proof that the levels of fertility prevailing in the 1860s are not themselves the outcome of an earlier, perhaps slower, decline. For certain sectors of the population (such as religious minorities or social elites) the decline may have started well before unification without showing up in the aggregate data for the country as a whole, or for its regions or provinces.

The first chapter of the book, therefore, deals with fertility before unification, and exploits the large volume of published and unpublished material available for the half-century from Napoleonic times to 1861. This material, although invaluable, makes the application of sophisticated methodology and uniform systems of analysis impossible; the information originates from seven or eight politically independent states with primitive and changing procedures for gathering demographic statistics. Even after 1861, boundary changes complicate the analysis.

For the first five or six decades of the nineteenth century, the analysis is based on material of uneven completeness and quality. The main aim is to give some insight into the regional variability of fertility in pre-unification Italy and to search for urban-rural or social differentials that may carry through into the post-1861 period. The findings will at best indicate the possibilities for more systematic research among the dispersed, but rich, historical sources.

1.2 *Organization of the Statistical Services and Nature of the Sources*

The first six decades of the nineteenth century may be roughly subdivided into two periods: the first, prior to 1815, marked by the direct or indirect influence of the Napoleonic Empire; the second, from 1815 to 1860, characterized by the return to the pre-Napoleonic situation and by the slow preparation for unification.[1] The French influence, important for so many aspects of the political, social, and cultural life of the Italian people, also affected the organization of the statistical system. The need for statistics and for quantitative and qualitative information concerning many aspects of demographic, economic, and social life was deeply felt by the authorities of the Empire, and the demand for data was continuous from the first years of the Consulate to the fall of Napoleon.[2] From 1800 on, several Italian regions fell under the direct rule first of the Republic and later of the Empire: Piemonte and Liguria, the Ducato di Parma, the Granducato di Toscana, and part of the Stato Pontificio (Umbria and Lazio); the remainder of Central and Northern Italy was organized under the Regno d'Italia (Kingdom of Italy), but the influence of the Empire was very strong and close. More than half the Italian population was, therefore, administered according to principles derived from the Code Napoleon. The existing statistical data make reference to the comuni and dipartimenti. The former was the traditional administrative subdivision, whereas the latter was altogether new to the Italian states. Of the rest of Italy, the largest part—the Regno di Napoli (Sicilia excluded)—fell under French political influence and participated, to a certain extent, in the administrative innovations introduced by the Code Napoleon.[3] Only the islands, Sicilia and Sardegna, remained untouched by innovation.

[1] For a historical outline of the development of the statistical organization from the Napoleonic times to unification, see U. Giusti, *Pagine di storia della statistica italiana: Dalla metà del secolo XVIII fino alla formazione del Regno*, in ISTAT, *Decennale*, Roma, 1936, pp. 5-18.

[2] C. Corsini, "Le migrazioni stagionali di lavoratori nei dipartimenti italiani nel periodo Napoleonico (1810-12)," in *Saggi di Demografia Storica*, Dipartimento Statistico Matematico, Firenze, 1969, pp. 98-101.

[3] R. Zangheri, *La popolazione Italiana in età Napoleonica*, Bologna, 1966, p. 4. The book is a useful guide to the demographic sources of the Napoleonic times. See also, E. Sonnino, "Le rilevazioni demografiche di stato in periodo napoleonico e postnapoleonico fino all'unificazione," in Comitato Italiano per lo Studio della Demografia Storica, *Le fonti della demografia storica in Italia*, Roma, 1973.

The French influence marks an innovation from the point of view of statistics for three reasons:

(1) because the civil authorities are substituted for the clergy in the responsibility for data collection
(2) because the curiosity of the ruler is not satisfied by the mere collection of data on population, births, deaths, and marriages, but demands information concerning pauperism, migration, health, criminality, and many other aspects of social life
(3) because a new dimension and scope is given to statistical surveys, which, earlier, were restricted to the narrow limits of the parish, the diocese, or, at most, the state, but now are referred to new, broader political areas.

With the Restoration in 1815, the prerogatives of the clergy in the collection of vital data were restored, and remained more or less untouched until unification. But the Napoleonic influence was not lost. In some of the states, most notably Regno di Sardegna and Granducato di Toscana, centralized systems for data collection, and in some instances for their publication and analysis, were set up. In Toscana, beginning in 1817, a centralized bureau (*Ufficio di Stato Civile*) was organized, to which copies of the individual records of birth, death, and marriage were transmitted monthly by the parishes (about 2500 in number) of the Granducato.[4] The individual records for the period 1808–1865 are kept in Firenze's National Archive.

In Piemonte, a Central Commission for Statistics was created in 1836 and for several years issued directives for the collection and elaboration of demographic data. This Commission supervised the three censuses of 1838, 1848, and 1858 and their publication, and also ordered several surveys in the field of demographic statistics. A few important publications testify to this activity.[5] In Lombardia and Veneto, the Austrian administration continued the brilliant statistical tradition initiated in Lombardia in the eighteenth century, and population and vital statistics were collected annually for the various administrative areas and trans-

[4] A. Zuccagni-Orlandini, *Ricerche Statistiche del Granducato di Toscana*, Firenze, 1848, I: 489.

[5] *Informazioni Statistiche raccolte dalla Regia Commissione Superiore per gli Stati di S. M. in Terraferma*, Torino, Vol. I, 1839 (1838 Census); Vol. II, 1843 (vital statistics 1828-1837); Vol. III, 1847 and Vol. IV, 1849 (medical statistics); Vol. V, 1852 (1848 Census).

mitted to Vienna. Few data were published at the time, in accord with the secrecy with which the Austrian Empire surrounded all statistical data.[6] In the Stato Pontificio no systematic collection of vital statistics was undertaken, except in the city of Roma.[7] A census for the entire state was taken in 1853.[8] Finally, in the Regno delle due Sicilie, statistical tables drawn from parish registers, concerning the size and distribution of the population and vital statistics, were collected and occasionally published in an aggregate form. The reliability of these statistics, given the successive manipulations of the parish data, is seriously questioned. More care was exercised in Sicilia, administratively autonomous from the rest of the kingdom, where a *Direzione Generale della Statistica*, created in 1832, collected and partly published the vital statistics of the island from the 1830s until unification.[9]

With the exception of the French period—a secular intermission in a clergy-dominated system of data collection—almost the whole body of statistical material is drawn from parish sources: records of baptisms, burials, and *status animarum*, the annual count of the parish population made by the priest at Easter. The quality of this vast statistical material, for the most part still buried in the archives, is unequal, and continuous critical caution is required in its analysis, partly because of the varying degree of care employed by the priests in the registration of vital events (which depended on the control exercised by the higher authorities and, also, on the cultural level of the clergy) and partly because of the varying criteria employed by the central authorities in the collection and aggregation of the parish data. Mistakes were frequent in the aggregation of the statistics, often because of the omission of particular sectors of the population (religious minorities, institutional populations, and foreigners). The time reference of the data is also sometimes uncertain.

But it must be remembered that a thick network of parishes covered

[6] M. Romani, "Il movimento demografico in Lombardia dal 1750 al 1850," *Economia e Storia* II, no. IV (1955): 413.

[7] F. Bonelli, *Evoluzione demografica ed ambiente economico nelle Marche e nell'Umbria nell'Ottocento*, Torino, 1967, pp. 1ff. P. Castiglioni, *Della popolazione di Roma dalle origini ai nostri tempi*, Roma, 1878, pp. 158ff.

[8] Ministero del Commercio e dei Lavori Pubblici, *Statistica numerativa della popolazione dello Stato Pontificio, dell'anno 1853*, Roma, 1857. A. Bellettini, "Contenuto e tecnica degli ultimi Censimenti dello Stato Pontificio," mimeograph, Gruppo di Demografia Storica, Bologna, 1972.

[9] Giusti, *Pagine*, pp. 5-18. Maggiore-Perni, *La popolazione di Sicilia e di Palermo nel secolo XIX*, Palermo, 1897.

the country, that the control of the clergy on the population was strict, and that very few vital events could pass unnoticed and unregistered.[10] In no respect can the statistical material of many premodern European populations be considered parallel with that of the developing nations of our time; and once collected and handled with careful critical sense, this material can give a good picture of the demographic situation of the country during the first sixty years of the century.

1.3 *Population Growth during the First Part of the Nineteenth Century*

A comprehensive history of the Italian population during the first part of the nineteenth century has still to be written. Although many monographs have been published—some of them very good—for the various states, a systematic study is lacking. Among the existing works, the most comprehensive is the rich monograph written by Castiglioni[11] as a historic introduction to the publication, in 1862, of the results of the censuses taken in 1857–1858 in several states of the North. In his work, the pre-unification statistical material—censuses and counts of the population of all kinds—is carefully collected, analyzed, and compared, of course, with the many limitations imposed by the rough techniques of analysis of the time. But Castiglioni purposely excluded from his analysis the vast and complex sector of vital statistics, and therefore this work is only indirectly useful for our purposes. It is, however, interesting to have a general idea of the growth of the population during the pre-unification period. Travaglini has critically analyzed, and partly corrected and integrated, Castiglioni's estimates; his series on the growth of the Italian population within the 1914 boundaries is given in Table 1.1. The rate of increase is, during the period considered, around .6 percent, almost identical to the rate of growth in the hundred years following unification, and not much higher than that experienced during the same period by Portugal (.4 percent) and Spain (.5 percent). Recurrent crises of mortality marked the history of the Italian population during the period under consideration—particularly the epidemic of typhus in 1817, and of cholera in the 1830s and again in the 1850s. The wars

[10] C. A. Corsini, "Libri dei matrimoni e della nascite," in Comitato Italiano, *Le fonti della demografia storica.*

[11] P. Castiglioni, *Introduzione storica dei Censimenti delle popolazioni italiane dai tempi antichi all'anno 1860*, Censimento degli antichi Stati Sardi (1.1.1858) e Censimento di Lombardia, di Parma e Modena, Ministero di Agricoltura, Industria e Commercio, Torino, 1862, Vol. I.

TABLE 1.1

TOTAL POPULATION: 1801 TO 1861

Date	Population (000)	Intercensal annual rate of increase (percent)
1801	17,860	--
1811	18,257	0.22
1821	19,000	0.41
1831	21,089	1.10
1841	22,355	0.60
1851	24,162	0.81
1861	25,017	0.35

SOURCE: V. TRAVAGLINI, La popolazione Italiana nel secolo anteriore all'unificazione del Regno, Padova, 1933, p. 42.

NOTE: Data are for boundaries of 1914.

of 1848 and 1859–1860 and the still recurrent food scarcities also had an effect on growth. The effects of extraordinary mortality were, however, much less disastrous than they were in the preceding centuries. In Toscana, where the average mortality rate during the first 60 years of the century was around 30 per thousand, mortality exceeded 40 per thousand in only two years (1817 and 1855). On the other hand, the political and economic crisis of the first two decades of the century depressed the marriage rate and, consequently, the birth rate; a strong recovery of marriages around 1820 caused an accelerated increase in births during the 1820s (the rate of increase of the population, according to Travaglini's estimate, reached the level, exceptional for Italy, of 1.1 percent during the 1821–1831 decade) followed by a slow decrease and a period of relatively low birth rate from the late 1830s to the early 1850s.

However, a general picture of population dynamics during the first part of the century is not yet possible, nor is it our task to fill this still considerable gap in the demographic history of the country.

1.4 *Some Characteristics of Premodern Fertility in Some Italian Villages*

Experience shows that premodern levels of fertility have, in many countries, a relatively high geographical variability. The extensive application of the techniques of family reconstruction to the demographic history of parishes and villages in many European countries has made possible an analysis of fertility patterns, to a degree of detail that is not possible with data from aggregate vital statistics. Age-specific or duration-specific fertility rates (by age at marriage), average intervals between births, age at birth of the last child, and other refined measures of fertility are commonly derived by the nominative system of family reconstruction. This reference to isolated parochial studies—generally in the period from the seventeenth to the early nineteenth century—may seem far from the scope of our study, which aims to describe the trends of Italian fertility in the last 150 years. In fact, only a few thousand families have been integrally reconstituted in the many villages for which this kind of analysis has been attempted.[12] Variation in fertility patterns may be imputed, in the first place, to the scarcity of cases on which the analysis has been based and to the fact that there has been no firm evidence that the families reconstituted are statistically representative of the universe (the parish or the groups of parishes). Variation may be also imputed to the peculiar characteristics of the various parishes studied. It is therefore difficult to assess in what proportion, and to what extent, fertility differentials can be accepted as typical.

We believe, however, that it may be useful to give the reader a brief survey of the levels of fertility in a few Italian villages for which nominative reconstitution has been attempted. The age-specific legitimate fertility rates for the five villages considered are reported in Table 1.2, together with the Hutterite fertility schedule, which will be employed later as a model of very high fertility, probably close to the maximum experienced by any sizeable population.

The fertility of the five villages is sensibly lower than that of the Hutterites, but within the normal range found in the studies concerning populations of the seventeenth to nineteenth centuries, and still apparently untouched by voluntary control of fertility. The average hypothetical number of children[13] per woman marrying at the age of 20 or 25 is 1/5 to 1/3 lower than that of the Hutterites.

Table 1.3 offers a few other indicators of fertility and nuptiality. The mean number of children per married woman, all ages at marriage, does not exceed six, including in the average all those marriages terminating

[12] M. Livi-Bacci, "Una disciplina in rapido sviluppo: la demografia storica," *Quaderni Storici* 17 (1971): 279-298.

[13] Sum of the age-specific marital fertility rates from age 20 (or 25) to age 50.

TABLE 1.2

AGE-SPECIFIC MARITAL FERTILITY OF SELECTED ITALIAN VILLAGES, 17TH-19TH CENTURIES, COMPARED WITH AGE-SPECIFIC MARITAL FERTILITY OF HUTTERITES, 1921-1930

Village	Date	Marital fertility rate by age at marriage							Hypothetical number of children per woman by age at marriage	
		Less than 20	20-24	25-29	30-34	35-39	40-44	45-49	20	25
Casalvecchio	1711-1750	.238	.370	.405	.337	.296	.235	.088	8.7	6.8
Empoli	1650-1700	.435	.434	.437	.384	.332	.165	.029	8.9	6.7
Fiesole	1630-1660	--	.466	.408	.353	.234	.144	.015	8.1	5.8
Pitigliano	1807-1866	.323	.471	.370	.354	.281	.177	.014	8.3	6.0
Ponte Buggianese	1700-1800	--	.332	.340	.323	.262	.167	.017	7.2	5.5
Hutterites	1921-1930	--	.550	.502	.447	.406	.222	.061	10.9	8.2

SOURCES: Empoli: P. MANETTI, Aspetti della fecondita' in Empoli dal 1650 al 1700, unpublished thesis in Demography, Faculty of Economics, University of Florence, 1969-70, p. 48; Fiesole: C. A. CORSINI, Problemi delle Ricerche di demografia storica, Società Italiana di Statistica, Proceedings of the XXVI meeting, Florence, 1969, Vol. III, p. 1084; Casalvecchio: S. FEDELE, Struttura e movimento della popolazione in una Parrocchia della Capitanata in "Quaderni Storici", VI, 17, 1971. Pitigliano and Ponte Buggianese, unpublished data, Dipartimento Statistico, University of Florence.

NOTE: Data for Pitigliano is for Jewish population only.

TABLE 1.3

MEAN NUMBER OF CHILDREN BY AGE AT MARRIAGE, MEAN AGE AT MARRIAGE, AND MEAN AGE AT BIRTH OF LAST CHILD, SELECTED ITALIAN VILLAGES: 17TH-19TH CENTURIES

Village	Date	Mean number of children by age at marriage						Mean total children	Mean age at marriage	Mean age at birth of last child	N
		Less than 20	20-24	25-29	30-34	35-39	40-44				
Empoli	1650-1700	7.1	6.5	5.2	3.4	4.0	--	6.0	23.8	35.1	256
Fiesole	1630-1660	6.0	5.9	5.6	3.3	3.0	--	5.6	23.7	36.7	176
Ponte Buggianese	1700-1800	6.3	5.7	3.9	2.7	3.0	--	4.6	26.6	35.9	302
Valdibure	1700-1800	6.8	6.3	5.0	4.5	3.7	1.3	5.2	26.5	37.5	153
Pitigliano	1807-1866	6.4	4.9	4.4	[a]	1.8[a]	[a]	5.0	25.3	--	96

SOURCE: Table 1.2 and unpublished data, Dipartimento Statistico, University of Florence.

NOTE: Data for Empoli and Fiesole are for families with at least one child.

[a] Mean for ages 30-44.

before the end of the reproductive period of the wife (45 years). If only "completed" marriages were to be taken into account (that is, those marriages terminating after the 45th birthday of the wife) the mean number of children would be raised by one to one and a half.[14] The mean age at birth of the last child was around 36-37 years, but wives of "completed" marriages had their last children two or three years later.

The mean birth interval was generally between 24 and 30 months, as can be seen from the data in Table 1.4.

TABLE 1.4

MEAN NUMBER OF MONTHS BETWEEN BIRTHS, BY PARITY, SELECTED ITALIAN VILLAGES: 17TH-19TH CENTURIES

Village	Date	Parity				
		1-2	2-3	3-4	4-5	5-6
Fiesole	1630-1660	25.9	29.5	30.6	32.1	31.9
Ponte Buggianese	1700-1800	33.1	31.5	31.2	36.8	36.7
Valdibure	1700-1800	24.9	29.2	30.7	32.4	31.6

SOURCES: Table 1.2 and unpublished data, Dipartimento Statistico, University of Florence.

After the first child, birth intervals range from two and one-half to three years. The length of breastfeeding probably plays a major role. Corsini has shown that birth intervals among wet nurses were five months longer than among other women.[15]

Given the small number of cases and the different periods and areas considered, these data certainly do not pretend to represent legitimate fertility in Italy as a whole. But the evidence collected is consistent with the impression, derived from other sources as well, that premodern fertility (combined with the patterns of marriage and widowhood that prevailed) produced only moderate numbers of children per family, with an average family size normally above five children but generally below six.

[14] In Empoli and Fiesole, the mean number of children, completed marriages, is 7.3 and 6.6, as against 6.0 and 5.6 for all marriages.

[15] C. A. Corsini, "Ricerche di demografia storica nel territorio di Firenze," *Quaderni Storici* 17 (1971): 395-397.

1.5 *Birth Rate of the Italian Dipartimenti during Napoleonic Times*

The centralized administrative system during Napoleonic times makes possible some knowledge of the level of the birth rate between 1807 and 1813. More exactly, the data concerning the population and the vital statistics of the dipartimenti incorporated, after 1806, in the French Empire, can be traced in scattered official publications and in the National Archives in Paris. These dipartimenti covered the greater part of Piemonte, Liguria, part of Emilia (roughly corresponding to the province of Parma), almost all of Toscana (with the exception of the nominally independent Ducato di Lucca), and Umbria and Roma with the Lazio. The total population this area was between 4 and 4.5 million, or about 1/4 of the total population of the time. The rest of Northern and Central Italy constituted, as said before, the Regno d'Italia, subdivided into 24 dipartimenti, with 6 million inhabitants, almost 1/3 of the total population.

The 1810–1812 birth rate for the 24 dipartimenti within the Regno d'Italia is reported in Table 1.5 and the 1807–1812 birth rate for the 15 dipartimenti within the French Empire is reported in Table 1.6. The quality of data is uncertain, since we do not know the procedure followed for their collection. In some cases, the passage of registration from the clergy to the civil bureaucracy may have resulted in the deterioration of their quality. The reservations advanced in Section 1.1 apply, of course, and more strongly, to this period's statistics. They apply especially to the evaluations of the total population, which, in the absence of a general census, depended on the care with which the *status animarum* were compiled in each parish. In the absence of a systematic matching between the aggregate data and the individual parish returns, it is impossible to judge their reliability. They are, however, the only element at hand and the birth rate patterns derived seem consistent with later levels.

In the dipartimenti of Northwestern Italy (part of the Empire) the general birth rate was 36.3 per thousand. Only one dipartimento, the Ombrone (later, provinces of Siena and Grosseto) had a birth rate above 40 (44.8), a rate, incidentally, found again at later dates. Otherwise, variability was limited, with the lowest rates (33-34) to be found in Liguria; this is, again, a result consistent with later findings.

The birth rate was higher in the Regno d'Italia—39.2 per thousand in 1810–1812. Variability was also a bit higher; a large portion, includ-

TABLE 1.5

BIRTH RATE, DIPARTIMENTI WITHIN REGNO D'ITALIA: 1810-1812

Dipartimento	Capital city	Birth rate
Adda	Sondrio	34.6
Adige	Verona	41.4
Adriatico	Venezia	35.7
Agogna	Novara	39.3
Alto Adige	Trento	40.0
Alto Po	Cremona	44.4
Bacchiglione	Vicenza	41.3
Basso Po	Ferrara	44.3
Brenta	Padova	41.9
Crostolo	Reggio	36.8
Lario	Como	40.3
Mella	Brescia	35.5
Metauro	Ancona	38.2
Mincio	Mantova	40.9
Musone	Macerata	36.2
Olona	Milano	44.7
Panaro	Modena	38.3
Passariano	Udine	31.4
Piave	Belluno	45.7
Reno	Bologna	37.5
Rubicone	Forli	37.6
Serio	Bergamo	39.0
Tagliamento	Treviso	36.4
Tronto	Fermo	31.5
Regno d'Italia		39.2

SOURCE: G. FERRARIO, Statistica Medico Economica di Milano, Vol. II, Milano, 1840-1850, P. 303.

ing the greater part of Veneto and part of Lombardia, had a birth rate standing at fairly high levels (40-45). Given the peculiar territorial subdivision of the Napoleonic times, which renders unclear any comparison with later findings based on the traditional administrative areas, we may only say that—at least as far as the high fertility areas are concerned—there is a certain consistency with later patterns.

TABLE 1.6

BIRTH RATE, ITALIAN DIPARTIMENTI WITHIN FRENCH EMPIRE: 1807-1812

Dipartimento	Capital city	Birth rate
Sesia	Vercelli	38.9
Dora	Ivrea	36.1
Po	Torino	36.0
Stura	Cuneo	37.3
Marengo	Alessandria	37.2
Montenotte	Savona	36.0
Genova	Genova	33.5
Appennini	Chiavari	33.7
Taro	Parma	--
Arno	Firenze	35.7
Mediterraneo	Livorno	35.2
Ombrone	Siena	44.8
Isola d'Elba	Portoferraio	--
Roma	Roma	36.4
Trasimeno	Spoleto	--
Total		36.3

SOURCES: The population of the Dipartimenti has been drawn from C. A. CORSINI, Le migrazioni stagionali dei lavoratori nel Dipartimenti Italiani del periodo Napoleonico (1810-12), in "Saggi di Demografia Storica", Dipart. Statistico Matematico, Florence, 1969, p. 106.
The births of the Dipartimenti have been kindly communicated by C. A. CORSINI, and extracted from the National Archives of Paris (F20.465 to F.20.470).

NOTE: The birth rates are based on the average number of births of 1807-1812, with the exception of Stura and Genova (1807-1811), Arno and Ombrone (1809-1812), Mediterraneo (1810), Roma (1811), Marengo (1807-1809 and 1811-1812).

The distribution of the 36 dipartimenti for which data are available according to the level of the birth rate is shown in Table 1.7; the strong concentration in the class 35-40 is as expected.

1.6 *Birth Rate of Provinces in Pre-unification States during the 1830s*

The gradual organization of the statistical services in the pre-unification states greatly increased with the passage of time the possibilities of reliable territorial analysis. Our effort has been directed, therefore, toward establishing the geography of natality during the 1830s, to achieve

TABLE 1.7

DISTRIBUTION OF 36 DIPARTIMENTI BY LEVEL OF BIRTH RATE: CIRCA 1810

Birth rate	Distribution Number	Percent
Less than 35.0	5	14
35.0 - 39.9	20	55
40.0 - 44.9	10	28
45.0 and more	1	3
Total	36	100

SOURCE: Composed from data presented in Tables 1.5 and 1.6.

an intermediate point of reference between the Napoleonic times—examined before—and the early post-unification situation. The quality of the available data has certainly changed for the better, but is still uneven in different areas. The best data are those for Piemonte and Liguria (Regno di Sardegna) and for Toscana.

For Piemonte and Liguria, the Commission created in 1836 (mentioned earlier) ordered a systematic collection of vital statistics from the parish books for the decade 1828–1837. The work was done, and published in 1842.[16] The Commission also supervised the census of 1838, which, together with the population count of 1824, provides a sound, although not perfect, basis for the computation of birth rates.

We have already noted how, in Toscana, the vital statistics were centralized in Firenze; Bandettini has carefully collected and elaborated the series, which refers to the actual provincial boundaries from 1809 on.[17] Parochial *status animarum* were annually compiled in each parish and transmitted to the same *Ufficio di Stato Civile* of Firenze, and in 1841 a census was taken.[18]

In Lombardo-Veneto, under Austrian rule, vital statistics were collected annually, but little work has been done to test their quality, which, given a strong statistical tradition, is probably acceptable.

In the Stato della Chiesa, vital statistics are available only for the

[16] *Informazioni Statistiche.*

[17] P. Bandettini, *L'evoluzione demografica della Toscana,* Torino, 1960.

[18] P. Bandettini, *La popolazione della Toscana alla metà dell'Ottocento,* Roma, 1956.

city of Roma and for Bologna. We have, however, estimated the birth rate through stable techniques of analysis based on the age structure provided by the 1853 census and the 1833–1853 rate of growth.

The quality of the data for Regno delle due Sicilie is presumably poorer, with the exception of Sicilia, where *Direzione Generale della Statistica* did some good work of collection and elaboration. For the rest of this kingdom, we may only say that the few tests made on the data for Calabria, extensively analyzed by Izzo,[19] have left us dubious about their quality.

In Table 1.8, we have reported the birth rate for 78 provinces, covering the whole of Italy, with the exception of the Ducato di Modena. In the same table, we have given some detailed information about the sources for the data, and indicated the years of reference, centered, for the greatest part, on the 1830–1840 decade. The matching of this table with Tables 1.5 and 1.6 and with Maps 1.1 and 1.2 shows that, roughly speaking, the geography of the birth rate remained approximately the same. Northwestern Italy (Piemonte and Liguria) had lower fertility than the Northeast (Lombardia and Veneto). Most provinces of Veneto had a birth rate above 40 per thousand, as in the early and late periods of the century. In the South, the eastern provinces of Abruzzi Citra, Molise, Capitanata, Terra di Bari, Terra d'Otranto, and Basilicata had higher birth rate levels, on the average well above 40 per thousand; in Sicilia, the south (Caltanissetta and Noto) had the highest birth rate. These provinces also show birth rates above average at the end of the century.

It must be noted that, in addition to the differing quality of the material, limitations to statistical comparability also occur as a result of the varying periods to which the data reported in Table 1.8 belong. The difference in dates presumably has little effect on the distribution of the provinces, as shown in Table 1.9, according to the level of the birth rate; but the distribution may well be biased by inaccurate data. More than half the provinces had a birth rate between 35 and 40 per thousand. Similar results had been obtained for the Napoleonic period.

In Table 1.10, we have reported the birth rate of 10 regions for which, with some approximation, there is a coincidence between the pre-unification and post-unification boundaries.

Everything considered, territorial fertility seems to retain characteris-

[19] L. Izzo, *La popolazione della Calabria nel secolo XIX*, Napoli, 1966.

TABLE 1.8

BIRTH RATE, BY STATE AND ADMINISTRATIVE SUBDIVISION: CIRCA 1830-1840

State	Subdivision	Birth rate	Date
PIEMONTE[a]		37.8	Births, 1828-1837; population, 1824 count of population and 1838 census
	1 Aosta	33.7	
	2 Torino	36.7	
	2a Ivrea	36.4	
	2b Torino	35.3	
	2c Pinerolo	37.9	
	2d Susa	35.9	
	2e Biella	40.5	
	3 Cuneo	38.3	
	3a Alba	34.6	
	3b Saluzzo	37.9	
	3c Mondovi	36.9	
	3d Cuneo	42.4	
	4 Novara	39.9	
	5 Alessandria	37.4	
	5a Casale	38.6	
	5b Asti	35.9	
	5c Alessandria	37.2	
	5d Tortona	35.6	
	5e Voghera	40.6	
	5f Acqui	35.8	
R. LOMBARDO		40.1	1830-1833
	6 Sondrio	39.1	
	7 Como	39.2	
	8 Bergamo	37.7	
	9 Milano	44.2	
	10 Brescia	35.0	
	11 Pavia	43.4	
	12 Lodi/Crema	41.4	
	13 Cremona	44.0	
	14 Mantova	37.7	
R VENETO		43.5	1830-1839
	15 Belluno	49.3	
	16 Friuli	38.8	
	17 Treviso	43.2	
	18 Vicenza	45.1	
	19 Venezia	41.6	
	20 Padova	46.2	
	21 Polesine	46.6	
	22 Verona	42.3	

State	Subdivision	Birth rate	Date
TOSCANA		37.8	1830-1839
	36 Lucca	32.3	
	37 Massa	35.3	
	38 Pisa	37.3	
	39 Pistoia	37.4	
	40 Firenze	39.2	
	41 Arezzo	37.2	
	42 Livorno	36.8	
	43 Siena	41.8	
	44 Grosseto	43.5	
ABRUZZI		36.2	
	45 Abruzzi Ult. I	31.7	1830-1841
	46 Abruzzi Ult. II	32.0	1830-1831; 1833-1835; 1839-1840
	47 Abruzzi Cit.	38.4	1830-1841
	48 Contado Molise	40.6	1830-1831; 1833-1835; 1840
CAMPANIA		35.2	
	49 Terra di Lavoro	33.8	1830-1840
	50 Napoli	40.1	1830; 1832-1834; 1832-1834; 1836-1840
	51 Principato Ultra	32.5	1830; 1833; 1836; 1839-1840
	52 Principato Cit.	32.5	1830-1833; 1835; 1837-1838, 1840
PUGLIA		42.6	
	53 Capitanata	44.8	1830; 1834-1835; 1840
	54 Terra di Bari	42.4	1830-1831; 1834-1835; 1840
	55 Terra d'Otranto	41.0	1830-1831; 1834-1835; 1840

	23 Oneglia	33.9	1828-1837; population, 1824 count of population and 1838 census				1840, 1841
	23a Nizza	34.8					
	23b San Remo	33.3		CALABRIA		36.8	
	23c Oneglia	33.0			57 Calabria Cit.	37.6	1830-1831; 1833-1834; 1839-1840
	24 Genova	36.7					
	24a Albenga	34.3			58 Calabria Ult. I	36.2	1830-1831; 1833-1834; 1837-1840
	24b Savona	37.7					
	24c Novi	35.8					
	24d Bobbio	35.6			59 Calabria Ult. II	36.3	1830-1831; 1833-1834; 1839-1840
	24e Genova	37.2					
	24f Chiavari	36.1					
	24g Levante	38.0					
				SICILIA		37.4	
25 DUCATO DI PARMA		39.3	1830-1833		60 Trapani	36.2	1832-1840
					61 Palermo	36.0	1831-1840
26-27 DUCATO DI MODENA		--			62 Messina	35.0	1832-1840
					63 Girgenti	38.0	1831-1840
					64 Caltanissetta	44.1	1832 1840
STATO PONTIFICIO		37.3	1833-1853[b]		65 Catania	37.3	1832-1840
					66 Noto	39.8	1832-1840
	28 Bologna	33.0	1843	67 SARDEGNA		34.0	Births, 1836; population, 1837 estimate
	29 Ferrara	--					
	30 Ravenna	--					
	31 Ancona	--					
	32 Perugia	--					
	33 Macerata	--					
	34 Fermo	--					
	35 Roma (city)	30.8	1830-1839				

SOURCES: Piemonte and Liguria: Births and 1838 population -- Informazioni Statistiche raccolte dalla Regia Commissione Superiore per gli Stati di S.M. in Terraferma; 1824 population -- G. Muttini Conti, La Popolazione del Piemonte nel Secolo XIX, Turin, 1962, pp. 16-17.

Lombardia: G. Ferrario, Statistica Medico-Economica di Milano, Vol. II, Milan, 1840-1850, pp. 314 and 316.

Veneto: Tafeln zur Statistik der Oesterreichischen Monarchie. Unpublished data supplied by Dr. A. Schiaffino, University of Bologna. Published statistics for years 1821-1823 can be found in A. Quadri, Atlante di LXXXII Tavole Sinottiche relativo al prospetto Statistico delle Provincie Venete, Venezia, 1827.

Ducato di Parma: L. Serristori, Statistica dell'Isola di Sicilia e del Ducato di Parma, Firenze, 1836.

Bologna: A. Bellettini, La popolazione della campagne bolognesi alla metà del Sec. XIX, Bologna, 1971, pp. 88-89, 92.

Roma: P. Castiglioni, Della popolazione di Roma dalle origini ai nostri tempi, Rome, 1878.

Toscana: P. Bandettini, L'evoluzione demografica della Toscana, Turin, 1960.

Campania, Abruzzi, Puglia, Basilicata, Calabria, and Sicilia (Regno delle due Sicilie): Unpublished data drawn from the volume now under press: F. Assante, D. Demarco, L. Izzo, La popolazione del Mezzogiorno d'Italia dal 1815 al 1890. Data reproduced by kind permission of the authors.

Sardegna: Calendario Generale del Regno di Sardegna 1838, Cagliari, no date.

[a] Data include stillbirths, which were underreported and amounted to only 1 percent.

[b] Stable techniques; $c_x(1853)$ = 5, 10, 20, 30, 40, 50, and 60. Median estimate, r = 1833-1853.

[c] Population does not include clergy, army, etc. Diocese of Ales (39,508 inhabitants) not included.

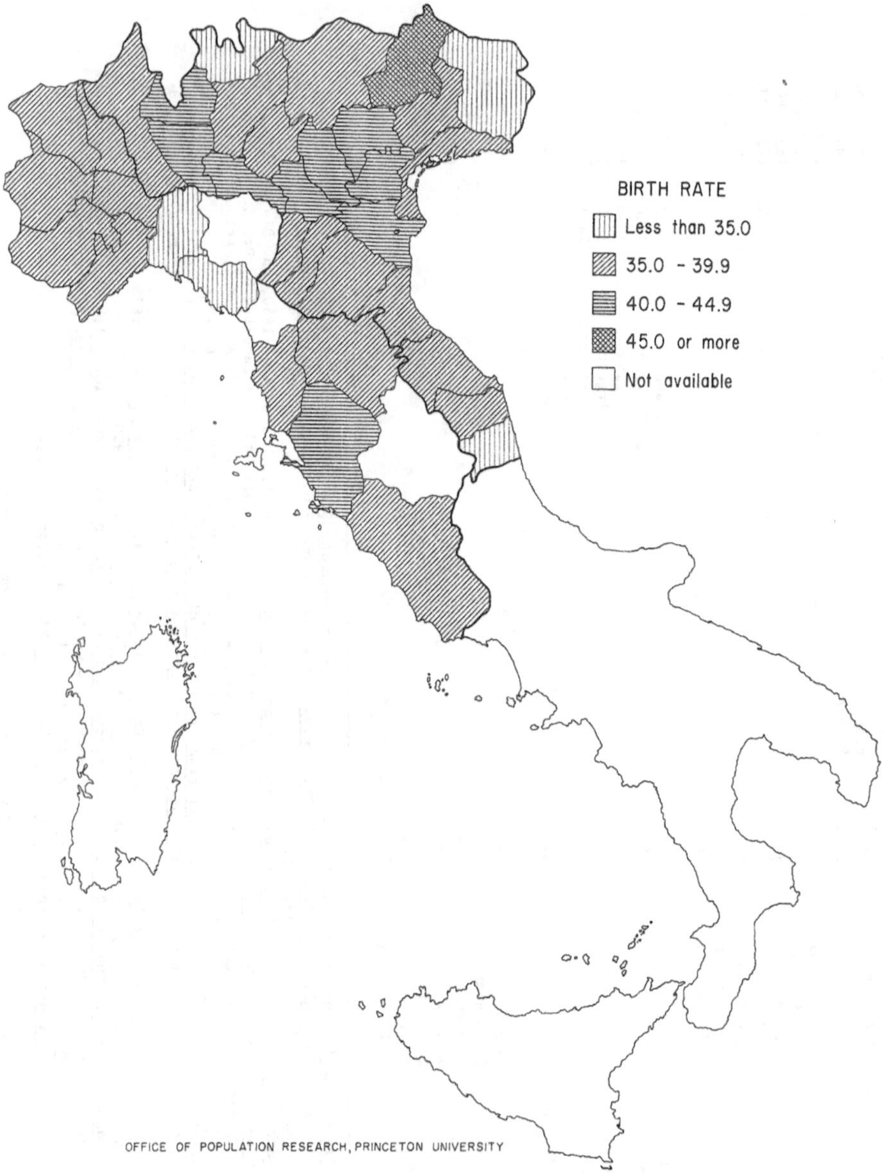

Map 1.1 Birth Rate, Italian Dipartimenti within French Empire, 1807-1812, and Regno d'Italia, 1810-1812

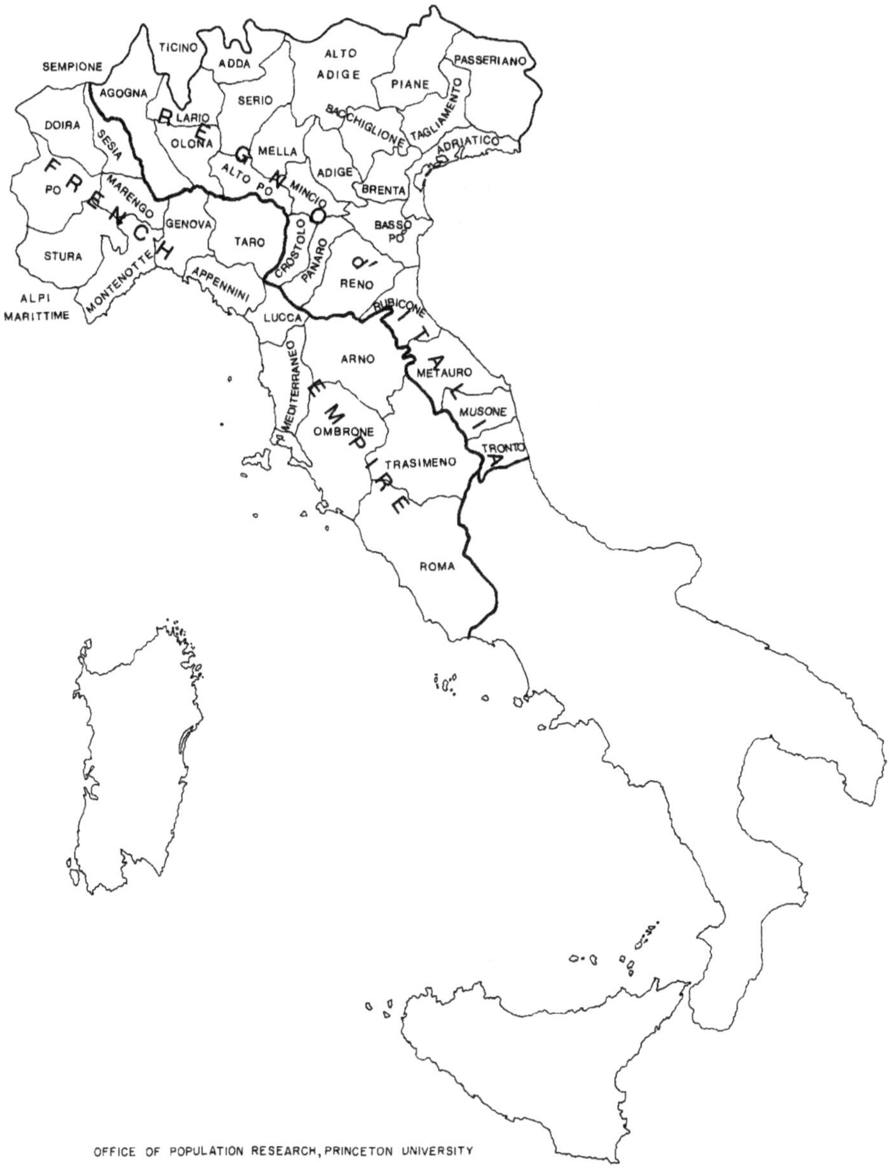
SEMPIONE
TICINO
ADDA
ALTO ADIGE
PASSERIANO
PIANE
AGOGNA
LARIO
SERIO
BACCHIGLIONE
TAGLIAMENTO
DOIRA
SESIA
OLONA
MELLA
ADRIATICO
ALTO PO
ADIGE
MINCIO
BRENTA
PO
MARENGO
GENOVA
TARO
BASSO PO
CROSTOLO
PANARO
STURA
RENO
APPENNINI
MONTENOTTE
ALPI MARITTIME
LUCCA
RUBICONE
ARNO
MEDITERRANEO
METAURO
MUSONE
OMBRONE
TRONTO
TRASIMENO
ROMA
FRENCH
EMPIRE
REGNO d'ITALIA
OFFICE OF POPULATION RESEARCH, PRINCETON UNIVERSITY

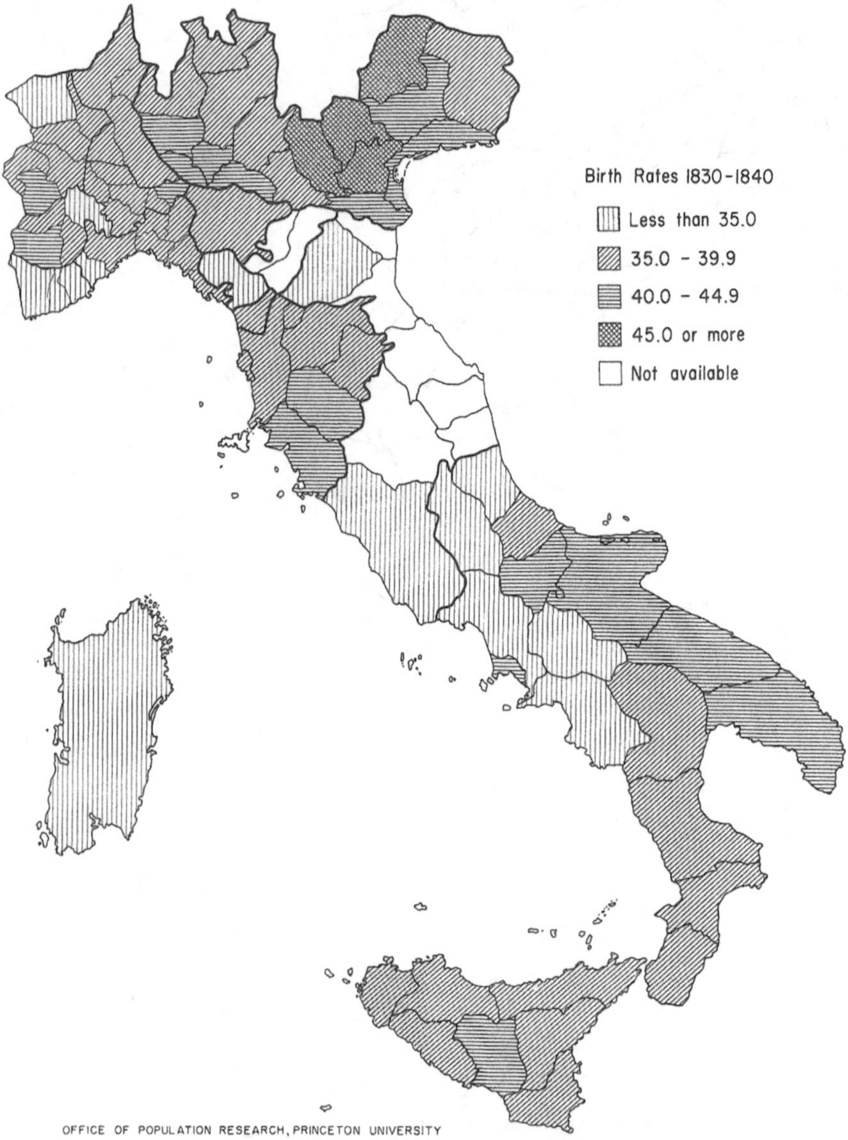

Map 1.2 Birth Rate, by State and Administrative Subdivision: Circa 1830-1840
Note: See Table 1.8 for names of geographic areas

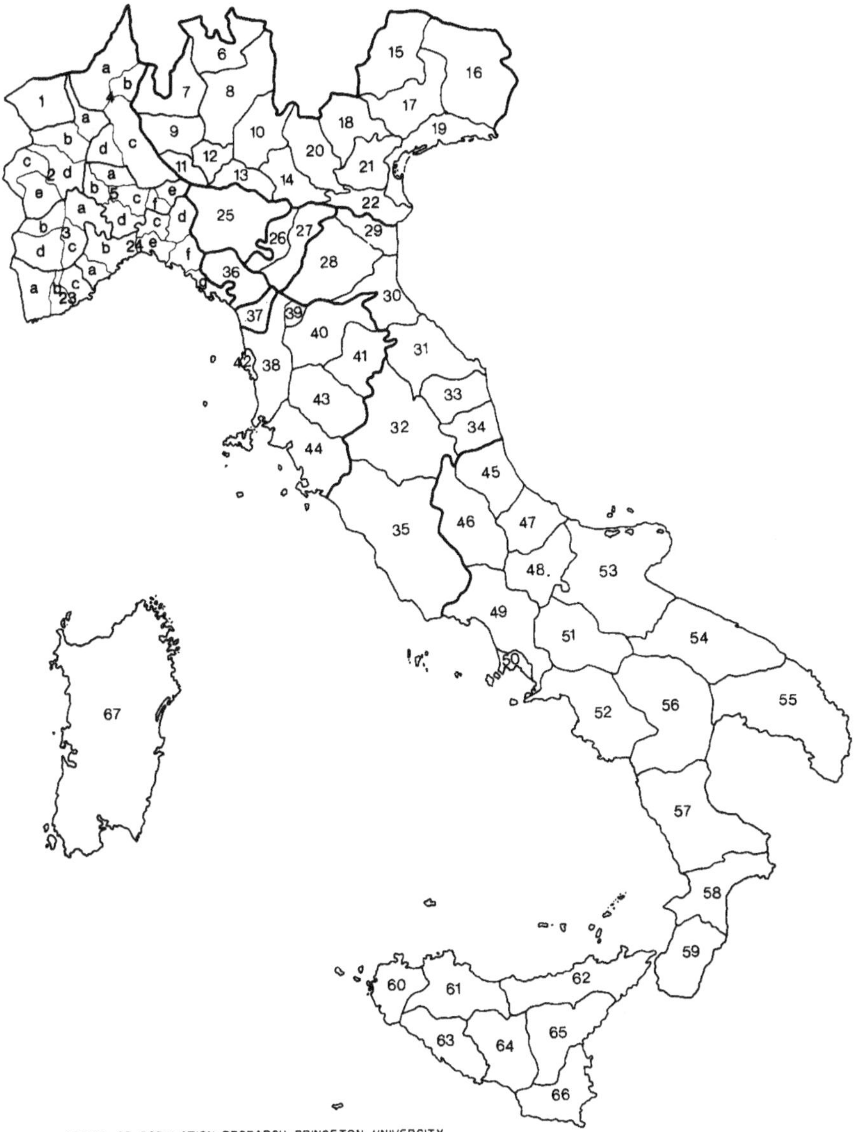

OFFICE OF POPULATION RESEARCH, PRINCETON UNIVERSITY

TABLE 1.9

DISTRIBUTION OF 79 PROVINCES BY LEVEL OF BIRTH RATE: CIRCA 1830-1840

Birth rate	Distribution: Number	Distribution: Percent
Less than 35.0	15	19
35.0 - 39.9	42	53
40.0 - 44.9	18	23
45.0 and more	4	5
Total	79	100

SOURCE: Composed from data presented in Table 1.8.

tics unchanged through time, so that, at least until the 1880s, there is a certain stability in the birth rate patterns.

1.7 *Fertility of Toscana in the Early Nineteenth Century*

The paucity and imperfection of available statistical material for Italy makes it difficult to go beyond raw measures such as the birth rate, or

TABLE 1.10

BIRTH RATE, SELECTED REGIONS: 1830s AND 1862-1866 TO 1880-1882

Region	1830s	1862-1866	1870-1877	1880-1882
Piemonte	37.8	36.2	35.7	34.7
Liguria	36.0	35.4	34.5	32.3
Lombardia	40.1	37.6	37.6	36.3
Veneto	43.5	--	37.6	34.5
Toscana	37.8	40.0	38.2	34.4
Campania	35.2	38.1	37.1	36.6
Abruzzi	36.2	37.6	36.8	38.2
Puglia	42.6	42.1	40.7	42.4
Basilicata	38.7	41.7	39.9	42.3
Sicilia	36.8	38.4	38.6	37.0
Mean	38.4	38.9	37.9	37.2

SOURCE: Composed from data presented in Tables 1.8 and 2.4.

NOTE: Boundaries of these regions remained almost the same throughout the given dates.

at most, the general fertility rate. However, for Toscana and, as we will see in the following section, for Piemonte and Liguria, a few more refined measures can be computed to yield additional information.

In Toscana it is possible to calculate, for each province, a very rough measure of legitimate fertility by dividing the number of legitimate births by the total number of married women. The obvious drawback of this measure derives from its including in the computation all those married women whose age is above the end of their reproductive period. However, for the nineteenth century, this limitation is not extremely serious; given the high rate of widowhood and the fairly young age-composition of the population, the proportion of the married women above 50 years of age did not exceed 25-30 percent. This measure is, for our purposes, more flexible than the birth rate or the general fertility rate, and more apt to describe trends in marital fertility.

Table 1.11 contains the crude marital fertility rate for seven of the nine provinces (modern boundaries) from 1814–1816 to 1876–1885. Overall, the provinces show a relatively low level of fertility in 1814–1816; a very high level in 1816–1825, which continuously declines until 1846–1855; a recovery in the following decade; and a new fall afterwards. If we started at 1816–1825, it would appear that the Tuscan provinces experienced an almost continuous decline of fertility until the end of the century. But the exceptional increase of marriages after 1817, strongly affecting the duration-structure of the existing marriages, is certainly responsible for part of the increase. But if we take as a starting point 1814–1816, a period with an unusually low number of births as a consequence of the fewer marriages of the Napoleonic period, we take a more conservative and prudent view of the trends, as is the case of the lower part of Table 1.11, in which we have reported the relative values of the crude marital fertility rates. Even taking as a reference the very low—probably abnormally low—level of 1814–1816, in two provinces (Livorno and Grosseto) fertility falls below 100 in 1836–1845; another province (Siena) can be added to the list in the following decade. In 1866–1875, all provinces, with the exception of Arezzo and Pistoia, have reduced their levels of fertility below the 1814–1816 values. On the other hand, taking a less conservative and cautious view, if we take as a reference the fertility levels of the 1816–1825 or even 1816–1835 (and it is difficult to label as "abnormal" or "exceptional" a twenty-year period of time) all provinces show reduced levels of fertility from 1836 on. Even the 1856–1865 decade, which marks a recovery, albeit

TABLE 1.11

GROSS MARITAL FERTILITY RATE, BY PROVINCE, TOSCANA: 1814-1816 TO 1876-1885

Province	1814-1816	1816-1825	1826-1835	1836-1845	1846-1855	1856-1865	1866-1875	1876-1885
	Actual levels							
Arezzo	185.1	231.8	223.3	199.5	194.8	210.4	190.8	176.5
Firenze	191.2	233.2	220.8	198.4	199.4	209.3	176.5	172.3
Grosseto	248.0	261.2	247.9	243.7	242.3	233.0	217.3	206.1
Pisa	190.4	211.6	220.7	203.9	212.1	199.1	173.5	153.3
Livorno	210.2	227.2	218.6	207.2	193.6	198.9	189.6	172.9
Pistoia	187.2	205.3	225.2	200.7	192.7	216.6	192.8	192.3
Siena	210.4	233.4	228.5	212.0	207.2	207.5	186.1	172.8
Total	198.3	229.0	222.8	204.5	201.4	208.7	185.1	175.0
	Relative levels (1814-1816 set at 100)							
Arezzo	100	125.2	120.6	107.8	105.2	113.7	103.1	95.4
Firenze	100	122.0	115.5	103.8	104.3	109.5	92.3	90.1
Grosseto	100	105.3	100.0	98.3	97.7	94.0	87.6	83.1
Pisa	100	111.3	115.9	107.1	111.4	104.6	91.1	80.5
Livorno	100	108.1	104.0	98.6	92.1	94.6	90.2	82.3
Pistoia	100	109.7	120.3	107.2	102.9	115.7	103.0	102.7
Siena	100	110.9	108.6	100.8	98.5	98.6	88.5	83.2
Total	100	115.5	112.4	103.1	101.6	105.2	93.3	88.3

NOTE: Gross Marital fertility rate refers to legitimate births per 1,000 married women.

temporary, of fertility, shows levels on the average 7-8 percent lower than the reference period.

The existence, for Toscana, of a continuous series of vital statistics, allows the computation of a perhaps more sophisticated measure of fertility. In Appendix B we show how, with the help of a standardized distribution of births by duration of marriage, it is possible to obtain a fairly good approximation of the mean number of children per marriage. In practice, the number of legitimate births of a given year is divided by a weighted average of the marriages of the preceding years; the weights are proportional to the fertility rates by duration of marriage of a standard population. The result, *F*, is an estimate of the gross productivity of marriages, or, in other words, of the mean number of children per marriage.[20]

The results for Toscana are presented, by five-year averages, in Table 1.12, together with the corresponding birth rates, 1820 to 1899. The

TABLE 1.12

NUMBER OF CHILDREN PER MARRIAGE (F) AND BIRTH RATE, TOSCANA: 1820-1824 TO 1895-1899

Date	Actual levels		Relative levels (1820-1824 set at 100)	
	F	Birth rate	F	Birth rate
1820-1824	5.64	43.2	100.0	100.0
1825-1829	5.52	42.6	97.9	98.6
1830-1834	5.33	39.3	94.5	91.0
1835-1839	5.12	36.2	90.8	83.8
1840-1844	5.06	34.3	89.7	79.8
1845-1849	5.06	35.4	89.7	81.9
1850-1854	4.90	35.8	86.9	82.9
1855-1859	4.74	36.0	84.0	83.3
1860-1864	4.69	38.7	83.2	89.6
1865-1869	4.77	39.6	84.6	91.7
1870-1874	4.67	37.5	82.8	86.8
1875-1879	4.62	36.7	81.9	85.0
1880-1884	4.44	34.7	78.7	80.3
1885-1889	4.50	35.5	79.8	82.2
1890-1894	4.45	33.7	78.9	78.0
1895-1899	4.23	31.6	75.0	73.1

NOTE: From 1820-1824 to 1860-1864, all legitimate births; after 1865, legitimate live births.

different trend of the birth rate and of *F* can be immediately appreciated. The average number of children per marriage declines almost continuously from 1820–1824 to the end of the century. *F* is above 5.5 during the 1820–1829 decade; it falls below this level in 1830–1840, below 5.0 in 1850–1854, and below 4.5 in 1880–1884. It reaches 4.2 during the

[20] M. Livi-Bacci, "The Fertility of Marriages in Tuscany during the 19th Century; Results and Methodology," in *Saggi di Demografia Storica*, Dipartimento Statistico Matematico, Firenze, 1969, pp. 53-64.

last five years of the century. The decline is almost uninterrupted, except for two slight recoveries in 1865–1869 and 1885–1889. On the whole, from the beginning to the end of our period, *F* declines by 1.4 points, or by 25 percent. The trend of the birth rate is quite different, with long-term fluctuations, from a maximum of 43 per thousand during the 1820s to a minimum of 34 in the early 1840s, up again to 40 in the late 1860s, and then almost continuously down until the end of the century.

The question now arises whether the decline in births per marriage is due to change in the behavior of couples or to other factors independent of their individual decisions.

The level of *F* is affected by:

(1) Changes in the frequency of marriage terminations (because of death, divorce, and migration) before the end of the fertile period
(2) Changes in the age at marriage
(3) Changes in the timing of births, not affecting the final family size
(4) Changes in the attitudes of individual couples

Let us neglect the third factor, because changes in timing may be responsible for short-term fluctuations of *F*, but certainly not for long-term, gradual changes. We will focus our attention on the first two factors before discussing the possibility of changes in attitudes.

A change in marriage terminations can have not only a substantial but also a misleading effect on *F*. Divorce and migration can be set apart as causes of termination; the first because it did not exist, the second because it is difficult to measure and had negligible influence on the Tuscan population. We have attempted to estimate the depressing effect on *F* of the termination of marriages because of the death of one (or both) partners. The estimate is based on two levels of mortality: that prevailing in the first 70-80 years of the century ($e^o_0 = 35$) and that at the turn of the century ($e^o_0 = 45$). The estimate also includes a simplifying hypothesis that all brides married between 20 and 25 years of age, and all grooms between 25 and 30. We have then estimated the number of surviving marriages at duration 1, 2, 3 . . . 30 years, by multiplying the male and female probabilities of surviving for the same intervals of time.[21]

[21] For this evaluation, we have employed the model *South* tables drawn from A. J. Coale and P. Demeny, *Regional Model Life Tables and Stable Populations*, Princeton, 1966.

When marriages increase by 1 percent every year (as they did in Toscana during the nineteenth century), the underevaluation of *F* is 9.7 percent with an expectation of life of 45 years and 13.4 percent with an expectation of life at 35 years. When marriages are stationary, underestimation is respectively 10.2 percent and 14.1 percent.

In our case, *F* declined 25 percent from 5.64 in 1820–1824 to 4.23 in 1895–1899; allowing for mortality (expectation of life of 35 and 45 years respectively at the beginning and at the end of the century), the two levels would be 6.43 and 4.65, with a decline of 28 percent. Allowing for the decline of mortality would magnify the decrease of *F* by about 3 points.

The second factor affecting *F* is modification in the age at marriage. When fertility is high, and close to "natural patterns," an increase in the age at marriage causes a decrease in the final family size. Assuming an average legitimate fertility rate of .400 in the age group 20-29, a decrease in *F* of one child (as from 1820–1824 to 1860–1864) could be explained by an increase in the mean age at marriage of 2.5 years. Unfortunately, Italian statistics on the age at marriage start in 1865. The mean age at marriage of brides (including remarriages) is very stable, and oscillates between 25 and 26 years until World War I when it declines by about one year. This long-term stability does not imply a constant mean age at marriage before 1865.

There are two elements that make us believe that during the first part of the nineteenth century the age at marriage did not change drastically, at least enough to justify the fall of *F*. The first element, illustrated in Table 1.13, is that the percentage of females, aged 14 and more, who were married, remained stable from 1815 to 1881. The 1831 peak is probably the result of the very high marriage rate of the 1820–1829

TABLE 1.13

PERCENTAGE FEMALES MARRIED, TOSCANA: 1815 TO 1881

Date	Percentage	Date	Percentage
1815	48.3	1851	49.2
1821	48.8	1861	49.2
1831	52.9	1871	49.6
1841	49.4	1881	49.9

NOTE: Data refer to females 14 years and older.

decade (8.5 per thousand compared with 7.1 for 1810–1819 and 6.7 for 1830–1839). In any case, the percentage married slightly increases over time, instead of showing the substantial decrease that would have been induced by a rise in age at marriage. The second element is that the percentage single after age 45 remained constant. This is important because, setting apart the negligible influence of changes in the age structure and in widowhood (the fall of mortality takes place at the end of the century), a constant proportion married could be consistent with an increase in age at marriage if there is a substantial fall in the proportion remaining single. Data from the 1871 census, illustrated in Table 1.14, show that this was not the case. The rise of 2 points from the 1782–1791

TABLE 1.14

PERCENTAGE FEMALES SINGLE, TOSCANA: COHORTS OVER 45 IN 1871 CENSUS

Age	Approximate date of birth	Percentage
45-49	1822-1826	11.4
50-54	1817-1821	11.5
55-59	1812-1816	11.7
60-64	1807-1811	10.8
65-69	1802-1806	10.4
70-74	1797-1801	10.6
75-79	1792-1796	10.4
80-89	1782-1791	9.4

to the 1822–1826 cohort may well be explained by factors related to the selectivity of mortality by marital status or to old-age marriages. Although we badly need more detailed data, it seems to us that any evidence of an increase in the age at marriage fails to show up in the available statistics. We thus conclude that the decline of *F* cannot be explained by changes in this factor.

This leaves us with the last factor affecting *F*. Our discussion so far has strongly indicated that the evident decline of family size after 1820 cannot be explained either by changes in mortality or by modifications in the age at marriage. Thus, it is likely that a change in the attitude of the couples was the cause of the declining family size in the first part of the century. This demonstrates also that the computation of the number of children per marriage radically changes the picture of fertility trends offered by the birth rate series.

1.8 *Fertility of Piemonte and Liguria*

It is possible to compare the crude levels of marital fertility of 1836–1837 with the post-unification patterns for the provinces of the two regions. In Table 1.15 it is shown that there are no appreciable differences

TABLE 1.15

GROSS MARITAL FERTILITY RATE, BY PROVINCE, PIEMONTE AND LIGURIA: 1836-1837 TO 1880-1882

Region	Province	Actual levels 1836-1837	1862-1863	1870-1872	1880-1882
Piemonte		203.2	204.1	197.8	190.9
	Alessandria	184.9	180.9	181.7	179.2
	Novara	214.0	217.4	204.2	192.8
	Cuneo	213.3	221.0	212.5	202.7
	Torino	202.7	203.3	197.1	181.5
Liguria		187.3	197.9	188.5	171.7
	Genova	189.6	202.0	191.2	174.7
	Porto Maurizio[a]	173.5	176.4	173.6	155.8
		Relative levels (1836-1837 set at 100)			
Piemonte		100.0	100.4	97.3	93.9
Liguria		100.0	105.7	100.7	91.7

NOTE: Gross marital fertility rate refers to legitimate births per 1,000 married women.

[a] Oneglia in Table 1.8.

between the two periods. The decline does not start earlier than the 1870s. We have also computed the same rates for smaller administrative units, the 28 circondari. The comparison between 1836–1837 and 1880–1882 shows a general, although moderate, decline between the two periods. The distribution of the circondari according to the size of the decline appears on Table 1.16.

There are at least three major areas where the decline approaches 15 percent: (1) across the provinces of Torino, Novara, and Alessandria, including the contiguous circondari of Biella, Ivrea, Aosta, Pallanza, and Vercelli; (2) south of the Po, including Voghera and Tortona; and (3) the eastern portion of Liguria, bordering on France, which includes San Remo, Porto Maurizio, and Albenga.

TABLE 1.16

DISTRIBUTION OF 28 CIRCONDARI BY PERCENTAGE CHANGE IN GROSS MARITAL FERTILITY BETWEEN 1836-1837 AND 1880-1882, REGNO DI SARDEGNA

	Distribution	
Percentage change	Number	Percent
Positive change	4	14
0 to -5	4	14
-5 to -10	9	32
-10 to -15	8	29
-15 to -20	3	11
Total	28	100

The data, however, are too few, and the measures too raw, to enable us to attempt a geographical outline of fertility decline. We may only say that, unlike Toscana, Piemonte and Liguria between the 1830s and the 1890s exhibit no signs of substantial changes in fertility patterns.

1.9 *Urban-Rural Differentials*

Textbooks of demography frequently point out the earlier and faster decline of fertility in urban areas. The general hypothesis is that fertility control and acceptance of family planning attitudes are more likely to spread in the urban areas, where the socioeconomic status of the population is higher and where easy communications and faster circulation of information make the population—or some of its sectors—more receptive to new ideas and attitudes. Moreover, it has also been pointed out that the different economic structure of the urban areas makes the task of having and rearing children harder since children in cities become economically active at later ages. The hypothesis of an earlier reduction in fertility in urban than in rural populations seems plausible, and evidence in its favor has indeed been found in some (but not all) other European countries. However, it is not a simple matter to determine whether the hypothesis applies to pre-unification Italy for several reasons. First, the higher mobility of the population in urban areas and the peculiarities of certain sectors of this population (the high proportion of servants, institutional population, short time visitors, religious and foreign minorities, etc.) tend to distort the value and the precision of traditional measures of fertility. Second, cities in Italy often had an extremely high number of foundlings and of illegitimate births. The presence in the cities of charitable institutions for foundlings and motherless children in general is, by itself, an attraction from the rural areas.[22] These factors, and many others that it would be useless to review, weaken the relationship that ought to link the numerator of the traditional rates (births) to the denominator (or the population exposed to the risk of producing births). In addition, the refined nominative technique of family reconstitution that could give a precise picture of fertility have not yet been applied to urban populations because of the many technical obstacles posed by the size and the high mobility of the urban populations.

The few and scattered data available for the first part of the nineteenth century give some information on urban fertility: on birth rates, general and marital fertility, and, in some cases, the unweighted ratio of legitimate births to marriages.

Table 1.17 shows the urban-rural differentials for Torino and Genova. In each case, the rural areas (rest of province) have a higher marital fertility than the city. The difference is conspicuous in Torino (59 per-

TABLE 1.17

GROSS MARITAL FERTILITY RATE AND BIRTHS PER MARRIAGE, URBAN/RURAL, TORINO AND GENOVA: CIRCA 1837

Area	Rate (1836-1837)		Births per marriage (1828-1837)	
	Torino	Genova	Torino	Genova
Province	189.9	192.3	4.19	4.81
City (urban)	142.7	178.1	3.01	4.36
Rest of province (rural)	210.8	200.0	4.79	5.08
Ratio of rural to urban	147.7	112.3	159.1	116.5

NOTES: Gross marital fertility rate refers to legitimate births per 1,000 married women.
Births per marriage refers to number of births divided by number of marriages.

[22] Many legitimate children born outside Firenze were taken to the city's baptistry. In 1785-1786, of 6.959 children baptized, 9.3 percent were foundlings, and 12.5 percent were legitimate children born outside Firenze. In the same years, 2,075 foundlings were accepted by the charitable institution *Spedale degli Innocenti*, many coming from the countryside. In 1785-1794, in the baptistry of Bologna, 22.9 percent of all children baptized were born to parents living in the countryside.

cent) and still substantial for Genova (16 percent). Structural factors might possibly account for the lower fertility of Genova, but this cannot be the case for Torino. A 50 percent difference between the fertility of the city and of the rest of the province cannot reasonably be imputed to the age structure of the married population.

In his two monographs on nineteenth-century Bologna, Bellettini makes it possible to observe substantial urban-rural differentials. The result is presented in Table 1.18. In 1811–1812, general and legitimate fertility is 25 to 30 percent higher in the rest of the province than in the

TABLE 1.18

GENERAL FERTILITY AND MARITAL FERTILITY RATES, URBAN/RURAL, DIPARTIMENTO DEL RENO: 1811-1812

Area	General fertility rate	Marital fertility rate
Dipartimento	163.4	270.9
City of Bologna (urban)	137.0	206.2
Rest of Dipartimento (rural)		
Plain	176.3	282.3
Hills	158.4	294.5
Mountain	162.0	314.9
Ratio of rural to urban	124.7	144.0

SOURCE: A. BELLETTINI, La popolazione del Dipartimento del Reno, Bologna, 1965, pp. 169, 173.

NOTES: General fertility rate refers to live births per 1,000 women aged 15-45.
Marital fertility rate refers to legitimate live births per 1,000 married women aged 15-50.

city. Later, in 1847, the differences remain conspicuous; the birth rate in the "rest of the Dipartimento" is 14 to 33 percent higher and the general fertility rate 15 to 40 percent. These data are shown in Table 1.19. In Firenze, thanks to the careful collection of data made by Zuccagni-Orlandini, we can follow the fertility of the city and of the rest of the province from 1818 to 1845. As shown in Table 1.20, the fertility of the rest of province remains 26 to 39 percent higher than that of the city. Here again, the differences are so large that it would be against

TABLE 1.19

BIRTH AND GENERAL FERTILITY RATES, URBAN/RURAL, PROVINCE OF BOLOGNA: 1847

Area	Birth rate	General fertility rate
Province	33.0	135.1
City of Bologna (urban)	26.8	108.2
Rest of Province (rural)		
Plain	34.2	139.1
Hills	30.6	124.7
Mountain	35.5	151.6

SOURCE: A. BELLETTINI, La popolazione delle campagne Bolognesi alla metà del secolo XIX, Bologna, 1971, pp. 88-89 and 92.

NOTE: General fertility rate refers to live births per 1,000 women aged 15-50.

common sense to impute them to structural factors. Data for Roma and Napoli are scant. In Roma, the number of births (1851–1855) per 1,000 married women (1853 census) was 197.2; this would be reduced by at least 5 to 10 percent if only legitimate births were taken into account. In the period 1840–1849, the ratio of births to marriages was 3.71. Both figures are moderate, but we have no evidence that the levels of the countryside were higher, although we suspect it.

TABLE 1.20

GROSS MARITAL FERTILITY RATE, URBAN/RURAL, FIRENZE: 1818-1825 TO 1836-1845

Area	1818-1825	1826-1835	1836-1845
Province	249.0	235.1	208.0
City of Firenze (urban)	182.6	169.2	165.0
Rest of province (rural)	233.2	220.8	198.4
Ratio of rural to urban	136.4	138.9	126.1

SOURCE: A. ZUCCAGNI ORLANDINI, Ricerche statistiche sul Granducato di Toscana, Tomo I, Florence, 1848.

NOTE: Gross marital fertility rate refers to legitimate live births per 1,000 married women.

In the 1845–1846 census in Napoli,[23] 186.8 legitimate births per 1,000 married women and 4.07 births per marriage were counted, compared to 234.7 and 5.17 for the entire "Napoletano" (10 years earlier). Here again, given the imprecise terms of reference, it is difficult to deduce the existence of urban-rural differentials, although the evidence points in this direction.

TABLE 1.21

POPULATION OF MAJOR CITIES: FIRST HALF 19TH CENTURY

City	Date	Population
Torino	1838	117,000
Genova	1838	97,000
Bologna	1811	79,000
Firenze	1830	93,000
Roma	1853	176,000
Napoli	1846	412,000

As shown in Table 1.21, the total population of all these cities, with the exception of Napoli, was modest. The available data suggest that the inhabitants of most of these cities, and probably of many others for which we lack statistical evidence, had lower marital fertility than the rural populations. As for the reasons for this lesser productivity, we have no decisive proof of the existence of positive birth control; it could be due to structural factors. Even if raw, however, the measures reported consistently show lower levels for the urban areas, and it is highly improbable that only structural factors are at play in determining the differences. Our impression is that further and deeper research would confirm our provisional finding that urban women had—other factors made equal—fewer children than their rural counterparts.

1.10 *The Fertility of a Religious Minority: The Italian Jews*

It is extremely interesting to observe the behavior of sectors of the population having common characteristics that mark them off from the rest of society. When dealing with aggregate data, this is as close as we can get to the results that can be obtained by nominative analysis, in

[23] *Censo della città di Napoli al 1º Gennaio 1845 con notizie statistiche*, Officio del Censo, Real Ministero di Stato della Polizia Generale, Napoli, 1846.

which the characteristics of each individual are observed. We have, therefore, devoted some effort to the study of two special groups, a religious minority and the aristocracy, to discover any unusual characteristics in their demographic behavior.

The demographic development of the Jewish communities followed patterns completely different from those of the rest of the population.[24] Early in the nineteenth century, there were about 30,000 Jews in Italy, concentrated in a few urban communities and forced to reside within the narrow walls of the ghettos. With a marked professional specialization in commerce and trade and a very high degree of endogamy, members of the Jewish communities had, in Italy as abroad, a unique social life. Their restricted contacts with non-Jews and their strict social and moral codes maintained their individuality for centuries. The process of emancipation, initiated during the French period at the beginning of the nineteenth century and reinforced by the waves of liberalization at mid-century, weakened the physical and social cohesion of the Jews. When the doors of the ghettos opened, the Jewish population started migrating, intermixing, and then intermarrying with the Catholic population and losing, little by little, its ethnic, social, and economic attributes. The process was completed by the last part of the nineteenth century. After that time it becomes difficult to follow the demographic development of the Jewish population, both because of its mobility and because of mixed marriages. But until the mid-nineteenth century, the close control of the communities by the various pre-unification states and the rigid organization of the communities makes possible and rewarding the study of the demography, and of the other aspects, of the Jewish population.

From a demographic point of view, mortality declined earlier among the Jews than in the general population, and the same is true of fertility. Although literally locked nightly in the ghettos, they maintained a vast network of relations with the other Jewish communities of Italy and the Mediterranean. In this sense, although their short-range mobility was low, and sometimes nonexistent, they kept an open window on the

[24] The best study of the demographic and social development of the Italian Jewish communities is that of L. Livi, *Gli Ebrei alla luce della statistica*; Vol. I: *Caratteristiche antropologiche e patologiche, ed individualità etnica*, Firenze, 1918; Vol. II: *Evoluzione demografica, economica e sociale*, Firenze, 1920. See also: R. Bachi, "La demografia degli Ebrei Italiani negli ultimi 100 anni," *Atti del Congresso Internazionale per gli Studi della Popolazione*, Roma, 1934, VI: 79-152. For a general history of the Italian Jews, see: A. Milano, *Storia degli Ebrei in Italia*, Torino, 1963.

world. In Table 1.22, we give the birth rates in seven large Jewish communities from the end of the seventeenth century to the end of the nineteenth. These are drawn, for the most part, from the original research contained in Livi's classic book. While the data cover different time spans, they all point to an early decline of Jewish fertility, a decline that appears to be under way in all the communities by the beginning of the nineteenth century. The decline is more gradual for the community

TABLE 1.22

JEWISH BIRTH RATE, SELECTED COMMUNITIES: 1669-1675 TO 1901-1915

Date	Firenze	Livorno	Modena	Padova	Roma	Trieste	Verona
1669-1675	43.8[a]	54.8	--	--	--	--	--
1675-1700	45.9[b]	42.3	--	--	--	--	--
1701-1725	--	28.1	--	--	--	--	--
1726-1750	39.4[c]	27.5	--	--	--	--	--
1751-1775	30.6	25.2	27.1[g]	--	41.6[k]	--	--
1776-1800	26.7	21.6	28.5	--	44.1	51.0[n]	--
1801-1825	27.2[d]	22.6	27.0	23.9[i]	36.4	44.4	25.9[p]
1826-1850	24.3[e]	25.5	26.9	28.0	36.8	35.3	26.0[q]
1851-1875	--	29.5[f]	22.1[h]	26.7	35.3	29.6	22.9[r]
1876-1900	--	--	--	16.4	29.3[l]	20.7	16.6[s]
1901-1915	--	--	--	11.8[j]	27.6[m]	15.5[o]	13.4[t]

SOURCES: Firenze, Livorno, Modena, Padova, and Roma: L. LIVI, Gli Ebrei alla luce della statistica, Vol. II, "Evoluzione demografica, economica e sociale", Florence, 1920, p. 75.
Trieste: I. ZOLLER, La comunità Israelitica di Trieste, in "Metron", Vol. III, No. 4, 1924, p. 544.
Verona: R. BACHI, La demografia degli Ebrei Italiani negli ultimi 100 anni, in "Atti del Congresso Internazionale per gli Studi della Popolazione," Vol. VI, Rome, 1934, pp. 79-152.

[a] 1675.
[b] 1676-1685.
[c] 1741-1750.
[d] 1801-1807.
[e] 1826-1844.
[f] 1851-1860
[g] 1756-1775.
[h] 1851-1865.
[i] 1816-1825
[j] 1901-1912.
[k] 1771-1775.
[l] 1876-1807.
[m] 1904-1915.
[n] 1786-1800.
[o] 1901-1915.
[p] 1816-1825.
[q] 1826-1845.
[r] 1846-1875.
[s] 1876-1895.
[t] 1906-1915.

of Roma, whose social and economic level was much lower than that of the other communities.

Jewish fertility had been much higher than that of the Catholic population; levels of the birth rate around 50 per thousand were not uncommon prior to the nineteenth century. This may be in connection with the very low age at marriage, which many writers fix, on the average, at less than 20; this age was more than five years earlier than that of Catholic women. But toward the end of the eighteenth, and during the nineteenth century, particularly once emancipation had started, Jewish age at marriage tended to rise to the Catholic levels. This is probably a concomitant factor of the birth rate decline, which, however, fell well below the Catholic pattern in all of the communities except Roma. In most of the communities the rapidity and extent of the decline imply the action of voluntary factors in reducing marital fertility.

In Livorno and Firenze, it is possible to follow the development of both the Jewish and the total birth rate. This is presented in Table 1.23. The birth rate of the Jewish communities remained between 20 and 30

TABLE 1.23

JEWISH AND TOTAL BIRTH RATE, FIRENZE AND LIVORNO: 1801-1805 TO 1846-1850

	Firenze		Livorno	
Date	Jewish	Total	Jewish	Total
1801-1805	27.7	--	21.3	42.8
1806-1810	24.4[a]	39.0[d]	22.5	35.4[d]
1811-1815	27.6[b]	40.2	19.2	38.8
1816-1820	26.8	42.7	21.5	39.8
1821-1825	28.3	43.9	28.6	38.4
1826-1830	23.1	42.0	27.0	36.7
1831-1835	25.1	39.4	26.3	34.4
1836-1840	24.0	37.8	25.8	33.7
1841-1845	25.1[c]	37.5	23.7	35.6
1846-1850	--	--	24.5	36.3

SOURCES: Jewish birth rate - Table 1.22; total birth rate - P. BANDETTINI, L'evoluzione demografica della Toscana, Turin, 1960.

[a]1806-1807.

[b]1815.

[c]1841-1844.

[d]1810.

per thousand, but that of the total urban populations of Firenze and Livorno only occasionally fell below 35. The same differences can be found for other communities; in Mantova, in 1791-1795, the Jewish birth rate was 28.1 compared with 44.2 for the total population.[25] Almost a century later, in Trieste, the Jewish birth rate was 24.2 (1881–1885) and that of the entire population of the city was 34. The only exception is that of Roma, where the Jewish birth rate remained throughout the nineteenth century between 30 and 40; this level was the same or slightly higher than that of the Catholic population and was probably due to the poor social conditions of Roman Jews.

Summing up, and even taking into account the very peculiar situation of the Jewish communities, it is beyond doubt that in this small but socially important religious group, the birth rate started declining perhaps a hundred years before that of the rest of the population. It is also almost certain that the decline, although partially explained by a rise in the age at marriage, occurred, to a large extent, by the action of voluntary control within marriage. Better and more detailed data will clarify the terms of the problem, but not change the lines of its interpretation. For Livorno, for example, we are conducting an extensive analysis of the material referring to 5,000 Jews. The general legitimate fertility rate (births per married woman 15 to 50 years of age), around 1841, was .170, or less than one-half the maximum levels reached in populations not practicing birth control. This shows that fertility control was well on its way, as was the case in most of the other communities. The urban Jewish population, above average in education and income, and probably feeling the physical pressure of a limited environment, adopted neo-Malthusian habits anticipating, perhaps by a whole century, the rest of the population.

1.11 *The Fertility of Social Elites: The Aristocracy*

The studies of the French and the British nobility have shown that fertility control was adopted in these privileged elites well before it was in other sectors of the population. The analysis of such narrow groups in no way allows generalization about the population as a whole, but it is extremely interesting to know when, and how, they anticipated patterns of behavior widely adopted by later generations.

[25] See *Sommario della Popolazione della Città e Stato di Mantova dalla Pasqua 1790 alla Pasqua 1791, tratto dalle Tabelle trasmesse dai Reverendi Parrochi e compilato dall'Uffizio della Sanità,* 1790-1791, 1791-1792, 1792-1793, 1794-1795.

Two recent studies have made available some interesting, although limited, material. R. Litchfield, in a study of the aristocracy of Firenze, has analyzed the demography of 21 families of the nobility that gave birth to 2,427 children between 1600 and 1799.[26] The analysis of the fertility of the 86 marriages within these families is presented in Table 1.24.

TABLE 1.24

AGE-SPECIFIC MARITAL FERTILITY RATES OF ARISTOCRACY, FIRENZE: HUSBANDS BORN 17TH AND 18TH CENTURIES

Measurement	Age of mother	Date of husband's birth		
		1600-1699	1700-1799	1750-1799
Marital fertility	15-19	.508	.365	.300
	20-24	.453	.484	.540
	25-29	.416	.345	.313
	30-34	.264	.228	.204
	35-39	.200	.119	.031
	40-44	.030	.029	.000
	45-49	.009	.000	.000
Hypothetical number of children per woman by age at marriage	20	6.86	6.03	5.44
	25	4.60	3.61	2.74

SOURCE: R. B. LITCHFIELD, Caratteristiche Demografiche delle famiglie patrizie fiorentine dal XVI al XIX secolo, in "Saggi di demografia storica", Dipartimento Statistico Matematico, Florence, 1969, pp. 17-34.

By the second part of the eighteenth century, there was a clear tendency toward a reduction of fertility and family size. A hypothetical family size of 2.7 children for women marrying at the age of 25 reveals, beyond any reasonable doubt, the existence of voluntary control. The changing age pattern is also of a form that suggests voluntary control. The findings of Litchfield in Firenze are supported by the findings of Zanetti[27] on the families of the aristocracy of Lombardia. As shown in

[26] R. B. Litchfield, "Caratteristiche Demografiche delle famiglie patrizie fiorentine dal XVI al XIX secolo," in *Saggi di demografia storica*, pp. 17-34.

[27] D. Zanetti, *La demografia del Patriziato Milanese nei secoli XVII, XVIII e XIX*, Pavia, 1972, pp. 138-139.

Table 1.25, there is a substantial decline between the first and the second part of the eighteenth century; a slight upturn in the first part of the nineteenth and a further conspicuous decline in the second half of the century. Zanetti's data, as do Litchfield's, show that the nobility of Lombardia—or at least, those families of the nobility included in the study—practiced birth control before the nineteenth century. Similar patterns were found by Beltrami in the nobility of Veneto. The birth rate of this

TABLE 1.25

AGE-SPECIFIC MARITAL FERTILITY RATES OF ARISTOCRACY, LOMBARDIA: HUSBANDS BORN 18TH AND 19TH CENTURIES

Measurement	Age of mother	Date of husband's birth Pre1750	1750-1799	1800-1849	1850-1899
Marital fertility	15-19	.469	.459	.388	.421
	20-24	.543	.436	.414	.305
	25-29	.434	.269	.289	.224
	30-34	.350	.225	.218	.154
	35-39	.199	.140	.145	.093
	40-44	.082	.034	.060	.029
	45-49	.012	.000	.012	.000
Hypothetical number of children per woman by age at marriage	20	8.10	5.52	5.69	4.03
	25	5.39	3.34	3.62	2.50

SOURCE: ZANETTI, La demografia del patriziato Milanese nei secoli XVII, XVIII, XIX, Pavia, 1972, pp. 138-139.

group was 38.8 in 1563, 34.3 in 1581 and 1586, 27.6 in 1642, and only slightly above 20 at the end of the eighteenth century: 20.6 in 1766, 23.7 in 1780 and 20.0 in 1790.[28]

Here again it is worthwhile noting that statistical information, no matter how accurate and analytical, concerning a score of families is little more than a curiosity. But our task, in this book, consists in tracing the origin of new forms of behavior, and it is extremely interesting to find that these new forms were adopted by small, homogeneous elites well before they were adopted by the general population.

[28] D. Beltrami, *Storia della popolazione di Venezia dalla fine del Secolo XVI alla caduta della Repubblica*, Padova, 1954, p. 157.

Religious minorities and the aristocracy are, perhaps, two sectors of society in which family-planning attitudes have found early acceptance. It is very likely that the factors and motivations for these changing attitudes are not the same in the two groups, given their very different life and culture: that of the Jewish communities characterized by repression and oppression, that of the nobility marked by privileges. But the results have been analogous.

It is perhaps fair to say that these few families have told us more than their numerical share.

1.12 *Conclusion*

The political subdivision of Italy before unification in several states, each with its own statistical system, makes problematic any systematic attempt to outline the demographic development of the country from Napoleonic times to unification. A vast body of statistical material, partly unpublished, is available, and the modest work of collection and elaboration attempted in this first chapter provides a few guidelines for the interpretation of fertility patterns and trends during the period under consideration. The main findings may be summarized as follows:

(1) The few analytical nominative studies concerning some villages show that fertility, although largely uncontrolled, was moderate, probably due to social, cultural, and biological factors that like prolonged breastfeeding, tended to space birth.

(2) The geography of the birth rate during Napoleonic times, during the 1830s, and during the decade or two after unification shows a relative stability, a moderate variability, and a strong concentration of the birth rate in the 35-40 intervals.

(3) More detailed data available for Toscana seem to show that the mean number of children per marriage had been declining well before the mid-nineteenth century and that this decline is imputable neither to a decrease of the age at marriage nor to changes in mortality, and, thus, is very likely the consequence of voluntary control.

(4) During the first part of the nineteenth century, the fertility of the largest cities, although measured with very raw techniques, was generally lower than that of the contiguous nonurban populations, and these differentials were, in a few instances, quite conspicuous.

(5) The largest religious minority, the Jews, had evidently started a process of fertility control before the nineteenth century.
(6) The social elites, represented by the aristocracies of Lombardia, Veneto, and Toscana, also had begun fertility control before the nineteenth century.

In short, stable levels of fertility, existed, largely uncontrolled but moderate, with normal variability and persistent geographical features. Under this apparent uniformity small pockets of lower fertility are seen to be already well established. After national unification, these differentials, touching ever-widening sectors of the population, result in a visible and accelerating fertility decline.

CHAPTER 2: Regional Development of Fertility since Unification: 1861-1971

2.1 *General Traits of Population Growth*

Although this monograph is primarily concerned with fertility, an outline of other demographic components of population change after national unification provides a useful background.[1] The smooth and parallel transition of fertility and mortality from high to low levels protected the country from sudden accelerations and decelerations in the rate of population increase. In this respect, Italy resembles other Mediterranean countries, such as Spain, more than the countries of Northern and Central Europe. However, the smoothness of the transition on the national level hides profound regional differentials. These differentials were mainly due to fertility trends, and it is these trends that will be discussed at length in this and in the following chapters.

Map 2.1 shows the four major geographical areas (North, Center, South, and Islands) of Italy and Map 2.2 shows the regions within each of these areas. In Table 2.1, we present the total population, population density, and annual rate of increase from 1861 to 1971. Although impressive in absolute terms, the doubling of the population over the century-long period is less so when compared with the population increase in other European countries. The rate of increase has never surpassed 9 per thousand, and, excluding the 1911–1931 period, which was disturbed by World War I, it has remained between 6 and 8 per thousand, which is a moderate and steady level of population growth. Population density increased from 85 inhabitants per square kilometer in 1861 to 178 in 1971. While the latter figure is lower than that in Belgium, the Netherlands, Germany, and England, it has to be regarded as very high when consideration is given to the fact that more than one-third of Italy is mountainous and only 45 percent is suitable for farming.

The components of population growth are presented by decade in Table 2.2. The death rate fell below the 30 per thousand threshold sometime in the 1880s, below 20 in the 1900s, and below 10 after

[1] For a general description of Italian population trends during the last century, see the various essays in ISTAT, *Sviluppo della popolazione italiana dal 1861 al 1961,* Annali di Statistica 94, Roma, 1965. VIII: 17. See also Livi-Bacci, "Fattori Demografici dello Sviluppo economico," in G. Fua', ed., *Lo sviluppo economico in Italia,* Milano, 1969, Vol. II.

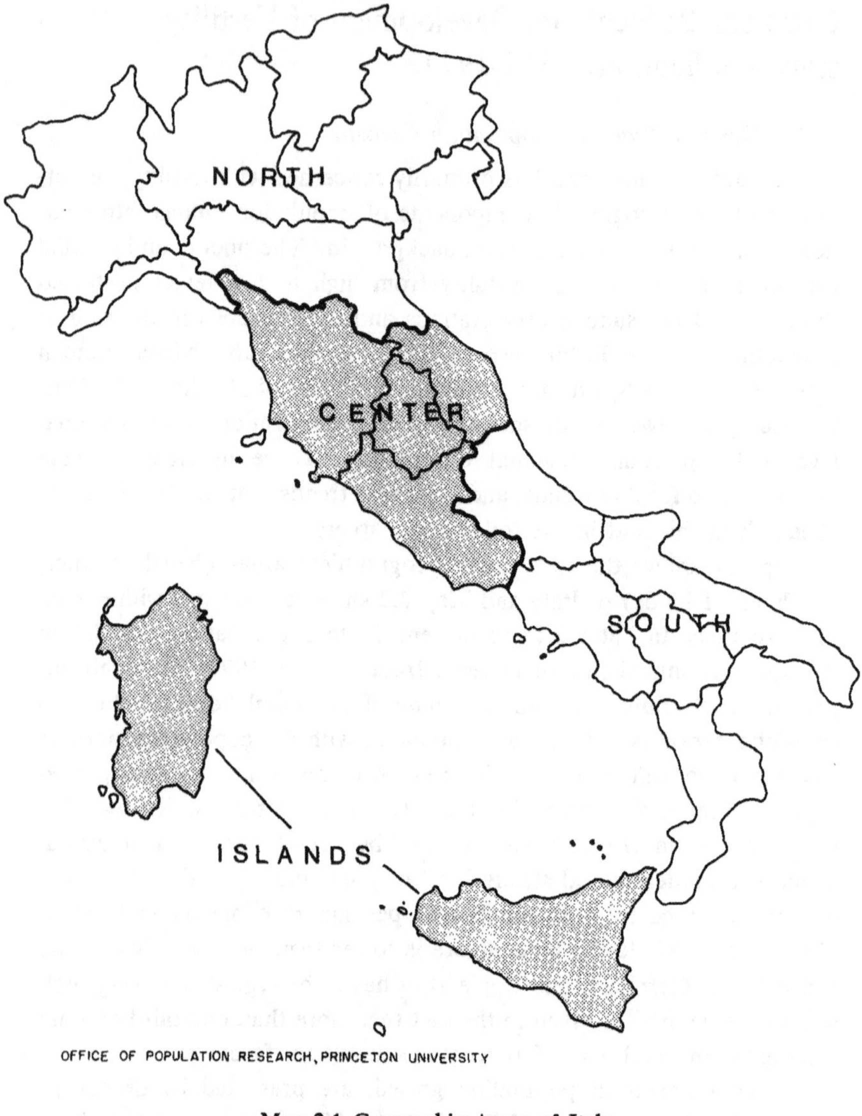

Map 2.1 Geographic Areas of Italy

World War II. In contrast, the birth rate did not begin to fall until the 1890s; prior to that, during the first three decades after unification, it remained at an almost constant level of 36 per thousand. The decline, once it began, was fairly rapid; the birth rate fell below 30 after World War I and below 20 after World War II, and reached a low of 18 in the

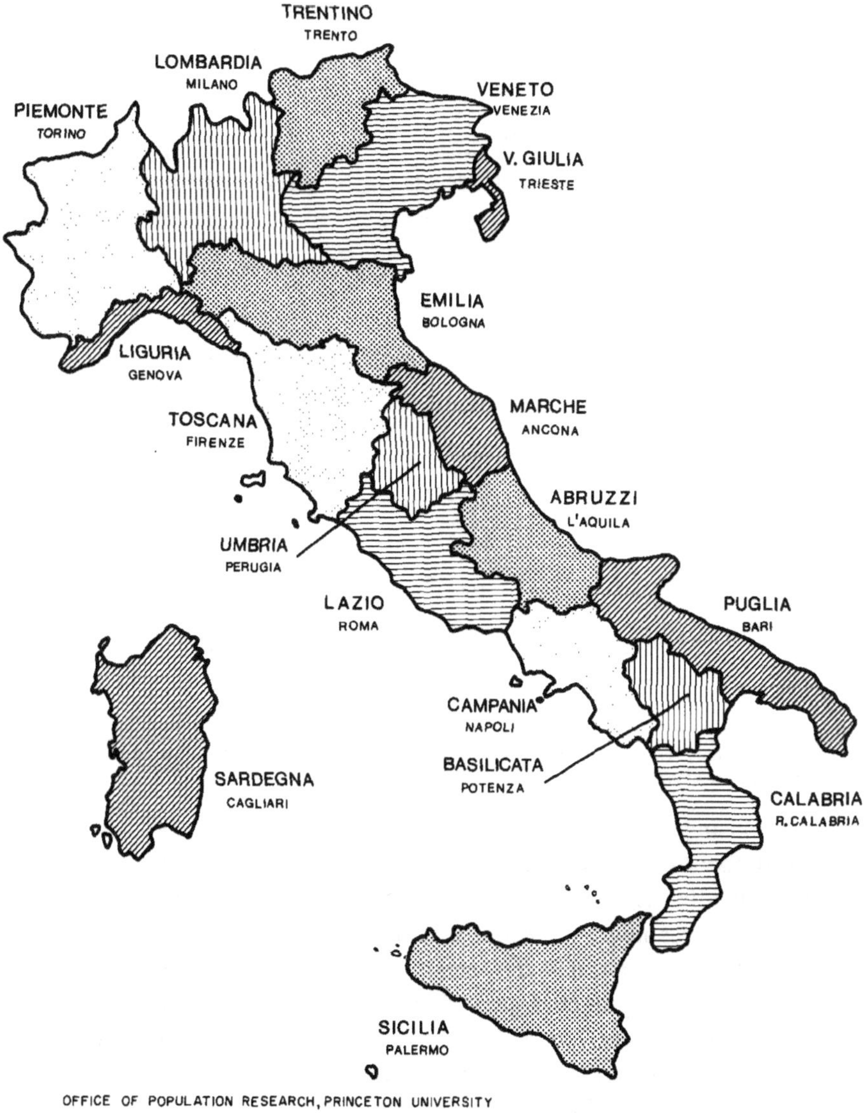

Map 2.2 Regional Areas of Italy
Note: Capital city of each region indicated in smaller type

1950s. The transition from high to low fertility and from high to low mortality has followed the pattern of the other Western European countries with a delay of only one or two decades.

TABLE 2.1

POPULATION DENSITY AND RATE OF INCREASE: 1861 TO 1971

Census date	Population (000) 1971 boundaries	Population (000) Census boundaries	Density (population per square kilometer)	Intercensal annual rate of increase (percent)
1861	25,756	21,777	85.5	--
1871	27,578	26,801	91.5	0.69
1881	29,278	28,460	97.2	0.60
1901	33,370	32,475	110.8	0.69
1911	35,695	34,672	118.5	0.65
1921	37,404	37,974	124.2	0.45
1931	40,582	41,177	134.7	0.87
1936	42,303	42,519	140.4	0.83
1951	47,159	47,159	156.5	0.70
1961	49,804	49,904	165.6	0.55
1971	53,770	53,770	178.5	0.75

NOTE: Intercensal annual rate of increase calculated on basis of 1971 boundaries, and de facto population.

Italian migration trends are, however, unique. From 1861 to 1971, official statistics put the total number of expatriations at about 26 million.[2] Slightly less than half of this figure went to overseas countries; of the overseas migrants, about 6 million went to the United States, 3 million to Argentina, and the remainder mostly to Brazil, Canada, and Australia. Net migration figures given in Table 2.2 put the net loss of inhabitants at about 8.6 million, or one-third of the total number of expatriations. The rate of overall migration rapidly increased until World War I. It fell sharply after the war due to the immigration restric-

[2] Commissariato Generale dell'Emigrazione, *Annuario Statistico dell'Emigrazione Italiana dal 1876 al 1925, con notizie sull'emigrazione negli anni 1869-75*, Roma, 1926. ISTAT, *Statistica delle migrazioni da e per l'estero*, various volumes, from 1925 to 1937; *idem, Annuario Statistico dell'Emigrazione 1955*, Roma, 1955; and *idem, Annuario di Statistiche del Lavoro e dell'Emigrazione*, each year, 1960 to 1971.

TABLE 2.2

POPULATION GROWTH, BIRTHS, DEATHS, AND MIGRATION: 1862 TO 1971

Date	Births (000)	Deaths (000)	Net migration (000)	Birth rate	Death rate	Natural increase rate	Net migration rate	Total increase rate
1862-1871	10,016	8,116	-78	37.4	30.3	7.1	-0.3	6.8
1872-1881	10,500	8,422	-378	36.9	29.6	7.3	-1.3	6.0
1882-1891	11,381	8,227	-845	37.2	26.9	10.3	-2.8	7.5
1892-1901	11,182	7,732	-1,378	34.2	23.7	10.5	-4.2	6.3
1902-1911	11,241	7,449	-1,417	32.2	21.3	10.9	-4.1	6.8
1912-1921	10,065	8,076	-903	27.2	21.8	5.4	-2.4	3.0
1922-1931	10,829	6,402	-898	27.5	16.3	11.3	-2.3	9.0
1932-1941	9,864	5,963	-242	23.0	13.9	9.1	-0.6	8.5
1942-1951	9,215	5,843	-631	20.1	12.8	7.3	-1.4	5.9
1952-1961	8,793	4,687	-1,305	18.0	9.6	8.4	-2.7	5.7
1962-1971	9,475	5,126	-483	18.2	9.8	8.4	-0.9	7.5

tions of the United States in the early 1920s, to the restrictive migration policy of the fascist regime from the late 1920s through the decade of the 1930s, and to the world depression. After World War II there was a new wave of transoceanic emigration until the mid-1950s; job opportunities in nearby European countries in the 1960s changed this trend, however, and the vast bulk now migrate within the European community.

Generally speaking, net emigration and migration rates have been higher during decades with high rates of natural increase. As a consequence, emigration has reduced the variation through time in the rate of increase of the population. Emigration was a very important phenomenon not only because it displaced many millions of Italians during the last century but also because it modified the demographic and social structure of many areas of the country. To the extent that emigration is a selective process with respect to the biological, psychological, and social characteristics of the population, it tends to modify, sometimes very deeply, the structure of the social body. The impact of large scale emigration on social life may vary, but it is always powerful. The structure of the family and the fertility of couples are certainly affected by migration; demographic techniques may eliminate some of the mechanical effects of migration on measures of fertility, but the indirect consequences cannot be easily identified and have to be evaluated carefully and critically.

The description of phenomena such as internal migration and urbanization would take more space than we can afford in a book that analyzes fertility. We may, however, give the following general outline.

(1) The regions of the North and of the Center have had, throughout most of the period under consideration, a much lower rate of natural increase than the regions of the South. In spite of this, their share of the total population has remained almost unchanged because of the strong migration from the South. This Southern migration has been both external and internal; in the latter case, migrants went to the Center (particularly Roma) and to the Northwest of the country. There have been other constant, although minor, migratory currents, such as those from the Northeast to the Northwest (from Veneto to Lombardia and Piemonte) and from the Center areas of Umbria and Marche to other regions of the Center and of the North.

(2) The process of urbanization has been very intense—as it has in almost all the developed world. We lack systematic studies, but the existing material is sufficient to give a fairly incisive view of the phenomenon. The classification of the population by number of inhabitants per comune shows that there was a rapid increase in the population living in larger comuni.

It should be noted that the size of a comune is only indirectly associated with the degree of urbanization. A small comune bordering on a large urban area may show all the characteristics peculiar to the urban area, and another comune that has a larger population but is not as densely settled may share most of the characteristics of a rural area. We are, however, close to the truth in assuming that the urban characteristics of the population increase or intensify (on the average) the larger the demographic size of the comune.

(3) The share of the total population living in comuni of 50,000 or more inhabitants increased from 11 percent in 1881, to 23 percent in 1931, and to 37 percent in 1971. The percentage of the population living in comuni with less than 10,000 residents

declined sharply. In 1881, two-thirds of the population lived in such comuni; by 1931, only one-half did, and today, the figure is little more than one-third. A further appreciation of the rapid urbanization of the country can be derived from observing the growth of the largest cities.[3] The 11 largest urban areas of the country (Torino, Milano, Genova, Venezia, Bologna, Firenze, Roma, Napoli, Catania, Messina, and Palermo) had a population of 2.6 million in 1871, or 10 percent of the total population. This figure grew to 6.9 million in 1951 (14.5 percent) and to 10.2 in 1971 (19.1 percent).

2.2 *Secular Trends in Fertility and Nuptiality*

2.2.1 When facing the task of an extensive and detailed analysis of a fertility decline, one must first confront the choice of appropriate measures. At least two requirements have to be satisfied: (1) the measures selected must be applicable to the whole period under consideration and to all areas for which the analysis is attempted; and (2) they must be sufficiently refined to eliminate the biases caused by changes in the age, sex, and marital status structure of the population. The choice is, of course, limited by the nature of census and vital statistics collected in the country. In Italy, the series of 10 official censuses (1861, 1871, 1881, 1901, 1911, 1921, 1931, 1936, 1951 and 1961) provide a breakdown of the population by sex, age, and marital status for the whole country, for each region, and, with only two exceptions (1901 and 1921), for each province. In the censuses of 1881 and 1911, these data are available also for smaller administrative areas (284 circondari). Birth statistics are available from 1861 through 1961 by region, province, and smaller administrative areas (circondari and comuni). The breakdown by age of mother and by duration of marriage is available only after 1930.

Bearing in mind the requirements indicated above and the nature of the data, one may find that an appropriate set of measures are those proposed by Coale. These measures provide indexes of fertility and nuptiality by means of indirect standardization and are used consistently in the analysis of fertility trends in the various countries covered by

[3] A. Golini, *Prospettive storiche e territoriali dell'accrescimento demografico dei centri urbani*, in M. Livi-Bacci, ed., *Le migrazioni interne in Italia*, Firenze, 1967, pp. 39-70.

the European fertility project. This set of related indexes has three main purposes:

(1) To present the fertility of a given population as a percentage of the highest fertility on record
(2) To minimize the dependence of fertility measures on the age structure of a population
(3) To provide measures that show the influence of marital status on fertility

The standard (and maximum) fertility schedule is the fertility of married Hutterite women (marriages of 1921-1930); it is a very high fertility level, probably close to the maximum attainable in a large population. In theory, the maximum is reached when an optimal state of health of the population is associated with the absence of conscious control of procreation within marriage and with a general attitude favorable to large families. Other populations have shown fertility levels close to those of the Hutterite women, but no instances are known of significantly higher patterns.

The related indexes are:[4] an index of overall fertility (I_f), an index of marital fertility (I_g), an index of illegitimate fertility (I_h), and an index of the proportion married (I_m). The relationship among the four measures is described by the following equation:

$$I_f = I_g \cdot I_m + I_h \cdot (1\text{-}I_m)$$

The four indexes have been computed for each census by region and

[4] The indices of fertility and nuptiality, standardized by age, adopted in our study can be defined as follows. Let us designate by the symbols f_i, g_i and h_i respectively the total, legitimate, and illegitimate births per woman in the ith age interval; by w_i, m_i and u_i respectively the number of total, married and unmarried women in the ith age interval; and by F_i the births per woman in the standard population (Hutterite women, marriages 1921-1930). We obtain the following expressions:

$$I_f = \frac{\Sigma f_i w_i}{\Sigma F_i w_i} \quad (1); \quad I_g = \frac{\Sigma g_i m_i}{\Sigma F_i m_i} \quad (2); \quad I_h = \frac{\Sigma h_i u_i}{\Sigma F_i u_i} \quad (3); \quad I_m = \frac{\Sigma F_i m_i}{\Sigma F_i w_i} \quad (4)$$

where the numerators of (1), (2), and (3) are, respectively, the actual number of total, legitimate, and illegitimate live births. The standard schedule is as follows: 15-19 = .300; 20-24 = .550; 25-29 = .502; 30-34 = .447; 35-39 = .406; 40-44 = .222; 45-49 = .061. See A. J. Coale, *Factors Associated with the Development of Low Fertility, an Historic Summary*, World Population Conference 1965, II: 205.

by province, ensuring a uniform territorial analysis of fertility and nuptiality. Whenever the data made it possible we used more refined techniques, including cohort analysis; we resorted to rougher indicators—as we did in the first chapter—whenever the paucity of data was balanced by the interest of the phenomenon.

TABLE 2.3

BIRTH RATE AND DEMOGRAPHIC INDICES (I_f, I_g, I_h, AND I_m): 1862-1866 TO 1968-1969

	Actual levels				
Date	Birth rate	Overall fertility (I_f)	Marital fertility (I_g)	Illegit. fertility (I_h)	Proportion married (I_m)
1862-1866	36.8	.399	.677	.044	.560
1870-1872	36.8	.389	.646	.050	.568
1880-1882	36.3	.384	.648	.063	.549
1890-1892	34.3	.376	.640	.055	.549
1900-1902	33.0	.369	.633	.048	.549
1910-1912	32.4	.346	.616	.037	.534
1921-1926	29.0	.304	.585	.029	.495
1930-1932	25.2	.255	.471	.027	.513
1935-1937	23.2	.236	.434	.022	.519
1950-1952	18.5	.192	.344	.014	.538
1960-1962	18.6	.200	.338	.011	578
1968-1969	17.7	.193	.307	.010	.616
	Relative levels (1862-1866 set at 100)				
1862-1866	100.0	100.0	100.0	100.0	100.0
1870-1872	100.0	97.5	95.4	113.6	101.4
1880-1882	98.6	96.2	95.7	143.2	98.0
1890-1892	93.0	94.2	94.5	125.0	98.0
1900-1902	89.7	92.5	93.5	109.1	98.0
1910-1912	88.0	86.7	91.0	84.1	95.4
1921-1926	78.6	76.2	86.4	65.9	88.4
1930-1932	68.4	63.9	69.6	61.4	91.6
1935-1937	62.9	59.2	64.1	50.0	92.7
1950-1952	50.2	48.1	50.8	31.8	96.1
1960-1962	50.4	50.1	49.9	25.0	103.2
1968-1969	48.1	48.4	45.3	22.7	110.0

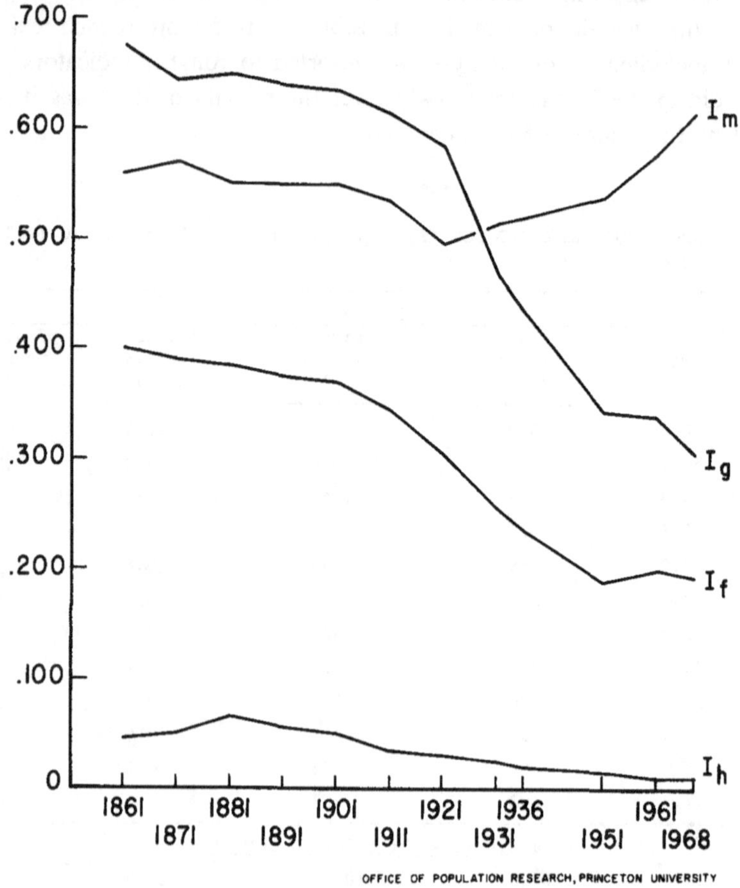

Figure 2.1 Demographic Indices: 1861-1968

2.2.2. Table 2.3 presents the secular trends of fertility and nuptiality; the data, supplemented by Figure 2.1, clearly show the decline of fertility.[5] The birth rate and the index of overall fertility (I_f) have a rather

[5] For the computation of the various indexes, it is necessary to have: (1) the age, sex, and marital status distribution of the population and (2) the annual number of live births by legitimacy. For the computation of the indexes of Table 3.3, we have used the census of 1861 and the average number of births of 1862-1866; 1871 (1870-1872); 1881 (1880-1882); 1901 (1900-1902); 1911 (1910-1912); 1921 (1921-1926); 1931 (1930-1932); 1936 (1935-1937); 1951 (1950-1952); 1961 (1960-1962). For the computation of the indexes of 1862-1866, the denominator of the expressions (1), (2), and (3) and both denominator and numerator of expression (4) (see above) have been centered at mid-period (June 30, 1864) by

similar trend; the decline becomes appreciable in the 1890s, proceeds at a steady rate until the early 1920s, accelerates thereafter until the early 1950s, and then recovers somewhat. In the whole period of one hundred years, each measure declined by 50 percent.

Marital fertility (I_g) shows a slow erosion until the end of the nine-

linear interpolation between the values computed for 1861 and 1871. The same procedure was followed for 1921-1926 where the estimates of the denominators of I_f, I_g, I_h, and I_m (and the numerator of I_m) have been made for December 31, 1923, interpolating between the values for 1921 and 1931. We have proceeded in a similar way for 1890-1892, interpolating between 1881 and 1901. For 1968-1969, the age, sex, and marital status distribution of the national population had been estimated by ISTAT (Istituto Centrale di Statistica) at the end of 1968. The computation procedures explained above have also been followed for the regional indexes reported in Tables 3.5, 3.6, 3.9, and, when applicable, to the provincial indexes contained in Tables 4.2 and 4.3.

The three-year averages (instead of averages over a longer period of years, i.e., 5 or 10) have been adopted for three reasons. First, since the age, sex, and marital status structure is known with a certain precision only at the census date, the longer the period for which the average of births is computed, the looser the correspondence between numerators and denominators, and the less exact the fertility measures. The second reason is technical: at the regional and provincial level, the many changes in the boundaries of the provincial or regional areas make it difficult to adjust the numerator (births) to the denominator (census population); the difficulty increases the longer the period (since the chances that changes in boundaries have occurred is higher). Third, the three-year periods considered do not seem (with a few exceptions) to fall in particularly disturbed periods. If we compare the annual number of births during each three-year period centered on the census date, and the eleven-year periods centered also on the census date, we find the following results:

Three-year averages		*Eleven-year averages*		*Difference (percent)*
1870-72	1,025	1866-76	1,020	+0.5
1880-82	1,060	1876-86	1,091	—2.8
1890-92	1,134	1886-96	1,140	—0.5
1900-02	1,101	1896-06	1,106	—0.5
1910-12	1,158	1906-15[a]	1,143	+1.3
1930-32	1,023	1926-36	1,019	+0.4
1935-37	971	1932-40[b]	993	—2.2
1950-52	904	1948-55[c]	894	+1.0
1960-62	926	1956-66	932	—0.6

a, b, and *c*: shorter periods to avoid war perturbations.
Source: Adjusted series (constant boundaries) drawn by: F. Giusti, *Bilanci demografici della popolazione italiana dal 1861 al 1961*, in ISTAT, *Sviluppo della popolazione*, p. 117.

If we except 1880-1882 and 1935-1937, the three-year averages are only 1 percent or less away from the corresponding averages calculated over longer periods. In 1880-1882, the influence of the very high mortality of 1880 was probably felt, and teenth century[6] (the data of 1862–1866 are not strictly comparable with those of later dates, since Veneto and Lazio were not yet part of the country); the decline continues with a slow pace until 1922–1926 (I_g had declined by 14 percent, compared with 24 percent for I_f), picks up momentum between the two wars, and continues, at a reduced rate, during the 1950s and the 1960s. The overall decline is around 55 percent.

Illegitimacy (I_h) is a small component of overall fertility; the increase in the latter part of the last century is artificial and due to the change in marriage legislation brought about by the law of 1865 (see Section 2.4.2). During this century, the decline has been uninterrupted, and I_h reaches negligible levels in 1968–1969; the overall decline is between three-fourths and four-fifths. Finally, the weighted proportion of married women, 15 to 50 years of age, shows less dramatic, but not less interesting, changes. There is a 12 percent decrease until 1921; this is partly due to changes in the structure of the population caused by emigration and by war deaths. After 1921, there is a continuous climb, which is particularly sharp in the last two decades.

During the three decades after unification, Italian married women experienced a legitimate fertility that was two-thirds the level of the Hutterite women, more or less the same pattern found in Spain and in Portugal. This fertility was generally stable and did not start to decline markedly until the last decade of the century (despite the fact, proved in the preceding chapter, that some sectors of the population undoubtedly practiced contraception during the nineteenth century). Thus, we may say that the fertility prevailing during the 1860s, 1870s, and 1880s

---

1935-1937 is disturbed by the Ethiopian war. For an analysis of fluctuations of births and fertility, see L. Livi, "La prolificità in rapporto alla produzione agricola in Italia dal 1861 al 1960," in *L'economia italiana dal 1861 al 1960*, Biblioteca of the journal *Economia e Storia*, Milano, 1961, pp. 62-78. See also: A. Santini, "Natalità, nuzialità e cicli brevi dell'economia: L'esperienza italiana tra il 1863 ed il 1965," *Genus* xxv, nos. 1-4 (1969).

Finally, the five-year average of 1862-1866 (census of 1861) is justified by the lack of data for 1861 and previous years and by the fluctuations of births in the first years after the unification. The six-year average 1921-1926 has been chosen in an attempt to eliminate the effects of the recovery of births after World War I.

[6] The reclassification of births by legitimacy to eliminate the artificial increase of illegitimacy caused by the law of 1866 would raise I_g in 1880-1882 (years in which illegitimacy reached a maximum) by 3.5 to 4 percent. Therefore the following decline until 1910-1912 (assuming that in those years the effects of the marriage law on illegitimacy had disappeared) would be about 10 percent instead of 6.5 percent.

represented a situation largely untouched by neo-Malthusian ideas and techniques (in other words, by voluntary control of fertility); we will define this as the predecline pattern of fertility. It is a rather moderate pattern, much below that observed in many other countries of Central or Northern Europe, and raises the question of the factors that depressed it far below the so-called natural levels. The problem cannot be solved now, but the elements that we will accumulate in this study may help give a tentative answer to this important question.

2.3 *Regional Trends of Overall and Marital Fertility*

Tables 2.4, 2.5, and 2.6 contain regional[7] birth-rates and the indexes of overall fertility (I_f) and marital fertility (I_g). It must be recalled that when illegitimacy is low (as it is in Italy throughout the whole period), overall fertility (I_f) depends almost completely on the levels of I_g and I_m.

With few exceptions, overall fertility has been higher in the South than in the rest of the country; until the end of the century, I_f exceeded .400 in Puglia, Basilicata, and Sicilia, while in the rest of the country that level is surpassed only once by Emilia (1862–1866) and Veneto (1870–1872) and twice by Toscana (1862–1866 and 1870–1872). The decline started in Piemonte, Liguria, and Toscana; in 1900–1902,

[7] Regional birth rates, I_f, I_g, I_h, and I_m are always referred to as the *current* boundaries at the time of the various censuses. Comparability through time is not perfect since regions have undergone some territorial modifications. The new regions of Valle d'Aosta and Molise, created respectively in 1947 and in 1963, have not been considered separately, and remain incorporated, in our tables, in Piemonte and Abruzzi. The province of Massa, which belonged to Emilia-Romagna until 1871, has always been considered, for our purposes, as belonging to Toscana. The province of Udine, which was separated from Veneto and aggregated to Friuli-Venezia Giulia in 1947, has been considered as part of Veneto also in 1951 and 1961.

The region of Venezia Giulia has undergone major changes. In 1947, the provinces of Pola and Fiume and part of the provinces of Gorizia and Trieste were annexed to Yugoslavia. Data for Venezia Giulia, therefore, are not comparable through time since the population lost to Yugoslavia accounted (1936 census) for 46 percent of the prewar population. Lazio, in 1923 and 1927, annexed territories detached from Umbria, Abruzzi, and Campania, and gained almost .5 million inhabitants, or about one-third of its 1921 population. Umbria lost 14 percent of its 1921 population; Abruzzi, 4 percent; and Campania, 9 percent. Another minor interchange affected Toscana and Emilia in 1933, with a loss for Toscana corresponding to 2 percent and an equal gain for Emilia. Other modifications affected only a few thousand inhabitants, and do not affect the comparability of regional data. For a detailed analysis of territorial modifications of regions, see A. Ferrantini, "Variazioni territoriali delle regioni," in ISTAT, *Sviluppo della popolazione*, pp. 205-215.

TABLE 2.4

BIRTH RATE, BY REGION: 1862-1866 TO 1960-1962

Region	Actual levels										
	1862-1866	1870-1872	1880-1882	1890-1892	1900-1902	1910-1912	1921-1926	1930-1932	1935-1937	1950-1952	1960-1962
Piemonte	36.17	35.70	34.74	31.47	29.13	24.15	18.79	16.65	14.64	11.25	12.98
Liguria	35.35	34.51	32.29	29.49	27.60	24.69	18.71	15.91	14.15	10.26	12.26
Lombardia	37.57	37.56	36.32	35.16	34.72	33.04	26.46	22.73	20.66	15.28	16.22
Trentino Alto Adige	--	--	--	--	--	--	28.07	22.44	20.08	18.55	19.23
Veneto	--	37.63	34.45	35.39	36.86	36.99	33.24	26.16	24.19	18.61	18.60
Venezia Giulia	--	--	--	--	--	--	26.89	20.31	18.72	11.38	13.21
Emilia	37.92	35.20	34.63	33.57	33.20	34.31	28.22	21.66	19.49	13.93	14.15
Toscana	40.03	38.18	34.39	32.08	30.52	29.25	25.04	19.29	17.51	13.03	13.47
Marche	36.56	33.53	35.32	33.54	32.46	34.24	30.86	25.39	23.40	17.14	15.95
Umbria	33.93	33.60	33.40	31.58	30.41	32.34	29.63	24.52	21.84	15.84	14.86
Lazio	--	35.39	32.99	30.92	29.55	31.15	27.97	25.48	23.80	17.99	19.05
Abruzzi	37.56	36.77	38.16	35.67	34.02	32.97	34.08	30.47	27.99	20.80	18.18
Campania	38.06	37.07	36.61	33.99	32.27	32.93	34.62	31.93	29.27	24.73	25.12
Puglia	42.13	40.69	42.43	39.10	36.72	37.71	36.22	33.12	31.00	25.65	24.47
Basilicata	41.71	39.90	42.25	38.74	35.87	36.61	37.88	35.74	34.02	27.06	24.70
Calabria	38.43	38.55	36.97	35.06	33.99	35.18	35.33	33.18	31.40	27.59	25.48
Sicilia	41.40	39.50	39.79	36.44	34.18	32.98	28.51	28.40	26.46	23.04	22.68
Sardegna	36.64	37.79	36.25	33.73	31.87	32.29	31.88	29.70	27.85	23.64	23.85
Italy	36.84	36.84	36.31	34.27	33.03	32.42	28.96	25.18	23.18	18.48	18.55

TABLE 2.4 - Continued

Region	Relative levels (1862-1866 set at 100)										
	1862-1866	1870-1872	1880-1882	1890-1892	1900-1902	1910-1912	1921-1926	1930-1932	1935-1937	1950-1952	1960-1962
Piemonte	100.00	98.70	96.05	87.01	80.54	66.77	51.95	46.03	40.48	31.10	35.89
Liguria	100.00	97.62	91.34	83.42	78.08	69.84	52.93	45.01	40.03	29.02	34.68
Lombardia	100.00	99.97	96.67	93.59	92.41	87.94	70.43	60.50	54.99	40.67	43.17
Trentino Alto Adige	--	--	--	--	--	--	100.00	79.94	74.54	66.08	68.51
Veneto	--	100.00	91.55	94.05	97.95	98.30	88.33	69.52	64.28	49.46	49.43
Venezia Giulia	--	--	--	--	--	--	100.00	75.53	69.62	42.32	49.73
Emilia	100.00	92.83	91.32	88.53	87.55	90.48	74.42	57.12	51.40	36.74	37.32
Toscana	100.00	95.38	85.91	80.14	76.24	73.07	62.55	48.19	43.74	32.55	33.65
Marche	100.00	91.71	96.61	91.74	88.79	93.65	84.47	69.45	64.00	46.88	43.63
Umbria	100.00	99.03	98.44	93.07	89.63	95.31	87.33	72.27	64.37	46.68	43.80
Lazio	--	100.00	93.22	87.37	83.50	88.02	79.03	72.00	67.25	50.83	53.83
Abruzzi	100.00	97.90	101.60	94.97	90.58	87.78	90.73	81.12	74.52	55.38	48.40
Campania	100.00	97.40	96.19	89.31	84.79	86.52	90.96	83.89	76.90	64.98	66.00
Puglia	100.00	96.58	100.71	92.81	87.16	89.51	85.97	78.61	73.58	60.88	58.08
Basilicata	100.00	95.66	101.29	92.88	86.00	87.77	90.82	85.69	81.56	64.88	59.22
Calabria	100.00	100.31	96.20	91.23	88.45	91.54	91.93	86.34	81.71	71.79	66.30
Sicilia	100.00	95.41	96.11	88.02	82.56	79.66	68.86	68.60	63.91	55.65	54.78
Sardegna	100.00	103.14	98.94	92.06	86.98	88.13	87.01	81.06	76.01	64.52	65.09
Italy	100.00	100.00	98.56	93.02	89.66	88.00	78.61	68.35	62.92	50.16	50.35

TABLE 2.5

OVERALL FERTILITY (I_f), BY REGION: 1862-1866 TO 1960-1962

	Actual levels										
Region	1862-1866	1870-1872	1880-1882	1890-1892	1900-1902	1910-1912	1921-1926	1930-1932	1935-1937	1950-1952	1960-1962
Piemonte	.375	.372	.369	.344	.319	.251	.184	.160	.148	.122	.145
Liguria	.375	.368	.339	.314	.293	.251	.179	.149	.134	.106	.135
Lombardia	.396	.389	.384	.383	.382	.343	.257	.211	.195	.155	.168
Trentino Alto Adige	--	--	--	--	--	--	.290	.230	.218	.206	.222
Veneto	--	.412	.379	.400	.419	.400	.348	.265	.251	.192	.197
Venezia Giulia	--	--	--	--	--	--	.273	.201	.189	.105	.130
Emilia	.401	.381	.370	.375	.380	.389	.300	.220	.194	.141	.152
Toscana	.426	.410	.371	.357	.345	.313	.255	.191	.173	.136	.148
Marche	.381	.352	.372	.373	.374	.375	.324	.262	.239	.172	.169
Umbria	.370	.363	.361	.361	.361	.318	.326	.267	.235	.160	.157
Lazio	--	.385	.350	.340	.333	.329	.283	.259	.234	.177	.193
Abruzzi	.393	.388	.393	.386	.378	.349	.369	.322	.298	.205	.194
Campania	.390	.387	.382	.372	.361	.357	.354	.338	.308	.252	.270
Puglia	.430	.423	.444	.430	.419	.406	.407	.358	.335	.272	.264
Basilicata	.417	.402	.429	.415	.399	.415	.419	.386	.370	.276	.266
Calabria	.379	.392	.373	.370	.367	.374	.388	.346	.329	.281	.279
Sicilia	.441	.421	.419	.398	.380	.356	.340	.304	.281	.239	.249
Sardegna	.377	.390	.388	.367	.349	.346	.343	.323	.309	.294	.272
Italy	.399	.389	.384	.376	.369	.346	.304	.255	.236	.192	.200

TABLE 2.5 - Continued

Region	Relative levels (1862-1866 set at 100)										
	1862-1866	1870-1872	1880-1882	1890-1892	1900-1902	1910-1912	1921-1926	1930-1932	1935-1937	1950-1952	1960-1962
Piemonte	100.00	99.20	98.40	91.73	85.07	66.93	49.07	42.67	39.47	32.53	38.67
Liguria	100.00	98.13	90.40	83.73	78.13	66.93	47.73	39.73	35.73	28.27	36.00
Lombardia	100.00	98.23	96.97	96.72	96.46	86.62	64.90	53.23	49.24	39.14	42.42
Trentino Alto Adige	--	--	--	--	--	--	100.00	79.31	75.17	71.03	76.55
Veneto	--	100.00	91.99	97.09	101.70	97.09	84.47	64.32	60.92	46.60	47.82
Venezia Giulia	--	--	--	--	--	--	100.00	73.63	69.23	38.46	47.62
Emilia	100.00	95.01	92.27	93.52	94.76	97.01	74.81	54.86	48.38	35.16	37.91
Toscana	100.00	96.24	87.09	83.80	80.99	73.47	59.86	44.84	40.61	31.92	34.74
Marche	100.00	92.39	97.64	97.90	98.16	98.43	85.04	68.77	62.73	45.14	44.36
Umbria	100.00	98.11	97.57	97.57	97.57	85.95	88.11	72.16	63.51	43.24	42.43
Lazio	--	100.00	90.91	88.31	86.49	85.45	73.51	67.27	60.73	45.97	50.13
Abruzzi	100.00	98.73	100.00	98.22	96.18	88.80	93.89	81.93	75.83	52.16	49.36
Campania	100.00	99.23	97.95	95.38	92.56	91.54	98.46	86.67	78.97	64.62	69.23
Puglia	100.00	98.37	103.26	100.00	97.44	94.42	94.65	83.26	77.91	63.26	61.40
Basilicata	100.00	96.40	102.88	99.52	95.68	99.52	100.48	92.57	88.73	66.19	63.79
Calabria	100.00	103.43	98.42	97.63	96.83	98.68	102.37	91.29	86.81	74.14	73.61
Sicilia	100.00	95.46	95.01	90.25	86.17	80.73	77.10	68.93	63.72	54.20	56.46
Sardegna	100.00	103.45	102.92	97.35	92.57	91.78	90.98	85.68	81.96	77.98	72.15
Italy	100.00	97.49	96.24	94.24	92.48	86.72	76.19	63.91	59.15	48.12	50.13

TABLE 2.6

MARITAL FERTILITY (I_g), BY REGION: 1862-1866 TO 1960-1962

Region	Actual levels										
	1862-1866	1870-1872	1880-1882	1890-1892	1900-1902	1910-1912	1920-1922	1930-1932	1935-1937	1950-1952	1960-1962
Piemonte	.642	.631	.642	.617	.592	.478	.374	.299	.264	.209	.228
Liguria	.658	.630	.615	.581	.551	.488	.368	.294	.261	.189	.222
Lombardia	.668	.657	.664	.674	.683	.619	.517	.407	.373	.286	.286
Trentino Alto Adige	--	--	--	--	--	--	.700	.528	.493	.430	.419
Veneto	--	.682	.651	.698	.743	.738	.704	.527	.492	.358	.340
Venezia Giulia	--	--	--	--	--	--	.518	.372	.335	.178	.212
Emilia	.648	.597	.595	.616	.638	.646	.535	.386	.340	.237	.237
Toscana	.733	.662	.634	.613	.595	.550	.473	.341	.308	.235	.233
Marche	.683	.620	.660	.645	.632	.652	.600	.475	.436	.299	.270
Umbria	.627	.600	.590	.590	.590	.614	.558	.439	.391	.256	.239
Lazio	--	.610	.539	.533	.528	.557	.517	.465	.426	.314	.356
Abruzzi	.669	.638	.644	.626	.609	.595	.666	.553	.504	.361	.316
Campania	.689	.667	.671	.652	.634	.667	.771	.647	.600	.496	.490
Puglia	.744	.701	.720	.697	.677	.703	.735	.643	.612	.501	.470
Basilicata	.678	.645	.642	.625	.606	.649	.716	.624	.590	.474	.425
Calabria	.640	.639	.610	.590	.573	.610	.704	.595	.566	.496	.463
Sicilia	.705	.696	.679	.647	.618	.606	.624	.531	.492	.416	.413
Sardegna	.642	.631	.648	.648	.647	.671	.714	.662	.632	.589	.547
Italy	.677	.646	.648	.640	.633	.616	.585	.471	.434	.344	.338

TABLE 2.6 - Continued

Region	Relative levels (1862-1866 set at 100) 1862-1866	1870-1872	1880-1882	1890-1892	1900-1902	1910-1912	1920-1922	1930-1932	1935-1937	1950-1952	1960-1962
Piemonte	100.00	98.29	100.00	96.11	92.21	74.45	58.26	46.57	41.12	32.55	35.51
Liguria	100.00	95.74	93.47	88.30	83.74	74.16	55.93	44.68	39.67	28.72	33.74
Lombardia	100.00	98.35	99.40	100.90	102.25	92.66	77.40	60.93	55.84	42.81	42.81
Trentino Alto Adige	--	--	--	--	--	--	100.00	75.43	70.43	61.43	59.86
Veneto	--	100.00	95.45	102.35	108.94	108.21	103.23	77.27	72.14	52.49	49.85
Venezia Giulia	--	--	--	--	--	--	100.00	71.81	64.67	34.36	40.93
Emilia	100.00	92.13	91.82	95.06	98.46	99.69	82.56	59.57	52.47	36.57	36.57
Toscana	100.00	90.31	86.49	83.63	81.17	75.03	64.53	46.52	42.02	32.06	31.79
Marche	100.00	90.78	96.63	94.44	92.53	95.46	87.85	69.55	63.84	43.78	39.53
Umbria	100.00	95.69	94.10	94.10	94.10	97.93	89.00	70.02	62.36	40.83	38.12
Lazio	--	100.00	88.36	87.38	86.56	91.31	84.75	76.23	69.84	51.48	58.36
Abruzzi	100.00	95.37	96.26	93.57	91.03	88.94	99.55	82.66	75.34	53.96	47.23
Campania	100.00	96.81	97.39	94.63	92.02	96.81	111.90	93.90	87.08	71.99	71.12
Puglia	100.00	94.22	96.77	93.68	90.99	94.49	98.79	86.42	82.26	67.34	63.17
Basilicata	100.00	95.13	94.69	92.18	89.38	95.72	105.60	92.04	87.02	69.91	62.68
Calabria	100.00	99.84	95.31	92.19	89.53	95.31	110.00	92.97	88.44	77.50	72.34
Sicilia	100.00	98.72	96.31	91.77	87.66	85.96	88.51	75.32	69.79	59.01	58.58
Sardegna	100.00	98.29	100.93	100.93	100.78	104.52	111.21	103.12	98.44	91.74	85.20
Italy	100.00	95.42	95.72	94.53	93.50	90.99	86.41	69.57	64.11	50.81	49.93

I_f had declined by 15 to 20 percent; in 1921–1926 the decline amounted to one-half in Liguria and Piemonte, two-fifths in Toscana, one-third in Lombardia, and one-fourth in Emilia, Lazio, and Sicilia. The lowest levels were recorded in 1950–1952, when I_f stood at about only one-fourth to one-third its original level in Venezia Giulia, Liguria, Piemonte, Toscana, and Emilia; at between one-third and one-half in the remaining regions of the Center and of the North; and at between one-half and two-thirds in the South, with the exception of Calabria and Sardegna, which had a lesser decline. A slight recovery took place during the following decade, particularly in those regions where I_f had fallen to the lowest levels. As the reader can see in Table 2.4, in four regions the birth rate had fallen to levels of 10 to 13 per thousand, corresponding to a net reproduction rate far below replacement.

Table 2.6 shows regional trends in marital fertility (I_g) and is the most interesting for our purposes. In 1862–1866, only three regions had an I_g above .700: Puglia (.744), Toscana (.733), and Sicilia (.705). After that period, only Puglia and Veneto exceeded, in a few instances, the level of .700 (excluding 1921-1926, marked by the transitory recovery after the war). Until the end of the century, variability was moderate (in 1862–1866 the high was .744 and the low .640), but after the turn of the century variability tended to increase, owing to the differential rate of change in I_g in the various regions.

To summarize the regional features of fertility decline, we may group regions as follows:

Piemonte, Liguria, and Toscana. These are the regions showing the earliest and most rapid decline. In Toscana and Liguria, a decline is in evidence from the earliest data in the series; in Piemonte, from 1880–1882. By 1910–1912, these regions had registered an I_g decline of 25 percent. Through 1960–1962, these regions consistently maintain the lowest I_g on record in Italy.

Other regions of the North and of the Center. In these regions, a sustained decline in fertility did not take place until after World War I. Lombardia and Lazio, however, represent an exception; here the onset of the fertility decline can be dated just prior to the war. The overall trends in the regions once belonging to the Papacy, however, are distorted by the effects of the introduction of civil marriage in 1866 (this point will be discussed later).

Regions of the South. Fertility decline was very slow to reach Southern Italy. In one area, Sardegna, a fertility decline did not start until as late as the 1940s. In the other regions of the South, the decline started between the two world wars. Sicilia represents an interesting exception. Starting from very high levels of marital fertility, this area showed a gradual but continual decline for over a century. In relative terms, I_g in 1960–1962 was 59 percent of the 1862–1866 level; yet it still remained one of the highest levels in the country.

The more relevant aspect of the overall fertility decline is the widening gap between the South and the rest of the country. Differences were trivial until the beginning of the twentieth century, but they rapidly increased to 50 percent and more from the 1930s to the present. The differential behavior of married women is a relevant factor of the widening gap between the social and economic level of the South and that of the rest of the country.

Experience shows that in many populations whenever a downward trend in fertility is caused by neo-Malthusian attitudes, or by the increasing use of contraceptive techniques, no fertility recovery takes place before very low levels are reached. In the Italian experience before World War I, this scheme applies only to Piemonte, Liguria, Toscana, Lombardia, and, in the South, to Sicilia. In Umbria, Lazio, and Emilia, a reduction of fertility between national unification and the end of the century does not appear to be a typical neo-Malthusian development because it was followed by a nontransient recovery before a new decline set in. In Southern Italy, the low levels of I_g in the two decades preceding World War I are apparently not due to the spreading of neo-Malthusian attitudes because there was a sharp recovery of I_g during the 1920s (only part of the recovery can be explained as a postwar reaction). Explanations of the early depression of marital fertility in Central and Southern Italy will be discussed later and will include the role of a new marriage law in the former area and of modifications of the structure of the population induced by emigration in the latter area.

2.4 *The Demographic and Sociological Significance of Nonmarital Fertility*

2.4.1. Illegitimacy has never had a major impact on the fertility of the Italian population. In Italy—as in most European countries—reproduction takes place mainly within marriage. This statement has become increasingly true over time: the ratio of I_h to I_g declined from a maximum of nearly 10 percent in 1880–1882 to only 3 percent in 1960–1962.

Generally an illegitimate birth is one that occurs out of wedlock. It is, therefore, the definition of marriage that determines the legitimacy of births. Until 1883, Italian statistics included a category for foundlings (*esposti*) in addition to legitimate births and illegitimate births. Foundlings were generally left in the *ruote* (literally "wheels") of the many charitable institutions for abandoned children, and were, in a large proportion, illegitimate. An unknown proportion of foundlings, however, were legitimate children whom the family could not support, and therefore had entrusted to the care of charitable institutions. In 1884, following the progressive abolition of the *ruote*, the category of foundlings (*esposti*) was abolished in official statistics, and children were classified only as legitimate and illegitimate. Illegitimate children were subdivided into illegitimate "recognized" and illegitimate "not recognized" by one or both parents. This last category included those foundlings whose legal status and origin was unknown, and it is likely that a small fraction of these were legitimate children.[8]

Statistics on illegitimacy were severely distorted by a new marriage law introduced shortly after unification. On January 1, 1866, civil marriage was introduced in all provinces of the kingdom; by February 1, 1871 it was enacted in Lazio and by September 1 of the same year in Veneto. The new regulation stated that a marriage, to achieve its legal status, had to be performed before the civil authority of the comune. A solely religious marriage, from 1866 on, did not have any legal standing. From the beginning, the new institution was poorly accepted by many sectors of the population[9] in which the custom of religious marriage had deep roots. In 1865 many couples (205,621) married under the old legal order, earlier than they otherwise would have, while in 1866 few couples (120,752) married under the new law. For many years after 1866, especially in those regions once subjected to the Papacy (Marche, Umbria, Lazio, and part of Emilia, or the provinces of the Romagna), the custom of getting married with only a religious ceremony persisted, sometimes in conscious opposition to the new legal order, sometimes because of ignorance of it. For example, from 1866 to 1880 in the province of Pesaro, 18,243 civil marriages were performed, compared to 23,025 religious marriages registered in the parish books. Thus, almost, 5,000 marriages, or more than 20 percent of the total, did not have the proper legal status; the children were, therefore,

[8] DIRSTAT, *Movimento dello stato civile, 1891*, Roma, 1892, pp. 23-31.

[9] E. Raseri, *I fanciulli illegittimi e gli esposti in Italia, Archivio di Statistica* VI, Roma, 1881, I: 6-24.

registered as illegitimate.[10] In the small comune of Sonnino (Lazio) during the decade 1871–1880, 401 religious marriages were performed and only 134 civil marriages.[11]

Examples such as the above led the Ministry of Justice to attempt a national comparison between civil marriages and religious marriages in the period 1866–1877. These statistics, together with the rapid rise in illegitimacy, constituted the evidence for a proposed law intended to prohibit the celebration of the religious marriage before the civil one. The data, presented in Table 2.7, were published by Bodio,[12] who also advanced some criticism on the techniques used in the collection of data, which underestimated religious marriages. Before the annexation of Veneto and Roma, civil marriages for all of Italy were 10 percent below

TABLE 2.7

CIVIL AND RELIGIOUS MARRIAGES: 1866 TO 1877

	Italy, without Roma and Veneto			Roma and Veneto		
Year	Civil	Religious	Difference	Civil	Religious	Difference
1866	120,752	147,218	-26,466	--	--	--
1867	148,147	171,099	-22,952	--	--	--
1868	160,419	182,123	-21,704	--	--	--
1869	182,810	202,036	-19,226	--	--	--
1870	168,067	183,431	-15,364	--	--	--
1871	172,557	191,917	-19,340	--	--	--
1872	181,861	194,125	-12,264	20,550	26,249	-5,749
1873	190,950	200,336	-9,386	23,956	28,822	-4,866
1874	183,910	174,916	+8,994	24,087	26,977	-2,890
1875	203,217	191,095	+12,122	27,269	29,580	-2,311
1876	200,686	191,606	+9,080	24,767	27,914	-3,147
1877	191,043	190,983	+60	23,929	26,785	-2,856

[10] Scelsi, *Statistica delle province di Pesaro e Urbino, Pesaro,* 1881, pp. 55-58, quoted by F. Bonelli, *Evoluzione demografica ed ambiente economico delle Marche e dell'Umbria nell'Ottocento,* Torino, 1967, p. 96.

[11] Raseri, *I fanciulli illegittimi,* p. 8.

[12] L. Bodio, *Sui matrimoni legali e sui matrimoni celebrati col solo rito religioso,* Annali di Statistica I, Roma, 1873, IV: 231. L. Bodio and F. Caligaris, *Sulla statistica dei matrimoni celebrati col solo rito religioso dal 1866 a tutto il 1873,* Annali di Statistica I, Roma, 1877, 9: 8; L. Bodio, *Sulla statistica dei matrimoni civili e dei religiosi,* Annali di Statistica II, Roma, 1880, 15: 281-288, esp. table on page 285.

the corresponding religious marriages; the difference changes its sign in 1874, owing to the "regularization" of many solely religious unions. In Veneto and Roma, where the new legislation was introduced in 1871, the difference between civil marriages and religious marriages, in the six years from 1872 to 1877, amounts to 13 percent. Unfortunately we have no data for the following period, and cannot say if the recovery of civil marriages in the years 1874–1876 was a transient phenomenon. The general opinion, however, is that the phenomenon of solely religious marriages continued, albeit with a very low frequency, until the Concordat in 1929. A large proportion of the illegitimate children were, in due course, legitimated through subsequent civil marriage of the couple or by royal decree. In Table 2.8 the ratio of "legitimated" children to total illegitimate births is shown for the provinces once belonging to the

TABLE 2.8

RATIO OF LEGITIMATED CHILDREN TO ILLEGITIMATE BIRTHS, PROVINCES FORMERLY OF THE PAPACY AND OF THE REST OF ITALY: 1885-1887 TO 1906-1908 AND 1919-1923 TO 1953

Date	Papal provinces	Other provinces	Italy
1885-1887	.194	.150	--
1891-1893	.377	.211	--
1895-1896	.449	.259	--
1897-1899	.477	.272	--
1900-1902	.540	.290	--
1903-1905	.557	.300	--
1906-1908	.579	.312	--
1919-1923	.306	.244	.259
1931	.544	.332	.375
1953	.534	.436	.450

Papacy and for the rest of the country. Benini, from whose work these data have been drawn, observed that the higher proportion of legitimated children in the provinces of the Papacy was a consequence of the many solely religious marriages.[13] Unfortunately the data on legitimized children cannot be used for the correction of the series, because we know neither the year of birth nor, what is more important, whether the

[13] R. Benini, "La demografia italiana nell'ultimo cinquantennio, in *Cinquant' anni di vita italiana*, Hoepli, Milano, 1911, Vol. III.

parents had experienced a religious marriage or were unmarried at the time of the birth of the child. In the latter case, the child is illegitimate according to both civil and canon law.

As indicated above, the phenomenon of "illegitimate" births issued by solely religious marriages continued until the Concordat between the church and the state concluded in 1929. According to the laws of May 27 and June 24, 1929, religious marriages had full civil consequences, and from that year the artificial inflation of illegitimacy came to an end.[14] There was still another change in the criteria of data collection: data on illegitimate births, until 1927, were communicated by each comune to the Central Statistical Office; from 1927 on it was ISTAT itself that proceeded directly to the classification of births on the basis of the individual form. The previous system is believed to have underestimated illegitimate births.[15]

Summing up, there are four main factors affecting the comparability of statistics on illegitimate births:

(1) The introduction of civil marriage in 1866 (Lazio and Veneto: 1871)
(2) The change in the classification of children as legitimate, illegitimate, and foundlings in 1883
(3) The change in the criteria of data collection in 1927
(4) The Concordat, in 1929, giving full civil effects to religious marriages.

2.4.2. Given the noncomparability of the data, the interpretation of nonmarital fertility trends is awkward. I_h, although a necessary help in explaining the trends of overall and marital fertility, is very unsatisfactory if illegitimacy per se is under investigation and especially if a measure of the fertility of the unmarried is sought. The basic problem consists of the definition of the universe of women exposed to the risk of conceiving an illegitimate child. Usually, this universe is made to coincide with all unmarried women in fecund ages, by analogy with the techniques employed in measuring legitimate fertility. This has an important drawback: while practically all married women are at risk of conceiving a legitimate child (in other words, have sexual intercourse with their husbands), only an unknown fraction of unmarried women are at risk of

[14] ISTAT, *Movimento della popolazione secondo gli atti dello stato civile negli anni 1929 e 1930*, Roma, 1933, p. 27.

[15] ISTAT, *Movimento*, p. 61.

having an illegitimate birth. This unknown fraction is probably very variable in space and time, and certainly on the increase during the period under observation. Thus the conclusion must be drawn that all measures of illegitimate fertility based on the total number of unmarried women are unsuitable for the interpretation of demographic tendencies.

Moreover, although it may be tempting to assume that the decline of illegitimacy, like that of legitimacy, is due to contraception,[16] this is not possible for several reasons. First, there is the role of marriage as a legitimizer of already conceived children. Little is known about the frequency of marriage of a pregnant girl before the birth of the child. Other factors remaining constant, if this level increases, the level of illegitimacy will fall. Shorter, Knodel, and van de Walle have shown that in Sweden the probability of a pregnant girl marrying before the birth of her child has been increasing.[17] The evidence for Italy, though very scanty, points in the same direction. For example, births of first order according to duration of marriage have been tabulated from a reconstitution of families in two areas of Toscana (Fiesole and San Godenzo).[18] Before 1700, the proportion of such births within the first 8 months of marriage was 6.6 percent; in 1700–1749 it was 7.3 percent, and in 1750–1799, 4.8 percent (6.0 percent for the whole period). The corresponding proportions of brides who were pregnant at the time of marriage were 6.1 percent, 6.6 percent, and 4.2 percent (5.3 percent for the whole period).

A second piece of evidence comes from a survey made at the beginning of this century. Mortara in his study on premarital conception made a special survey of birth statistics in six large cities;[19] data on the proportion of brides who were pregnant at the time of marriage are presented in Table 2.9. Approximately 12 to 16 percent of all brides were pregnant, more than twice the levels of eighteenth-century Toscana. Mortara did not find any association between age and frequency of premarital conceptions.

More evidence was made available during the 1930s, when legitimate births were classified according to the duration of marriage. In that period the proportion, for the whole country, of first births within 8 months

[16] E. Shorter, J. Knodel and E. van de Walle, "The Decline of Non-Marital Fertility in Europe, 1880-1940," *Population Studies* xxv, no. 3 (Nov. 1971): 392.

[17] *Ibid.*, p. 385.

[18] Unpublished data kindly supplied by C. A. Corsini, Dipartimento Statistico Matematico, University of Florence.

[19] G. Mortara, "I concepimenti antenuziali," *Giornale degli Economisti e Rivista di Statistica* XXII, Vol. XLIII (1911): 56-68.

of marriage was 25 percent, or in 22.5 percent of all marriages the bride was pregnant. Data for the last 30 years are not available.

The evidence could support the hypothesis of an increasing secular trend of the frequency of premarital conceptions; if other factors had remained constant (they have not), the fall of illegitimacy could be imputed to this factor.

TABLE 2.9

PERCENTAGE OF BRIDES PREGNANT, SELECTED CITIES: CIRCA 1900

City	Date	Percentage
Bologna	1906	15.5
Firenze	1910	14.0
Genova	1908	16.5
Messina	1894	16.3
Milano	1910	11.8
Palermo	1906	14.0

This fact leads to another consideration that we will develop on the basis of the 1930 statistics. In 1930, 65,428 legitimate births of the first order occurred within 8 months of the date of the marriage, or 25.8 percent of all births of the first order and 22.2 percent of all marriages.[20] The total number of illegitimate births was, in the same year, lower (54,695). In that year, therefore, 120,123 births, 11 percent of all births, were conceived out of wedlock.

Of these, 65,428 were born legitimate because the mother was married before giving birth to the child, and another 15,000–20,000[21] were subsequently legitimated through the marriage of the mother, presumably with the father of the child. Therefore, for about two-thirds of the unmarried conceiving out of wedlock, the relationship with the (presumed) father of the child was so strong that a marriage (hurried or delayed) followed. A measure of the risk of pregnancy out of wedlock (and of its reciprocal, or the efficiency of contraception) ought to in-

[20] F. Savorgnan, "La statistica delle nascite legittime secondo l'ordine di generazione," in ISTAT, *Movimento della popolazione 1929 e 1930*, Roma, 1933, p. 117.

[21] While it is known, for each year, the number of legitimated births, their dates of birth are unknown. Mortara, for Bologna and Messina, has found that the average age of legitimated children was 3-5 years. The mean number of children legitimated by marriage was 1.29 in Florence, 1.43 in Bologna, and 1.88 in Messina. See Mortara, "I concepimenti," pp. 62, 63, and 65.

clude at the numerator all births conceived out of wedlock, and a good analysis of the fertility of the unmarried ought to be based on the three components just examined: (1) legitimate births, conceived out of wedlock; (2) illegitimate births, legitimated through marriage following the birth of the child; and (3) truly illegitimate births.

A further consideration is that nothing is known either about the "denominator" (the number of women at risk) of illegitimate fertility measures, or about the nature of the risk involved and, therefore, about the possible motivations for controlling fertility. We may only advance the hypothesis that the proportion of women at risk of becoming pregnant has increased over time. However, the universe of women at risk is composed of nonhomogeneous subgroups as far as motivation for control and knowledge of contraception are concerned. There are women entertaining stable relationships that lead to premarital conception and eventually to marriage. The motivation for control is probably strong because of the negative reactions of the family and society, but knowledge about methods may be limited. There are women who cannot get married, but have a marital-like relationship; their motivation for control and their knowledge will be the same as for normally married women. There are other women—prostitutes, for instance—with high motivation and knowledge, but also with high exposure to risk. There are other women (generally very young) with no or little knowledge and high motivation. Other examples could be found. Even if it were possible to know the "aggregate" of the unmarried women at risk, the interpretation of fertility trends would be difficult owing to the difference of knowledge and motivation among the various subgroups.

The parallel decline of marital and nonmarital fertility may be, therefore, fortuitous, and it may be the combined consequence of: (1) an increase of premarital conceptions leading to marriage before the birth of the child (a factor that tends to lower illegitimate fertility calculated in the traditional way); (2) an increasing contraceptive knowledge (same consequence as 1); (3) an increasing universe at risk (inverse effect); and (4) a changing structure of that universe (undeterminate effect). Our conclusion is that little can be inferred from the observation of a declining illegitimacy (traditionally measured) about the patterns of diffusion of fertility control. Moreover, the Italian situation (which we suspect to be true also for other countries) is affected until the 1920s by the noncomparability of the time series of illegitimate births.

Regional trends of I_h can be followed in Table 2.10. In 1862–1866 variability is substantial, going from a minimum of .022 (Sardegna) to a maximum of .068 (Sicilia). The effects of the 1866 marriage law are evident in the rise of I_h in the following years, particularly in the regions of the Center. In 1880–1882, I_h had risen to levels between .100 and .160 in Emilia, Marche, Umbria, and Lazio; a substantial increase can also be observed in Toscana and in Sardegna. After the beginning of the twentieth century, the situation slowly returned to normality, and I_h gradually decreased in all regions. In 1960–1962 the minimum level was .004 in Marche and the maximum was .018 in Calabria and Trentino. Even in these latter regions, the ratio of I_h to I_g was only 4 percent, compared with 3 percent for the total population.

It is interesting to note that the tendency (illustrated in Table 2.8) of areas with higher illegitimacy to have also a higher incidence of legitimated births by subsequent marriage is confirmed by later data and by more detailed territorial statistics. The fact that until the beginning of this century more boys than girls (far above the biological sex ratio at birth) were legitimated has also very interesting implications.[22]

From 1931 statistics cease to be biased, and trends can be compared and analyzed with more confidence. I_h falls everywhere, and the 1961 level goes from a minimum of one-fifth of the 1930–1932 level in Marche and Umbria to a maximum of two-thirds in Piemonte. The average fall in the North and in the South is approximately the same, and little can be inferred from the regional data about the factors causing the decline of nonmarital fertility.

2.5 *New Estimates of Marital Fertility*

2.5.1. The rise of illegitimacy at the end of the nineteenth century in the regions of the Center and the unbalanced sex composition of the population until World War I pose the question of the comparability of I_g and I_h trends with those of other regions. As we have just discussed, a large but unknown share of the children classified as illegitimate were borne by parents married solely with a religious ceremony. It is almost certain, however, that the great majority of the parents of these children were classified as married in the 1871 as well as in later censuses. Therefore, in the computation of I_g, the numerator is underestimated and needs correction. Fitting a straight line between the level of illegitimacy in

[22] From 1896 to 1907, 114 boys were legitimated for every 100 girls. This ratio fell to 107 from 1908 to 1913. See DIRSTAT, *Movimento della popolazione secondo gli atti dello stato civile nell'anno 1913*, Roma, 1915, p. xlvi.

TABLE 2.10

ILLEGITIMATE FERTILITY (I_h), BY REGION: 1862-1866 TO 1960-1962

Region	Actual levels										
	1862-1866	1870-1872	1880-1882	1890-1892	1900-1902	1910-1912	1921-1926	1930-1932	1935-1937	1950-1952	1960-1962
Piemonte	.041	.030	.029	.024	.020	.017	.010	.015	.014	.008	.009
Liguria	.033	.033	.036	.034	.033	.025	.016	.018	.015	.009	.010
Lombardia	.046	.032	.025	.022	.020	.022	.018	.019	.016	.009	.008
Trentino Alto Adige	--	--	--	--	--	--	.025	.030	.029	.019	.018
Veneto	--	.028	.051	.050	.049	.046	.049	.033	.026	.016	.010
Venezia Giulia	--	--	--	--	--	--	.053	.046	.037	.019	.014
Emilia	.036	.079	.117	.105	.094	.090	.069	.049	.034	.018	.012
Toscana	.053	.086	.079	.065	.052	.038	.023	.017	.013	.008	.007
Marche	.027	.087	.103	.090	.075	.053	.033	.020	.013	.006	.004
Umbria	.055	.097	.144	.122	.099	.046	.039	.036	.022	.010	.007
Lazio	--	.080	.157	.145	.135	.092	.042	.035	.027	.016	.013
Abruzzi	.035	.041	.045	.039	.033	.019	.020	.024	.022	.012	.008
Campania	.039	.037	.037	.035	.032	.023	.021	.025	.022	.016	.013
Puglia	.046	.040	.048	.041	.034	.025	.022	.023	.019	.013	.009
Basilicata	.050	.025	.063	.049	.033	.019	.019	.022	.022	.015	.010
Calabria	.066	.070	.075	.067	.058	.046	.033	.041	.039	.026	.018
Sicilia	.068	.065	.080	.065	.052	.030	.020	.024	.019	.016	.012
Sardegna	.022	.066	.087	.065	.047	.029	.018	.026	.022	.019	.011
Italy	.044	.050	.063	.055	.048	.037	.029	.027	.022	.014	.011

TABLE 2.10, continued

Region	Relative levels (1862-1866 set at 100)										
	1862-1866	1870-1872	1880-1882	1890-1892	1900-1902	1910-1912	1921-1926	1930-1932	1935-1937	1950-1952	1960-1962
Piemonte	100.00	73.17	70.73	58.54	48.78	41.46	24.39	36.53	34.15	19.51	21.95
Liguria	100.00	100.00	109.09	103.03	100.00	75.76	48.48	54.55	45.45	27.27	30.30
Lombardia	100.00	69.57	54.35	47.83	43.48	47.83	39.13	41.30	34.78	19.57	17.39
Trentino Alto Adige	--	--	--	--	--	--	100.00	120.00	116.00	76.00	72.00
Veneto	--	100.00	182.14	178.57	175.00	164.29	175.00	117.86	92.86	57.14	35.71
Venezia Giulia	--	--	--	--	--	--	100.00	86.79	69.81	35.85	26.42
Emilia	100.00	219.44	325.00	291.67	261.11	250.00	191.67	136.11	94.44	50.00	33.33
Toscana	100.00	162.26	149.06	122.64	98.11	71.70	43.40	32.08	24.53	15.09	13.21
Marche	100.00	322.22	381.48	333.33	277.78	196.30	122.22	74.07	48.15	22.22	14.81
Umbria	100.00	176.36	261.82	221.82	180.00	83.64	70.91	65.45	40.00	18.18	12.73
Lazio	--	100.00	196.25	181.25	168.75	115.00	52.50	43.75	33.75	20.00	16.25
Abruzzi	100.00	117.14	128.57	111.43	94.29	54.29	57.14	68.57	62.86	34.29	22.86
Campania	100.00	94.87	94.87	89.74	82.05	58.97	53.85	64.10	56.41	41.03	33.33
Puglia	100.00	86.96	104.35	89.13	73.91	54.35	47.83	50.00	41.30	28.26	19.57
Basilicata	100.00	50.00	126.00	98.00	66.00	38.00	38.00	44.00	44.00	30.00	20.00
Calabria	100.00	106.06	113.64	101.52	87.88	69.70	50.00	62.12	59.09	39.39	27.27
Sicilia	100.00	95.59	117.65	95.59	76.47	44.12	29.41	35.29	27.94	23.53	17.65
Sardegna	100.00	300.00	395.45	295.45	213.64	131.82	81.82	118.18	100.00	86.36	50.00
Italy	100.00	113.64	143.18	125.00	109.09	84.09	65.91	61.36	50.00	31.82	25.00

1862–1866 (still untouched by the influence of the new law) and in 1910–1912 (when the effects of the law probably for the most part disappeared), we may tentatively estimate the levels of "true" illegitimacy at the intermediate dates. We have then revised I_g; the results are shown in Table 2.11.

Except for Toscana, where I_g declined uninterrupted from the beginning, the new estimates of I_g smooth out the deep depressions that appeared previously in the 1870s, 1880s, and 1890s. In none of the four regions once belonging to the Papacy, does I_g decline by as much as 10 percent until World War I. The low of 1900–1902 in Lazio (9 percent from the levels of 1870–1872), Marche, and Umbria is followed by a recovery in 1910–1912. In Marche and Umbria, the new

TABLE 2.11

MARITAL FERTILITY (I_g) CORRECTED FOR ILLEGITIMACY, REGIONS OF THE CENTER: 1862-1866 TO 1910-1912

Region	1862-1866	1870-1872	1880-1882	1890-1892	1900-1902	1910-1912
	Actual levels					
Emilia	.648	.621	.653	.655	.658	.646
Marche	.683	.680	.734	.692	.648	.652
Umbria	.627	.640	.690	.655	.593	.614
Lazio	--	.594	.609	.590	.540	.557
Toscana	.733	.688	.666	.632	.599	.550
	Relative levels (1862-1866 set at 100)					
Emilia	100	95.8	100.8	101.1	101.5	99.7
Marche	100	99.6	107.5	101.3	94.9	95.5
Umbria	100	102.1	110.0	104.5	94.6	97.9
Lazio	--	100.0	102.5	99.3	90.9	93.8
Toscana	100	93.9	90.9	86.9	81.7	75.0
	Relative levels based on data in Table 2.6 (1862-1866 set at 100)					
Emilia	100	92.1	91.8	95.1	98.5	99.7
Marche	100	90.8	96.6	94.4	92.5	95.5
Umbria	100	95.7	94.1	94.1	94.1	97.9
Lazio	--	100.0	88.4	87.4	86.6	93.8
Toscana	100	90.3	86.5	83.6	81.2	75.0

estimates raise I_g perhaps too much, and it may well be that the correction underestimates illegitimacy. Perhaps not all the couples married solely by a religious ceremony were counted as married by the census.[23] In any case, it is clear that once the distortion in illegitimacy is eliminated, the extended depression of I_g at the end of the nineteenth and beginning of the twentieth centuries disappears almost completely.

2.5.2. Fertility is generally measured by relating live births to a fraction of the female population. Although fertility measures that take account of the male population have been proposed in several instances, they have seldom been employed in empirical research. If male measures merely represented parallel alternatives to currently used measures, their neglect would not greatly affect fertility studies. But there are situations in which consideration of the male population introduces information not conveyed by female-based fertility measures. This is particularly true in areas where long-term male emigration takes place on a large scale, resulting in an unbalanced sex-ratio.

It is obvious that substantial emigration often tends to inflate the proportion of women in the population. As a consequence, a proportion, sometimes considerable, of young women do not get married or, if married, run the risk of a long-lasting physical separation from their husbands, similar to a precocious widowhood. The index of marital fertility we have been using, composed of all married women of childbearing age, naturally includes those who, although fecund, are not fertile because they are physically separated from their husbands. Unfortunately, Italian census statistics do not tabulate the number of married women by presence or absence of husband, and an indirect estimate must be attempted. Two different estimates can be made and, therefore, two new estimates of I_g. The first type of correction (already made in an earlier monograph),[24] consists of multiplying I_g by the ratio of married women aged 15-49 to married males 20-54. Since the difference in the mean age at marriage of females and males is, in the Italian population, close to five years, this ratio is close to one in normal times and exceeds one when there is a consistent emigration of males. This procedure leads to the same results that would be obtained by relating births

[23] Perhaps the hypothesis is sustained by the fall in the proportion married at 15-24 years in Umbria and Marche in 1871 and 1881.

[24] M. Livi-Bacci, "Il declino della fecondità della popolazione italiana nell'ultimo secolo," *Statistica* xxv, no. 3 (1965): 412-413.

to the number of married men in age groups corresponding to principal fertile ages of women. It suffers from the drawback that differences in age at marriage are never exactly five years; even when the average is five years, the combined distribution by age of husbands and wives show that many women, aged 15-49 years, are married to men younger than 20 or older than 55. Moreover, differences in the age at marriage oscillate from time to time and from region to region. A second, simpler correction is to multiply I_g by the ratio of all married women to all married males. Here the inconveniences described above do not exist. However, another drawback has to be pointed out: sex imbalances are more evident in the young age groups that are more hard hit by emigration and are also more fertile, while the ratio takes into consideration the whole population, regardless of age.

In Table 2.12, the values of the two ratios ($k = Fm_{15\text{-}49}/Mm_{20\text{-}54}$; $k' = Fm/Mm$, all ages) are reported for regions in which the level rose above 1.1 at some time during the 1861–1961 period.

TABLE 2.12

TWO RATIOS OF MARRIED FEMALES TO MARRIED MALES, REGIONS WITH UNBALANCED SEX RATIOS AND ALL ITALY: 1861 TO 1961

Region	Ratio	1861	1871	1881	1901	1911	1921	1931	1951	1961
Liguria	k	111.8	108.5	107.7	104.9	101.0	100.5	100.5	97.2	96.2
	k'	105.8	103.0	103.8	103.0	100.3	100.5	100.6	101.6	100.2
Veneto	k	--	102.1	102.5	103.5	111.2	98.7	107.2	100.0	97.4
	k'	101.5	101.5	101.6	103.4	109.6	101.1	107.3	103.3	101.7
Abruzzi	k	104.9	106.4	108.1	114.8	127.2	112.2	115.0	105.9	106.2
	k'	106.3	106.6	109.3	114.8	121.1	110.9	111.7	110.3	110.0
Basilicata	k	103.3	104.2	105.9	113.5	114.0	103.1	102.3	99.6	105.3
	k'	101.8	102.8	106.0	112.0	111.1	104.3	104.8	103.7	108.4
Calabria	k	104.8	104.6	104.3	122.0	130.2	111.1	120.2	108.3	109.7
	k'	101.7	102.2	103.6	116.4	120.3	108.8	113.1	111.2	111.9
Italy	k	102.9	102.6	101.4	103.7	106.3	101.2	103.4	99.0	98.1
	k'	101.5	100.5	101.2	103.5	105.4	101.8	103.2	102.5	102.0

NOTE: k = ratio of married females aged 15-49 to married males aged 20-54.
k' = ratio of all married females to all married males.

For Italy as a whole, both ratios show a moderate surplus of married women in the first three censuses; this surplus is significantly higher in 1901 and 1911 (due to heavy transoceanic emigration), and then returns to an almost normal situation. Among regions, the surplus reaches very high levels at the beginning of the century in the South, exceeding 20 percent in Calabria and Abruzzi. The increase of the ratios coincides with the depression of I_g in the South and probably explains it almost completely. When the excess of married females reached such high values, a correction of marital fertility rates is obviously necessary, since male deficits reduce the number of women exposed to the risk of procreation. In addition, in a population experiencing a large scale emigration, the probability of migration, or the will to migrate, or even the feeling of instability associated with a declining society could be associated with postponed marriages, temporary separations, and an accentuated resort to any folk method of birth control to avoid obstacles to mobility.

2.5.3. Correcting marital fertility for abnormal levels of illegitimacy and the effects of migration (using in the latter case the more conservative ratio of all married females per all married males) produces the data in Table 2.13. It is interesting to concentrate for a while on the differential timing of regional decline. Of the several methods that could be followed, we have chosen the two simple ones that have already been employed in the earlier monograph on Portugal.[25] In the first method, we assume that an irreversible process of fertility decline starts once fertility has dropped 10 percent below the initial plateau in a sustained decline (without later recovery). In the second method, we select the period in which marital fertility (I_g) falls (again, without later recovery) below .600. When marital fertility falls below .600, it is almost certain that the population has adopted efficient methods for the control of procreation, methods that are usually destined for further diffusion within the population.

In Table 2.14, the timing of the decline is shown following the two criteria. The picture is similar with each method. Following the 10 percent decline guideline, the timing of the decline is earliest in Liguria, Toscana, and Sicilia, while it is delayed in Sardegna. In each case, the regions of the South come last and, in several instances, no decisive decline can be identified before 1936. According to the first of the two criteria, 70 years elapse from the date of decline in Liguria and Toscana and that in Sardegna. The following chapters attempt to explain the reasons for this slow but continuous process of diffusion of fertility decline.

[25] M. Livi-Bacci, *A Century of Portuguese Fertility*, Princeton, 1971, p. 59.

TABLE 2.13

ADJUSTED MARITAL FERTILITY (I_g'), BY REGION: 1862-1866 TO 1960-1962

Region	Actual levels										
	1862-1866	1870-1872	1880-1882	1890-1892	1900-1902	1910-1912	1921-1926	1930-1932	1935-1937	1950-1952	1960-1962
Piemonte	.657	.643	.655	.631	.608	.494	.382	.304	.268	.228	.228
Liguria	.696	.649	.639	.601	.567	.489	.370	.296	.267	.226	.222
Lombardia	.669	.659	.648	.680	.691	.641	.526	.416	.382	.289	.286
Trentino Alto Adige	--	--	--	--	--	--	.703	.543	.493	.430	.420
Veneto	--	.688	.683	.712	.760	.809	.712	.565	.525	.358	.346
Venezia Giulia	--	--	--	--	--	--	.518	.383	.346	.227	.223
Emilia	.653	.629	.664	.668	.673	.653	.538	.393	.352	.240	.239
Toscana	.737	.690	.683	.647	.610	.565	.477	.348	.318	.235	.235
Marche	.711	.709	.763	.725	.685	.702	.621	.490	.455	.299	.275
Umbria	.628	.640	.693	.661	.601	.638	.562	.443	.399	.256	.243
Lazio	--	.594	.609	.590	.540	.562	.517	.467	.435	.358	.360
Abruzzi	.711	.680	.704	.701	.699	.720	.738	.618	.566	.361	.348
Campania	.689	.672	.680	.679	.678	.716	.797	.667	.627	.508	.509
Puglia	.744	.701	.720	.697	.677	.723	.743	.653	.630	.501	.490
Basilicata	.690	.663	.681	.682	.679	.721	.747	.654	.628	.474	.461
Calabria	.651	.653	.632	.649	.667	.734	.766	.673	.648	.515	.518
Sicilia	.705	.696	.679	.647	.624	.619	.624	.541	.512	.425	.422
Sardegna	.642	.631	.648	.648	.647	.672	.714	.663	.633	.589	.551

TABLE 2.13 continued

Region	Relative levels (1862-1866 set at 100)										
	1862-1866	1870-1872	1880-1882	1890-1892	1900-1902	1910-1912	1921-1926	1930-1932	1935-1937	1950-1952	1960-1962
Piemonte	100.0	97.9	99.7	96.0	92.5	75.2	58.1	46.3	40.8	34.7	34.7
Liguria	100.0	93.3	91.8	86.4	81.5	70.3	53.2	42.5	38.4	32.5	31.9
Lombardia	100.0	98.5	96.9	101.6	103.3	95.8	78.6	62.2	57.1	43.2	42.8
Trentino Alto Adige	--	--	--	--	--	--	100.0	77.2	70.1	61.2	59.7
Veneto	--	100.0	99.3	103.5	110.5	117.6	103.5	82.1	76.3	51.0	50.3
Venezia Giulia	--	--	--	--	--	--	100.0	73.9	66.8	43.8	43.1
Emilia	100.0	96.2	101.7	102.3	103.1	100.0	82.4	60.2	53.9	36.8	36.7
Toscana	100.0	93.6	92.7	87.8	82.8	76.7	54.7	47.2	43.2	31.9	31.9
Marche	100.0	99.7	107.3	102.0	96.3	98.7	87.3	68.9	64.0	38.8	38.7
Umbria	100.0	100.9	110.4	105.3	95.7	101.6	89.5	70.5	63.5	38.5	38.7
Lazio	--	100.0	102.5	99.3	90.9	92.1	84.8	76.6	71.3	58.7	60.6
Abruzzi	100.0	95.6	99.0	98.6	98.3	102.3	103.8	86.9	79.6	49.0	48.9
Campania	100.0	97.5	98.7	98.6	98.4	103.9	115.7	96.8	91.0	73.7	73.9
Puglia	100.0	94.2	96.8	93.7	91.0	97.2	99.9	87.8	84.7	64.7	65.9
Basilicata	100.0	96.1	98.7	98.8	98.4	104.5	108.3	94.8	91.0	63.9	66.8
Calabria	100.0	100.3	97.1	99.7	102.5	112.8	117.7	103.4	99.5	79.1	79.6
Silicia	100.0	98.7	96.3	91.8	88.5	87.8	88.5	76.7	72.6	60.3	59.9
Sardegna	100.0	98.3	100.9	100.9	100.8	104.7	111.2	103.3	98.6	91.7	85.8

TABLE 2.14

REGIONS GROUPED BY DATE OF DECLINE IN MARITAL FERTILITY (I_g): 1881-1891 TO 1951-1961

Date	Decline in marital fertility (I_g): 10% below 1862-1866 level	Decline in marital fertility (I_g): Below .600
1881-1891	Liguria, Toscana	Lazio
1891-1901	Sicilia	Liguria
1901-1911	Piemonte	Toscana, Piemonte
1911-1921	Lazio, Lombardia, Emilia, Marche, Umbria	Emilia, Umbria, Lombardia
1921-1931	Abruzzi, Puglia, Veneto, Trentino	Trentino, Marche, Sicilia, Veneto
1931-1936	--	Abruzzi
1936-1951	Campania, Basilicata, Calabria	Campania, Puglia, Basilicata, Calabria, Sardegna
1951-1961	Sardegna	--

2.6 *Regional Fertility and Family Size*

2.6.1. Indexes and rates of fertility do not give the whole picture of the complex phenomenon of procreation. The index of marital fertility, for instance, may be the same in two groups of women, one with a very low, the other with a very high, age at marriage. The ratio of their actual fertility performance within their married life to the Hutterite standard would, in both cases, be the same. But the number of children per woman, or per marriage, would be very different. For example, the I_g of Albania was .696 in 1955; and that of Ireland was .612 in 1960–1962, or 12 percent less; however, the birth rate of the latter country (21.2) was half the birth rate of the former (41.7).[26] Similar differences would also be found in the number of children per woman. This very exceptional example illustrates our point; let us for a moment suppose that a situation like that of Ireland and Albania existed somewhere before the onset of fertility decline, in a situation where reproduction was not yet largely affected by individual control. It follows that at equal levels of I_g there would be substantially different patterns of children per marriage; is it likely that these two populations—other factors held constant—would start controlling their fertility approximately in

[26] M. Livi-Bacci, *Sur les régions d'Europe ou la fécondité demeure élevée*, Conseil de l'Europe, Conférence Démographique Européenne, Strasbourg, 1966.

the same period and experience similar trends in marital fertility? Different answers could be given to this question. It could be argued that the population with the higher ratio of children per woman or per marriage would feel a stronger motivation to control procreation. On the other hand, control could spread more easily where the number of children per woman or per marriage is lower, and where the adoption of Malthusian ways of control (higher age at marriage) might imply a more rational attitude toward procreation.

Both of these hypotheses—and others—could be sustained with a variety of arguments. However, everybody will agree that the burden of children is, in any case, a relevant factor and, therefore, must be analyzed.

2.6.2. A substantial amount of information can be gathered from the 1931 census special report on fertility.[27] Included in this report was the distribution of married women by age, according to the number of children ever born; thus, the mean number of children per married woman (married once) in each age group can be easily computed. We will limit our analysis to those women who, by 1931, had already completed their fecund period, i.e. married women of 45-49, 50-59 and 60 years and over, born respectively in 1881–1886, 1871–1881, and before 1871.

The information that can be gathered from the census measures is of a different nature from that which can be deduced from current statistics. The mean number of children of a married woman after completion of her childbearing period is a final measure of fertility, and is affected by: (1) age at marriage; (2) selective factors associated with mortality (differential mortality of women with a given number of children, or differential mortality according to social class); and (3) selective factors associated with migration. In Table 2.15 is shown the mean number of children per married woman of three different cohorts, by region; only married women with living husband and married once are considered.

It should be noted that married women 45-49 years of age in 1931 spent part of the normally most fecund period during World War I. They were 29-33 years old at the beginning, and 33-37 at the end, of the war, when birth rates fell to a very low level. It is to be expected that for

[27] ISTAT, VII Censimento Generale della Popolazione, *Indagine sulla fecondità della donna*, Roma, 1936.

TABLE 2.15

MEAN NUMBER OF CHILDREN PER MARRIED WOMAN AGED 45-49, 50-59, AND 60 AND OVER, BY REGION: 1931 CENSUS

Region	Mean number of children ever had by cohort			Percentage difference between cohorts		
	45-49 (1881-1886)	50-59 (1871-1881)	60+ (1871+)	45-49 and 50-59	50-59 and 60+	45-49 and 60+
Piemonte	3.67	4.40	5.23	-16.6	-15.9	-29.8
Liguria	3.54	4.21	5.12	-15.9	-17.8	-30.9
Lombardia	4.86	5.58	6.04	-12.9	- 7.6	-19.5
Trentino Alto Adige	5.01	5.38	5.52	- 6.9	- 2.5	- 9.2
Veneto	6.07	6.19	6.10	- 1.9	+ 1.5	- 0.5
Venezia Giulia	4.89	5.55	6.18	-11.9	-10.2	-20.9
Emilia	5.12	5.62	5.80	- 8.9	- 3.1	-11.7
Toscana	4.15	4.67	5.31	-11.1	-12.1	-21.8
Marche	5.16	5.54	5.66	- 6.9	- 2.1	- 8.8
Umbria	4.97	5.18	5.36	- 4.1	- 3.4	- 7.3
Lazio	4.68	4.98	5.37	- 6.0	- 7.3	-12.8
Abruzzi	5.29	5.54	5.63	- 4.5	- 1.6	- 6.0
Campania	5.94	5.98	5.96	- 0.7	+ 0.4	- 0.3
Puglia	6.44	6.64	6.74	- 3.0	- 1.5	- 4.5
Basilicata	6.27	6.48	6.35	- 3.2	+ 2.0	- 1.3
Calabria	5.85	5.92	5.77	- 1.2	+ 2.6	+ 1.4
Sicilia	5.66	5.95	6.12	- 4.9	- 2.8	- 7.5
Sardegna	5.53	5.52	5.61	+ 0.2	- 1.6	- 1.4
Italy	5.11	5.53	5.84	- 7.6	- 5.3	-12.5

NOTE: Data are for women with husband present.

this reason the mean number of children for this cohort might be smaller than that for other cohorts.

For women born prior to 1871, over 60 years of age, the average number of children ever born was 5.84 for Italy, with a minimum in Liguria (5.12) and a maximum in Puglia (6.74). Other regions, like Piemonte (5.23), Toscana (5.31), Umbria (5.36), and Lazio (5.37) had a ratio substantially lower than the national average. In Toscana, Piemonte, and Liguria, the decline had already started in 1881–1906, when these cohorts had their most fertile period. In addition to Puglia, five other regions show an average number of children above 6.00:

Basilicata (6.35), Venezia Giulia (6.18), Sicilia (6.12), Veneto (6.10), and Lombardia (6.04). It is interesting to note that these are the regions that show the highest birth rates in 1810–1812 and 1830–1840, and the highest marital fertility until the beginning of this century.

The two cohorts (45-49 and over 60) had their most fertile period in 1881–1906 and in 1906–1921, so that differences in fertility between the two generations may be thought of as an indicator of the differences in reproductive behavior prevailing in the two periods. We may therefore group the regions according to the decreasing intensity of change:

Large decrease: Liguria (—30.9 percent), Piemonte, Toscana, Venezia Giulia, and Lombardia (—19.5 percent)
Intermediate decrease: Lazio (—12.8 percent), Emilia, Trentino Alto Adige, Marche, Sicilia, Umbria, and Abruzzi (—6.0 percent)
Small or no decrease: Puglia (—4.5 percent), Sardegna, Basilicata, Veneto, Campania, and Calabria (+1.4 percent)

The data of Table 2.15 fit well in the general framework of fertility decline as outlined in Section 2.3. The sharpest decreases occurred in Liguria, Piemonte, and Toscana.

Two final points. First, comparing the 5.84 mean number of children per currently married woman (or 5.64 for all ever-married women) with the 8.70 hypothetical (period) number of children of the Hutterite women (married at age 24) yields a ratio of .671 (or .649 for all ever-married women). This ratio is very close to the late-nineteenth-century level of I_g, which, on the average, stayed around .650, and proves the consistency between fertility measures drawn from vital statistics and fertility measures drawn from the census. The second point refers to the considerable variation in mean number of children among the older cohorts (born before 1871). The mean extremes were 5.1 in Liguria and 6.7 in Puglia. However, even if Liguria, as well as Piemonte and Toscana (all areas where fertility was already declining) were excluded, the variation is still considerable and amounts to 1.3 children. Within the South, for example, women from Puglia had 1.1 children more than women from Sardegna or Abruzzi. If we take another index for this period, such as the proportion of women having 10 children or more, we find 23.1 percent in Puglia against 13.0 percent in Sardegna and 12.0 percent in Abruzzi.

These data show that before the onset of the decline, the burden of families, in terms of children ever had, varied considerably from one area to another and, probably more so from one social stratum of the population to another.

Six children per woman are, undoubtedly, a heavy burden. But other populations have, in the past, borne a heavier charge.

2.6.3. Another way, based exclusively on vital data, of measuring family size is the computation of the mean number of children per marriage. This is a period measure, already described in Section 1.7, where its defects are also discussed. The measure is heavily influenced by the combined impact of changing age at marriage, of the amount of immigration or emigration, and of the frequency of termination of marriages primarily through the death of husband or wife. The measures reported in Table 2.16 are influenced by all these factors. Throughout the period examined (1880–1964), mortality declines. In some regions there is a strong emigration, in others, substantial immigration; age at marriage does not show dramatic changes but fluctuates throughout the period. The data are, however, interesting because even with all their imperfections and distortion they reflect the changing level of family size.

In 1880–1889, in 10 of the 15 regions examined, the mean number of children per marriage was between 4.4 and 4.7; the regions above this limit are those that consistently show the highest fertility: Sicilia and Puglia in the South; Lombardia and Veneto in the North. The similarity of trends between I_g and the mean number of children per marriage is demonstrated in Figure 2.2. Emigration depresses the level of children per marriage (as it does I_g) in most regions of the South before World War I. If we take, as a standard way of determining the date of the decline, the 10 percent fall criterion, we find a distribution analogous to that obtained with I_g but much less variable. In Piemonte, Liguria, Marche, Toscana, Abruzzi, and Sicilia the decline is on its way after 1900; in Lombardia, Veneto, Umbria, and Lazio, after 1915; in Puglia, after 1930; in Campania and Basilicata, after 1940; and in Calabria and Sardegna, after 1950.

During the predecline period, the mean number of children per marriage rarely exceeded 5; this number represents 1 to 1.5 children less than the census mean number of children per married woman (see Table 2.16). The difference is explained by the fact that the census figure refers only to those women surviving, with their husbands, until the end of their reproductive age. The high proportion of marriages terminating before the end of the reproductive life because of widow-

TABLE 2.16

MEAN NUMBER OF CHILDREN PER MARRIAGE, BY REGION: 1880-1889 TO 1960-1969

Region	1880-1889	1890-1899	1900-1909	1910-1914	1915-1919	1920-1929	1930-1939	1940-1944	1945-1949	1950-1959	1960-1969
Piemonte	4.47	4.23	3.82	3.21	2.40	2.37	1.99	1.89	1.73	1.66	2.11
Liguria	4.45	4.38	4.08	3.69	2.94	2.70	2.20	1.82	1.76	1.62	2.02
Lombardia	4.80	4.86	4.88	4.58	3.45	3.54	2.92	2.68	2.61	2.15	2.54
Trentino Alto Adige	--	--	--	--	--	--	--	3.32	3.31	2.92	3.01
Veneto	4.87	4.75	5.08	5.25	3.80	4.30	3.37	3.17	3.23	2.51	2.52
Venezia Giulia	--	--	--	--	--	--	--	2.27	2.18	1.75	1.86
Emilia	4.51	4.08	3.82	3.90	3.20	3.54	2.82	2.81	2.23	1.72	1.63
Toscana	4.43	4.17	3.94	3.70	2.80	2.96	2.29	2.15	2.13	1.72	1.82
Umbria	4.57	4.23	4.23	4.38	3.40	3.38	2.56	2.35	2.30	1.75	1.82
Marche	4.68	4.32	4.06	4.14	3.30	3.65	3.11	2.98	2.96	1.96	1.87
Lazio	--	4.15	3.79	3.79	3.18	3.45	3.61	3.20	3.31	2.48	2.55
Abruzzi	4.45	4.26	3.95	3.89	3.33	3.92	3.59	2.96	3.19	2.22	2.00
Campania	4.58	4.42	4.18	4.35	3.95	4.50	4.16	3.90	4.43	3.18	2.93
Puglia	5.12	5.18	4.99	5.03	4.38	4.64	4.43	4.25	4.21	3.47	2.94
Basilicata	4.23	4.17	3.96	4.23	3.74	4.33	4.33	4.09	3.67	3.12	2.81
Calabria	4.46	4.45	4.11	4.22	3.87	4.36	4.28	3.93	4.07	3.23	2.93
Sicilia	5.25	4.95	4.41	4.22	3.68	3.94	3.73	3.79	3.56	2.91	2.77
Sardegna	4.73	4.38	4.38	4.32	3.91	4.21	4.33	4.37	4.51	3.97	3.47

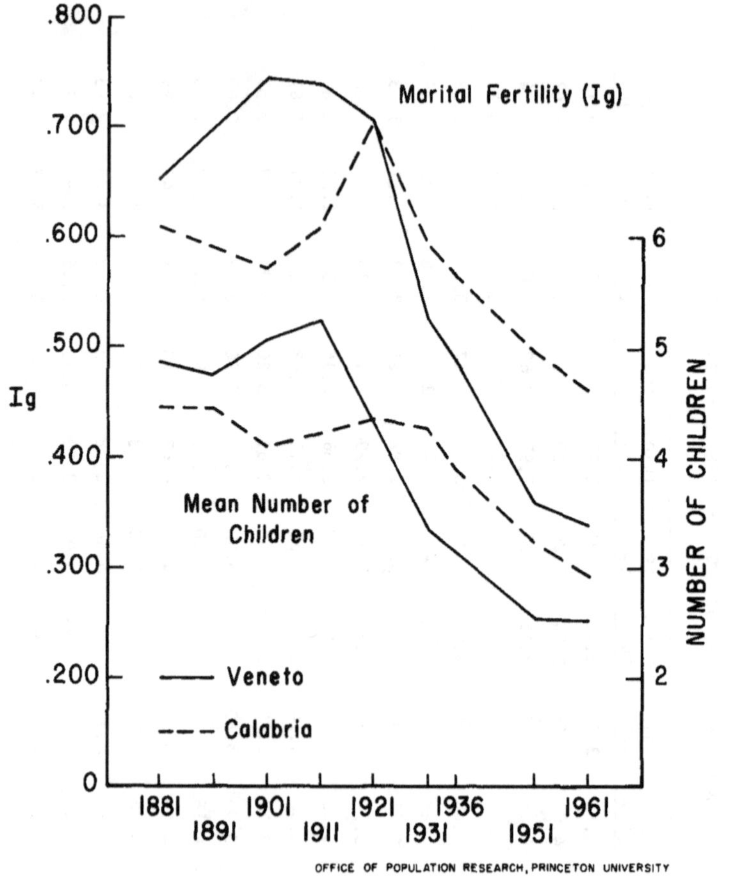

Figure 2.2 Marital Fertility (I_g) and Mean Number of Children, Veneto and Calabria: 1881 to 1961

hood or emigration accounts for the difference, which, of course, tends to be reduced for the younger generations because of the rapid fall in mortality.[28]

After 1930, only three regions in the Center and in the North (Trentino, Veneto, and Lombardia) failed to record a sustained decline in the

[28] We have shown elsewhere that according to the mortality of the times, of 1000 marriages, 623 survived at duration 30 in 1931, against 731 in 1951 and 761 in 1961. Therefore, when termination of marriage because of the death of one of the spouses is not taken into consideration, the mean number of children is underestimated. The difference was 8 percent with the 1931 mortality pattern, 3.5 percent in 1951, and 2.3 percent in 1961. It is certain that at the end of the nineteenth century the influence of mortality and emigration was much stronger than in 1931. See M. Livi-Bacci, *Recent Trends of Italian Fertility*, IUSSP General Conference, London, 1969, B.2.37.

number of children per marriage; in the South (with the exception of Abruzzi) the number fell slightly below 3.0 in the last 10 or 15 years.

2.7 *Cohort Analysis of Fertility Trends*

2.7.1. Cohort analysis offers new insights in the study of fertility trends, since the data are undisturbed by short time fluctuations and by changes in timing. The 1931 census gives the opportunity of following the performance of several female cohorts with completed fertility: those born before 1851 to those born in 1886–1891.

In Table 2.17 we have reported the mean number of children ever born (per ever-married woman), as well as the median number, the

TABLE 2.17

FERTILITY MEASURES OF EVER-MARRIED WOMEN, BY AGES 40-44 TO 80 AND MORE: 1931 CENSUS

Age at Census	Cohort	Number of Children Mean	Median	Percentage childless	Percentage with 7 or more children
80+	Pre1851	5.53	4.96	9.1	38.6
75-79	1851-1856	5.65	5.10	9.2	40.3
70-74	1856-1861	5.65	5.13	9.3	40.5
65-69	1861-1866	5.67	5.17	9.2	40.8
60-64	1866-1871	5.63	5.11	9.1	40.1
55-59	1871-1876	5.54	4.94	9.0	38.3
50-54	1876-1881	5.27	4.65	9.0	35.1
45-49	1881-1886	4.97	4.28	8.6	31.1
40-44	1886-1891	4.44	3.67	8.4	24.7

NOTE: Data for cohorts constructed from age reported at time of census.

proportion of women childless, and the proportion of women with seven or more children.[29] A reduced family size begins to be evident with the cohort of 1876–1881, a cohort whose period of maximum fertility occurred during the 15 to 20 years before World War I. Childlessness does not change much from one cohort to the other and remained around 8 to 9 percent. Among the early cohorts, the proportion of women with large families (seven or more children) remained at the 40 percent level; a sharp decline begins with the cohort born 1871–1876, falling to less than 25 percent in the 1881–1886 cohort.

[29] ISTAT, *Indagine sulla fecondità della donna*, p. 32. See also L. Galvani, "Altri aspetti della fecondità della donna italiana," *Notiziario Demografico*, June 1935.

Recently, the Dipartimento Statistico-Matematico of the University of Florence built a series of fertility tables by cohorts since 1930.[30] Tabulation of the distribution of births according to the age of the mother has allowed the computation of age-specific fertility rates, which, once cumulated, give the total fertility of each cohort. The available data have made possible the computation of the precise total fertility only for the cohorts born from 1915 to 1925; Santini has attempted an estimate of the total fertility of the truncated cohorts born between 1895 and 1915 (with the help of the information derived from the 1931 fertility survey) and between 1925 and 1940 (this latter cohort was at least 30 years old in 1970 and had achieved more than two-thirds of its total fertility).

TABLE 2.18

FERTILITY MEASURES, GENERAL FERTILITY RATE AND PARITY 7+ RATE: COHORTS OF 1891-1895 TO 1936-1940

Cohort	Absolute levels: General fertility	Absolute levels: Parity 7+	Relative levels (1891-1895 set at 100): General fertility	Relative levels (1891-1895 set at 100): Parity 7+
1891-1895	3,547[a]	448.4[a]	100.0	100.0
1896-1900	3,335[a]	368.0[a]	94.0	82.1
1901-1905	3,180[a]	348.9[a]	89.7	77.8
1906-1910	2,952[a]	272.2[a]	83.2	60.7
1911-1915	2,712	185.0	76.5	41.3
1916-1920	2,557	141.6	72.1	31.6
1921-1925	2,373	105.0	66.9	23.4
1926-1930	2,352[b]	96.1[b]	66.3	21.4
1931-1935	2,399[b]	92.8[b]	67.6	20.7
1936-1940	2,422[b]	87.6[b]	68.3	19.5

SOURCE: M. LIVI-BACCI and A. SANTINI, Tavole di fecondità della donna Italiana secondo le generazioni di appartenenza; Dipartimento Statistico-Matematico, Firenze, 1969, pp. 71 and 224.

NOTES: General fertility rate refers to children per 1,000 women. Parity 7+ rate refers to the number of women with 7 or more children per 1,000 women.

[a]Estimates on truncated cohorts (lower section) with the help of 1931 Census data.

[b]Estimates on truncated cohorts (higher section).

[30] M. Livi-Bacci and A. Santini, *Tavole di fecondità della donna italiana secondo le generazioni di appartenenza*, Firenze, Dipartimento Statistico-Matematico, 1969, pp. 71-224.

As shown in Table 2.18, total fertility (including still births) falls continuously from 3.55 children per woman born in 1891–1895 to 2.35 for women born in 1926–1930 (the latter cohort had the lowest fertility on record). Those initiating their reproductive life after World War II—the cohorts born after 1930—have shown a slight recovery; for example, the cohort of 1936–1940 has an estimated total fertility of 2.42. This recovery, however, is almost totally explained by the rise of nuptiality.

Figure 2.3 shows the long-term trend of cohort fertility followed through the 1931 census data[31] and through the total fertility presented in Table 2.18. While the two series are not strictly comparable, they do

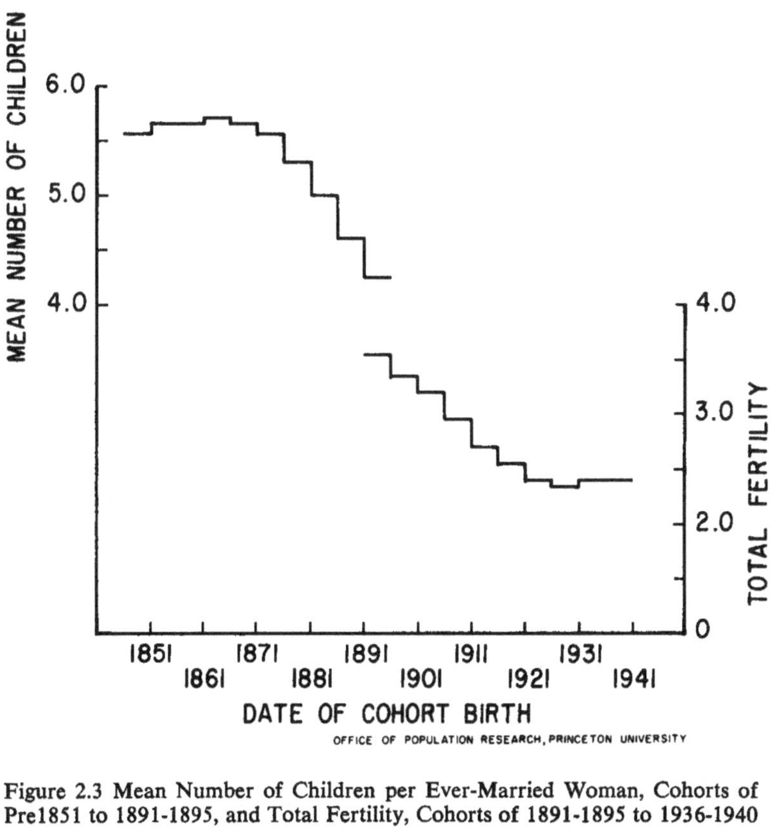

Figure 2.3 Mean Number of Children per Ever-Married Woman, Cohorts of Pre1851 to 1891-1895, and Total Fertility, Cohorts of 1891-1895 to 1936-1940

[31] For this purpose, we have estimated the final family size of those cohorts not yet 50 at the 1931 census, born in 1881-1886 (45-49 years), 1886-1891 (40-44), and 1891-1896 (35-39). We have completed their fertility using the age-specific schedule of legitimate fertility of 1931, 1936, and 1941 for ages from 35 to 50 years. The estimated final mean number of children for these cohorts is, respectively, 4.98, 4.61, and 4.26, against 4.97, 4.44, and 3.61 for the truncated cohorts.

clearly show a continuous fall among the 50 cohorts born from 1876–1881 to 1926–1930. This decline, as illustrated in Table 2.19 and Figure 2.4, took place at a steady rate. The rate of change remained within a

TABLE 2.19

MEAN NUMBER OF CHILDREN PER EVER-MARRIED WOMAN, COHORTS OF PRE1851 TO 1891-1895, AND TOTAL FERTILITY, COHORTS OF 1891-1895 TO 1936-1940

	Mean number of children			Total fertility	
Date	Absolute level	Percentage change	Date	Absolute level	Percentage change
Pre1851	5.53	--	1891-1895	3.55	--
1851-1856	5.65	+2.2	1896-1900	3.34	-6.0
1856-1861	5.65	0.0	1901-1905	3.18	-4.6
1861-1866	5.67	+0.4	1906-1910	2.95	-7.2
1866-1871	5.63	-0.7	1911-1915	2.71	-8.1
1871-1876	5.54	-1.6	1916-1920	2.56	-5.7
1876-1881	5.27	-4.9	1921-1925	2.37	-7.2
1881-1886	4.98	-5.7	1926-1930	2.35	-0.9
1886-1891	4.61	-7.9	1931-1935	2.40	+2.0
1891-1895	4.26	-7.6	1936-1940	2.42	+1.0

5 to 8 percent range per quinquennium from the 1876–1881 to the 1921–1925 cohort. No significant slowdown or acceleration can be detected throughout the period except changes that are imputable to the effects of exogenous factors such as the two world wars. The decline, once initiated, proceeds at a constant pace until very moderate levels of fertility have been reached.

2.7.2. The study of cohort fertility trends by region is possible for recent years.[32] Table 2.20 and Figure 2.5 contains total fertility values for the cohorts of 1906–1911 to 1926–1931. With regard to total fertility, women born in 1906–1911 show the highest regional variability, from a minimum of 1.5 for Liguria to a maximum of 4.3 for Basilicata.

Several regions fall below the level of 2.0 children per woman: Liguria and Piemonte with the 1906–1911 cohort; Toscana, with the 1911–

[32] Data for this section are based on M. Livi-Bacci and M. Ventisette, *Elementi per lo studio della fecondità regionale per generazioni, 1906-1946, Proceedings of the Twenty-seventh Meeting of the Società Italiana di Statistica*, Palermo, May 1972.

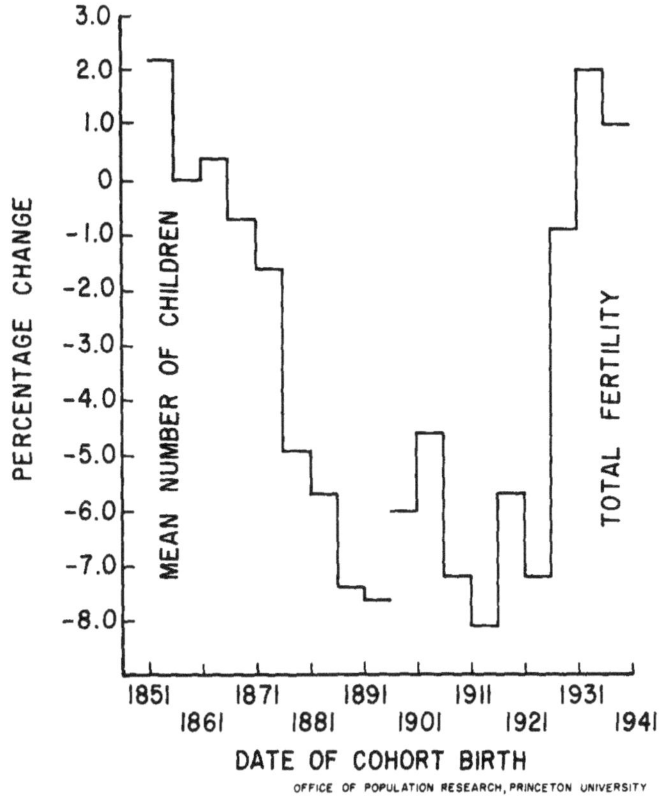

Figure 2.4 Percentage Change in Mean Number of Children per Ever-Married Woman, Cohorts of Pre1851 to 1891-1895, and Total Fertility, Cohorts of 1891-1895 to 1936-1940

1916 cohort; and Emilia, with the following. Lombardia, Umbria, and Marche will certainly remain below the 2.0 level with the generations born in 1921–1926 and 1926–1931. Had we available a series of cohort life tables, the computation of the net reproduction rate would have added Veneto, Lazio, and Abruzzi to the list of the regions with cohorts remaining below replacement. In all, there are 10 such regions, representing two-thirds of the total population.

The decline from one generation to the following with a more or less rapid pace, is evident also in the regions of the South, four of which still show (1906–1911 cohort) a total fertility above 4.0. In the 20 years separating the first cohort from the last cohort, total fertility declines, in the South, by almost one child per woman: most of the Southern

TABLE 2.20

TOTAL FERTILITY RATE, COHORTS OF 1906-1911 TO 1926-1931, BY REGION: 1971

Region	Cohort 1906-1911	1911-1916	1916-1921	1921-1926	1926-1931
Piemonte	1,699	1,620	1,623	1,535	1,513
Lombardia	2,236	2,091	2,030	1,885	1,788
Liguria	1,547	1,448	1,434	1,390	1,404
Trentino Alto Adige	2,601	2,629	2,666	2,493	2,367
Veneto [a]	2,882	2,692	2,562	2,323	2,151
Emilia	2,234	2,022	1,900	1,784	1,762
Toscana	2,054	1,929	1,850	1,748	1,666
Umbria	2,677	2,360	2,150	1,945	1,800
Marche	2,675	2,373	2,232	2,169	1,890
Lazio	2,705	2,454	2,330	2,192	2,102
Abruzzi	3,244	2,843	2,631	2,385	2,148
Campania	3,741	3,484	3,366	3,122	2,918
Puglia	4,096	3,777	3,602	3,244	2,892
Basilicata	4,304	3,892	3,695	3,235	2,842
Calabria	4,021	3,734	3,608	3,369	3,065
Sicilia	3,440	3,184	3,073	2,879	2,673
Sardegna	4,023	3,887	3,817	3,486	3,091

NOTE: Fertility rate for cohorts born in 1921-1926 and 1926-1931 is computed for women aged 45 and 40 years, respectively; however, among the Italian population, only 0.5 percent of children are born to women over 45 and 3.5 percent to women over 40.

[a]Including the province of Udine.

cohorts born in 1926–1931 (with the exception of the Abruzzi and Sicilia) will, at the end of their reproductive life, achieve a total fertility of 3.0 children or more.

2.8 *The Marriage Pattern*

2.8.1. In this section, the analysis will be limited to a recounting of the principal characteristics of nuptiality during the last century, a period in which the forces of stability have counteracted with success the factors of change, at least until World War II. Table 2.21 reports some indicators of nuptiality; and Table 2.22, the mean age at marriage. We have already observed (Section 2.2.2) that I_m remained at approximately constant levels, decreasing slightly, until 1921, and then recovered with an

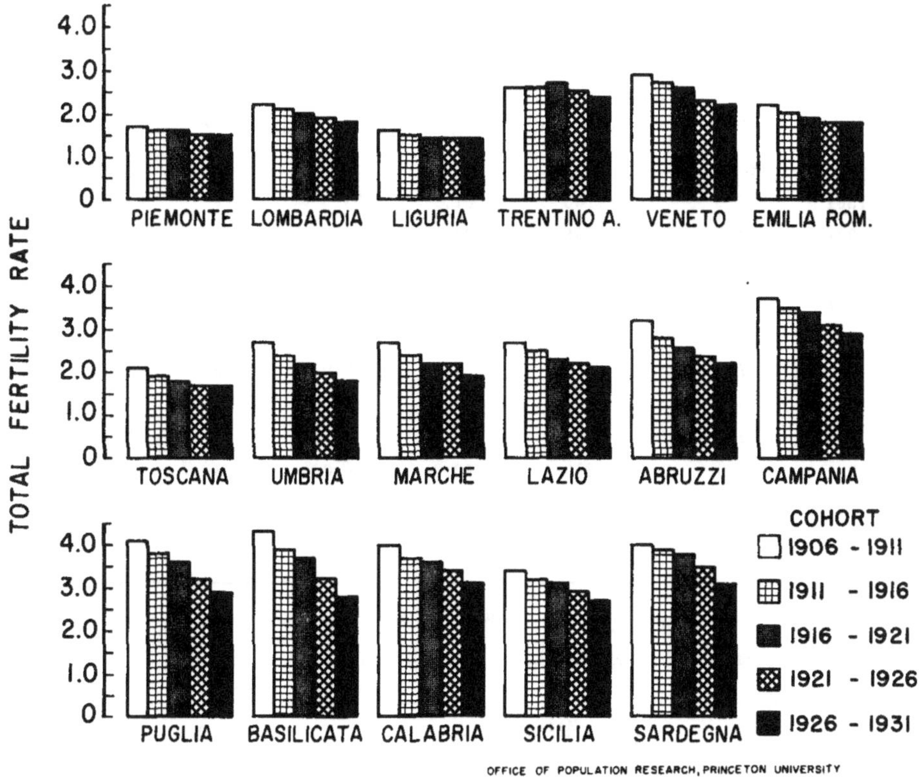

Figure 2.5 Total Fertility Rate, Cohorts of 1906-1911 to 1926-1931, by Region: 1971

accelerated pace during the last two decades. The factors of stability can be identified in the force of social norms and in the persistence of the traditional system regulating the process of choice, courtship, and marriage. Professional structure does not change very much until World War II; it is one of the factors of stability, reinforced by the rigidity of other regulations, such as the compulsory military service for males reaching age 21. The effects of the transoceanic emigration and of the war losses are evident in 1921, when I_m reaches the lowest point in a hundred years.

The mean age at first marriage for women remained slightly below 24 years until World War II, rose to about 25 years and fell to 24.3 years in 1965–1969. The proportion single at age 20-24 rose from slightly more than one-half of all women of that age in 1861 to about

TABLE 2.21

NUPTIALITY INDICES: 1861 TO 1961

Date	Crude nuptiality rate	Proportion married (I_m)	Percentage single by age			
			Males		Females	
			20-24	50-54	20-24	50-54
1861	7.8	.560	81.7	13.5	53.9	12.3
1871	7.4	.568	83.9	12.6	53.5	12.2
1881	7.7	.549	89.2	11.4	60.9	12.1
1891	7.4	.549	--	--	--	--
1901	7.2	.549	87.1	10.9	61.6	10.9
1911	7.6	.534	86.4	10.0	60.5	10.6
1921	8.8	.495	85.9	10.1	67.8	11.2
1931	6.8	.513	88.4	9.1	66.8	11.9
1936	7.6	.519	90.9	9.0	69.3	12.4
1951	7.2	.538	90.7	7.9	67.5	14.5
1961	7.8	.578	90.9	8.3	65.6	13.9

TABLE 2.22

MEAN AGE AT MARRIAGE, BY SEX: 1896-1900 TO 1966-1969

Date	Males		Females	
	Single	Widowers	Single	Widows
1896-1900	27.5	43.3	23.9	40.4
1901-1905	27.4	43.5	23.8	40.7
1906-1910	27.1	43.8	23.6	41.2
1911-1915	27.5	44.2	23.8	42.0
1916-1920	28.9	45.5	23.4	41.4
1921-1925	27.5	44.6	24.1	40.4
1926-1930	27.4	44.6	23.9	41.8
1931-1935	27.5	45.2	24.3	42.9
1936-1940	28.3	45.9	24.9	42.9
1941-1945	28.7	46.7	24.9	42.9
1946-1950	28.9	47.5	25.1	41.5
1951-1955	28.6	50.6	24.9	45.1
1956-1960	28.6	52.2	24.9	46.8
1961-1965	28.3	52.7	24.6	47.2
1966-1969	27.9	52.8	24.3	46.7

two-thirds in 1921, and remained approximately constant thereafter. The proportion single at age 50-54 was at a fairly constant level, with a minimum of 10.6 percent in 1911 and a maximum of 14.5 percent in 1951.

With the exception of the World War I years of 1914–1918, the mean age at first marriage for males remained at 27.5 years until the early 1930s; it then proceeded to rise to over 28.5 years by the late 1950s; since then it has fallen to 28. The proportion single at age 20-24 was also constant at about 85 to 90 percent from 1881 on, while the same proportion at age 50-54 fell from over 13 percent in 1861 to 8 percent in the last two censuses. The proportion single at age 50-54 for both sexes was about the same in the early censuses, but then fell for males and increased for females. This divergent tendency is due to the effects of transoceanic emigration, which led to shortages of males in the young and adult ages, and to the effects of war deaths. The largest difference is reached in 1951, when the proportion single among females is double that of men.

2.8.2. Data in Table 2.22 show an increase in the propensity to marry in the last decades. This fact is more clearly established by the data assembled by Santini for the female cohorts 1901 to 1941.[33] Table 2.23 reports the calculated proportion ever married at age 50 and the mean age at first marriage; data for the recent cohorts have been estimated on the basis of the truncated cohorts.

The proportion married remains between 84 and 86 percent in the first 20 cohorts; then it increases with an accelerated pace reaching (if Santini's estimate proves correct) 93.5 percent for the cohort born in 1941.

Cohort data seem to confirm the steady character of nuptiality patterns up to World War II, and the dynamic change of the last two decades brought about by a falling age at marriage and an increasing proportion married. This change conforms to that experienced in most of the western world, and partly justifies the slight recovery in cohort fertility observed after the early 1950s.

[33] A. Santini, *La nuzialità delle coorti femminili italiane, 1900-1941, Proceedings of the Twenty-seventh Meeting of the Società Italiana di Statistica*, Palermo, May 1972.

TABLE 2.23

PERCENTAGE FEMALES EVER MARRIED AT AGE 50 AND MEAN AGE AT FIRST MARRIAGE: COHORTS OF 1900 TO 1941

Cohort	Percentage married at age 50	Mean Age at first marriage	Cohort	Percentage married at age 50	Mean age at first marriage
1900	85.7	24.94	1921	86.1	24.93
1901	85.9	24.77	1922	86.0	25.11
1902	85.9	24.64	1923	85.6	25.13
1903	86.6	24.64	1924	87.0	25.13
1904	85.1	24.70	1925	87.3	25.06
1905	84.7	24.77	1926	87.8	25.06
1906	84.2	24.85	1927	87.7	25.02
1907	85.0	25.00	1928	88.3	25.03
1908	84.6	25.05	1929	88.6	25.01
1909	84.5	25.03	1930	88.4	24.73
1910	84.4	25.14	1931	88.9	24.75
1911	85.0	25.13	1932	88.8	24.63
1912	84.8	25.14	1933	88.3	24.48
1913	85.5	25.07	1934	90.5	24.46
1914	84.6	25.06	1935	89.5	24.37
1915	84.4	25.01	1936	90.1	24.27
1916	83.8	24.95	1937	89.1	24.20
1917	84.4	24.88	1938	92.1	24.09
1918	84.7	24.97	1939	91.3	24.04
1919	84.8	24.87	1940	92.1	23.96
1920	86.5	25.02	1941	93.5	23.84

2.8.3. Regional trends of I_m can be observed in Table 2.24. The proportion married (I_m) is a function of at least six variables:

(1) The mean age at marriage
(2) The proportion remaining single
(3) The frequency of separation and divorce
(4) The level of mortality
(5) The frequency of remarriage of the widowed and divorced
(6) The numerical balance between males and females

Of the six factors, (3) is negligible; (4) has affected all regions very much to the same extent; and the same can be said of (5). Factor (6) or the sex unbalance has affected the regions of the South much more than those of the rest of the country.

Regional differentials in I_m are small in 1861, ranging from a low in Campania of .539 to a high in Emilia of .597; though differences increase slightly over time, the overall pattern of relative homogeneity persists during the century-long period with I_m generally remaining between .500 and .600. The only region consistently above .600 is Basilicata. By 1921, all regions in the North have a level below .500; for most regions this pattern holds true until 1931. The depression of marriage levels in the North can be explained by war losses and by postponements because of war that were only partially recuperated after the war. Only Sardegna, from 1911 on, shows levels of I_m consistently below .500.

In the long run, however, two different trends can be observed in the North and in the Center, on the one hand, and in the South, on the other. In the North, the proportion married declined from 1871 to 1931 (excluding 1921, heavily affected by the war); then a recovery took place during the last 30 years. In the regions of the Center, I_m remains stable, increasing during the last 30 years. In the South, on the contrary, an increase of the propensity to marriage until 1901 was followed by a slight decrease due to the compounded effects of emigration and of the war, and then by stability. The increase of I_m takes place only during the last decade, between 1951 and 1961.

In short, levels of I_m are more stable in the Center and especially in the South than in the North. If we take the two largest regional populations, Lombardia in the North and Sicilia in the South, we may immediately appreciate the different patterns: in Lombardia I_m falls from .572 in 1871 to a low (1921 excluded) of .495 in 1931 and climbs to .576 in 1961. In Sicilia, I_m oscillates between a low (1921 excluded) of .552 in 1936 and a high of .592 in 1961.

In Tables 2.25 and 2.26 we have reported the mean age at first marriage and the proportion single at age 50-54, the factors that are responsible for a large part of regional differentials in I_m. Without going into a detailed analysis of the tables, we will point out that the propensity to marry seems to be higher at all times since the beginning of the century in the South than in the North. Southern women generally marry at a younger age with the exception of Campania and Sardegna, and they also have a lower proportion remaining single.

TABLE 2.24

PROPORTION MARRIED (I_m), BY REGION: 1861 TO 1961

Region	Actual levels										
	1861	1871	1881	1891	1901	1911	1921	1931	1936	1951	1961
Piemonte	.557	.570	.556	.539	.522	.508	.478	.511	.535	.567	.621
Liguria	.547	.562	.523	.512	.502	.488	.462	.474	.483	.539	.591
Lombardia	.562	.572	.562	.554	.547	.537	.479	.495	.501	.526	.576
Trentino Alto Adige	--	--	--	--	--	--	.393	.401	.407	.454	.508
Veneto	--	.586	.546	.540	.534	.512	.457	.470	.484	.515	.567
Venezia Giulia	--	--	--	--	--	--	.423	.474	.510	.540	.585
Emilia	.597	.584	.530	.528	.527	.537	.494	.508	.523	.560	.623
Toscana	.548	.563	.526	.533	.539	.538	.516	.538	.545	.566	.623
Marche	.540	.498	.483	.511	.538	.538	.514	.531	.535	.567	.621
Umbria	.550	.529	.487	.511	.534	.478	.553	.572	.577	.609	.645
Lazio	--	.575	.503	.503	.503	.509	.507	.520	.519	.540	.524
Abruzzi	.565	.581	.582	.590	.599	.573	.541	.564	.571	.553	.605
Campania	.539	.555	.545	.546	.547	.518	.484	.504	.494	.492	.538
Puglia	.550	.580	.588	.594	.598	.561	.541	.540	.533	.530	.552
Basilicata	.584	.608	.632	.635	.638	.628	.573	.604	.613	.509	.618
Calabria	.546	.566	.558	.580	.601	.581	.528	.550	.549	.543	.586
Sicilia	.585	.564	.566	.573	.579	.566	.530	.553	.552	.557	.592
Sardegna	.572	.573	.537	.519	.503	.493	.466	.467	.469	.483	.437
Italy	.560	.568	.549	.549	.549	.534	.495	.513	.519	.538	.578

TABLE 2.24, continued

Regio	Relative levels (1862-1866 set at 100)										
	1861	1871	1881	1891	1901	1911	1921	1931	1936	1951	1961
Piemonte	100.00	102.33	99.82	96.77	93.72	91.20	85.32	91.74	96.05	101.80	111.49
Liguria	100.00	102.74	95.61	93.60	91.17	89.21	84.46	86.65	88.30	98.54	108.04
Lombardia	100.00	101.78	100.00	98.58	97.33	95.55	85.23	83.08	89.15	93.59	102.49
Trentino Alto Adige	--	--	--	--	--	--	100.00	102.04	103.56	115.52	129.26
Veneto	--	100.00	93.17	92.15	91.13	87.37	77.99	80.20	82.59	87.88	96.76
Venezia Giulia	--	--	--	--	--	--	100.00	100.21	107.82	114.16	123.68
Emilia	100.00	97.82	88.78	83.44	88.27	89.95	82.75	85.09	87.60	93.80	104.36
Toscana	100.00	102.74	95.99	97.26	98.36	98.18	94.16	98.18	99.45	103.28	113.69
Marche	100.00	92.22	89.44	94.63	99.63	99.63	95.19	98.33	99.07	105.00	115.00
Umbria	100.00	96.18	88.55	92.91	97.09	86.91	100.55	104.00	104.91	110.73	117.27
Lazio	--	100.00	87.48	87.48	87.48	88.52	88.17	90.43	90.26	93.91	91.13
Abruzzi	100.00	102.83	103.01	104.42	106.02	101.42	95.75	99.82	101.06	97.88	107.08
Campania	100.00	102.97	101.11	101.30	101.48	96.10	89.80	93.51	91.65	91.28	99.81
Puglia	100.00	105.45	106.91	108.00	108.73	102.00	98.36	98.18	96.91	96.36	100.36
Basilicata	100.00	104.11	108.22	108.73	109.25	107.53	98.12	103.42	104.97	97.43	105.82
Calabria	100.00	103.66	102.20	106.23	110.07	106.41	96.70	100.73	100.55	99.45	107.33
Sicilia	100.00	96.41	96.75	97.95	98.97	96.75	90.60	94.53	94.36	95.21	101.20
Sardegna	100.00	100.17	93.88	90.73	87.94	86.19	81.47	81.64	81.99	84.44	85.14
Italy	100.00	101.43	98.04	98.04	98.04	95.36	88.39	91.61	92.68	96.07	103.21

TABLE 2.25

PERCENTAGE FEMALES SINGLE, AT AGE 50-54, BY REGION: 1861 TO 1961

Region	1861	1871	1881	1901	1911	1921	1931	1936	1951	1961
Piemonte	12.9	13.6	14.7	13.6	14.2	15.7	16.1	16.7	17.6	14.8
Liguria	13.4	15.8	15.4	14.1	15.6	16.4	16.8	17.0	18.0	16.3
Lombardia	10.4	10.9	12.4	12.7	12.5	13.0	13.4	13.8	15.9	14.9
Trentino Alto Adige	--	--	--	--	--	21.1	19.9	20.2	22.1	20.8
Veneto	--	9.8	10.0	10.2	10.5	11.3	11.8	12.7	16.8	15.8
Venezia Giulia	--	--	--	--	--	10.6	11.9	12.9	17.1	15.2
Emilia	9.1	9.3	10.2	10.8	10.0	10.3	10.4	11.3	13.6	13.1
Toscana	10.7	11.4	11.0	9.7	9.5	9.6	10.0	10.2	12.2	11.6
Marche	12.3	13.6	14.4	11.6	9.2	8.5	8.9	9.9	13.2	13.6
Umbria	11.0	11.8	11.8	10.9	8.3	8.1	7.9	8.0	8.5	8.9
Lazio	--	13.0	11.6	12.2	11.3	12.0	12.7	12.6	14.0	13.6
Abruzzi	8.5	8.8	8.5	6.4	5.6	6.0	6.8	7.8	10.2	11.2
Campania	16.2	15.0	13.8	10.2	10.8	10.8	12.3	12.7	13.5	13.9
Puglia	12.8	12.0	11.1	9.0	8.1	7.5	8.3	9.0	11.0	11.9
Basilicata	13.5	10.3	10.0	8.9	7.4	6.6	6.7	6.7	7.6	8.0
Calabria	15.4	15.8	13.5	11.6	9.9	9.4	9.6	10.4	13.4	13.7
Sicilia	15.6	15.1	12.0	10.2	9.4	9.5	9.8	10.4	12.9	13.1
Sardegna	8.4	9.2	8.2	9.1	9.9	11.1	12.2	12.7	15.9	16.6
Italy	12.3	12.2	12.1	10.9	10.6	11.2	11.9	12.4	14.5	13.9

TABLE 2.26

MEAN AGE AT FIRST MARRIAGE OF FEMALES, BY REGION: 1905-1907 TO 1968-1969

Region	1905-1907	1908-1910	1911-1913	1914-1916	1917-1919	1920-1922	1923-1925	1926-1928	1929-1931	1944-1946	1947-1949	1950-1952	1953-1955	1955-1958	1959-1961	1962-1964	1965-1967	1968 1969
Piemonte	23.3	23.4	23.5	24.7	25.7	24.6	24.4	24.2	24.3	26.0	25.7	25.5	25.3	25.1	25.0	24.8	24.6	24.4
Liguria	24.1	24.1	24.2	25.1	25.9	25.2	25.1	25.2	25.2	27.0	26.9	26.8	26.6	26.3	26.1	25.8	25.7	25.5
Lombardia	23.2	23.2	23.3	24.3	25.6	24.6	24.3	24.2	24.2	26.2	25.9	25.8	25.6	25.5	25.3	25.0	24.8	24.5
Trentino Alto Adige	--	--	--	--	--	--	26.2	26.0	26.2	27.3	27.3	27.0	26.9	26.7	26.4	25.9	25.6	25.4
Veneto	23.8	23.7	23.6	24.6	25.6	24.6	24.0	24.2	24.2	25.4	25.4	25.5	25.5	25.3	25.0	24.7	24.6	24.3
Venezia Giulia	--	--	--	--	--	--	24.5	24.2	24.3	24.9	25.3	25.4	25.4	25.3	25.0	24.7	24.6	24.3
Emilia	24.5	24.0	24.1	25.4	25.7	24.4	24.1	24.3	23.9	25.0	25.1	25.2	25.2	25.1	24.9	24.8	24.5	24.3
Toscana	24.1	23.9	23.8	25.3	25.8	24.5	24.3	24.0	23.9	24.8	25.0	25.1	25.2	25.1	25.0	24.8	24.6	24.4
Marche	24.6	24.0	23.9	25.8	26.5	24.3	23.7	23.6	23.4	24.5	24.5	24.5	24.5	24.5	24.3	24.5	24.3	24.1
Umbria	25.1	24.4	24.4	26.3	26.6	24.4	24.1	23.6	23.3	24.0	24.1	24.2	24.4	24.5	24.5	24.5	24.3	24.2
Lazio	25.6	24.9	25.1	26.7	26.8	25.0	24.5	24.4	24.3	24.9	25.0	25.0	25.0	24.9	24.9	24.8	24.6	24.5
Abruzzi	23.3	23.2	23.2	24.4	25.0	23.8	23.4	23.2	23.2	24.0	24.1	23.8	23.9	24.0	24.3	24.1	23.7	23.6
Campania	23.8	23.6	23.7	24.6	25.1	24.4	24.2	24.1	24.1	25.0	25.4	25.3	25.3	25.3	25.3	24.9	24.4	24.1
Puglia	23.0	23.0	23.1	23.6	24.2	24.0	23.5	23.2	23.2	24.1	24.6	24.3	24.3	24.3	24.7	24.2	23.8	23.6
Basilicata	22.0	21.8	21.8	23.1	24.0	22.8	22.4	22.2	22.2	23.7	23.6	23.4	23.3	23.6	23.8	23.7	23.1	23.9
Calabria	22.9	22.5	22.5	23.4	24.6	23.2	22.9	22.7	22.7	23.7	23.7	23.3	23.3	23.4	23.6	23.5	23.0	22.8
Sicilia	23.2	22.9	23.1	24.2	24.6	23.6	23.2	23.0	22.8	23.8	24.1	23.8	23.7	23.7	23.9	23.7	23.4	23.2
Sardegna	25.0	24.8	24.9	25.5	26.3	25.3	25.0	24.7	24.7	25.4	25.3	25.2	25.2	25.1	25.2	25.1	25.0	25.0
Italy	23.7	23.5	23.6	24.7	25.5	24.3	24.0	23.9	23.9	25.0	25.1	25.0	24.9	24.9	24.8	24.6	24.4	24.2

2.9 *Conclusion*

This chapter represents the frame of the book; we have tried to provide the reader with as complete a presentation as possible of various homogeneous series of fertility and nuptiality measures, at both the national and the regional level, covering the last hundred years. During this period, a transition from high and largely uncontrolled fertility to very low family size norms was accomplished. The extreme points of this transition are represented by the 6.7 children per married woman (cohorts born before 1871) in Puglia and the 1.5 children per married woman (cohorts born in the 1920s) in Liguria. The various standardized period measures have been supplemented, whenever possible, by cohort measures less affected by short-term fluctuations.

It is difficult to summarize all the findings concerning fertility and nuptiality, so great is the variability of these phenomena; we will only make a selection of the principal ones, and outline the problems that require further investigation.

First, the variability of regional fertility trends is striking. At the national level, the fertility transition took about 60 years, starting at the end of the nineteenth century and ending in the early 1950s. But the transition covers very different time spans in the regions. In the northwest and in the Center, the decline starts shortly after unification in 1861 and ends in the late 1940s after World War II; in the South, a clear and deliberate control of fertility became evident only during the 1930s, and, in some instances, at mid-century; now, at the beginning of the 1970s, fertility is still relatively high and fertility control not yet fully established.

The marriage pattern is more stable, although some secular changes have taken place and a certain regional variability has always been evident, especially because of the higher propensity to marriage in the regions of the South.

Second, the relatively low level of premodern fertility, before the onset of the decline, is an interesting feature of the Italian demographic history. Our index of marital fertility (I_g) stands at about two-thirds of the empirical maximum until the end of the century. While this level can also be found in Spain and in Portugal before the beginning of the decline, it was much lower than that in Central or Northern Europe. On the other hand, at the end of the transition, the largest part of the population of the North and of the Center reaches extremely low levels of fertility, well below replacement level.

Third, the transition was a gradual rather than an abrupt process. This is very well illustrated by cohort data. They show, at the national level, a continuous and steady decline of fertility from the cohorts born in the 1870s to the cohorts born in the 1920s. The steadiness of the decline is less evident in period measures that are subject to short-term fluctuations mainly caused by fluctuations in the timing of the reproductive process. Experience has shown in numerous instances that the decline, once firmly established, is an irreversible process until low levels of fertility are reached; it is, however, interesting to prove that the process is not only irreversible but also gradual. This fact seems to suggest the existence of a "diffusion" pattern, according to which an increasing proportion of the population is led to reduce family size.

CHAPTER 3: Urban-Rural Residence and the Decline in Fertility

3.1 *Special Characteristics of Urban Populations*

3.1.1. Residence in an urban environment is generally believed to be a factor in the decline of fertility. It is assumed that patterns of neo-Malthusian behavior are more easily developed in urban populations, where social and territorial mobility are greater and the standard of living and degree of education are generally higher than in other sectors of the population.

The validity of this hypothesis is, at least in part, supported by the analysis of the available statistical evidence concerning urban-rural differentials in Italy during the first part of the nineteenth century. Although the measures employed are rather gross owing to the nature of the available statistics, urban fertility appears to have been consistently lower than the fertility of the rest of the population. This chapter is primarily concerned with testing the validity of the general hypothesis stated above by drawing upon the richer statistical material of the last hundred years, and with the following:

(1) Ascertaining whether the fertility decline actually started in the urban areas, and whether it was more rapid in the urban, than in the rural, population

(2) Ensuring that the decline is related to the diffusion of voluntary birth control methods, and not to the effects of external factors such as sex composition, postponement of marriage, and so forth

(3) Examining the structural characteristics peculiar to urban populations that may affect (at least indirectly) the level of fertility, but whose exact impact cannot be appreciated with the traditional tools of demographic analysis

Everybody is aware of the great difficulties involved in the precise definition of "urban" and "rural" settlement. Such a definition, when based on statistical information, may take into consideration various parameters, such as the size of urban agglomerations, the occupational composition of the labor force, and the distance from, and the relations with, metropolitan areas. In our case, given the practical impossibility of designing a classification valid over a century-long period, the distinction between the urban and the rural population has been made according to the size of the smaller administrative units of residence, the comuni.[1] There are three weaknesses in this procedure:

(1) Comuni with a large population may simply have a large territory and may therefore have a low density and lack any genuine urban characteristics. On the other hand, comuni with a small population, but with a high density or a location near important centers, often do not have rural characteristics. For instance, many large comuni of the South, mainly in Puglia and Sicilia, are mere agglomerations of rural population, with few of those characteristics that are commonly related to the urban environment.

(2) Independent of size, the population of a comune may not be homogeneous, being partly urban and partly rural.

(3) When the boundaries of a comune are changed, and its population increases, or decreases, the comune may be shifted from one class to another, while no modifications have occurred in its social structure.

With regard to the first point, all comuni with more than 100,000 inhabitants contain relatively large cities, and have all the characteristics commonly attributed to urban areas. In 1901, 11 comuni (Torino, Milano, Genova, Venezia, Bologna, Firenze, Roma, Napoli, Catania, Messina, and Palermo) had more than 100,000 inhabitants; there is little doubt about the urban nature of these cities. Many had been urban in character since the Middle Ages; Napoli, Milano, Venezia, Roma, Messina, and Palermo each had more than 100,000 inhabitants in the second part of the sixteenth century.[2] Finally, in the various

[1] Other authors have studied the development of birth, death, marriage, and growth rates of the population living in classes of comuni of different size. Unfortunately, besides the difficulty of attributing "urban" or "rural" nature to the population living in comuni of different size, there is also the difficulty of interpreting the differences in birth rate trends and levels. See P. Fortunati, "Natalità, mortalità e nuzialità dei Comuni del Regno in ordine di intensità di popolazione," *Supplemento Statistico ai Nuovi Problemi di Politica, Storia ed Economia* III, no. 3 (1937). I. Scardovi, "Ricerche sperimentali intorno alle relazioni tra popolosità e movimento naturale della popolazione," *Statistica* IV, no. I, 1955. Idem, "Ricerche sulle manifestazioni demografiche differenziali dei Comuni italiani," *Statistica* XVIII, nos. 2 and 3, 1958. For a criticism of Fortunati's approach, see L. Livi, "Sui concetti di minimum di popolazione e di optimum strutturale," *Economia*, XVI, 22, no. 1 (1938), p. 86ff.

[2] G. Mortara, *Le popolazioni delle grandi città italiane*, Biblioteca dell' Economista V, Vol. XIX (1908).

schemes adopted or proposed for the classification of the population as urban and rural, the comuni with 100,000 and more inhabitants have always been classified as urban. Although the number of such comuni has quadrupled in this century (from 11 in 1901 to 21 in 1931, 32 in 1961, and 44 in 1971) little doubt can be cast upon the urban character of their populations at each point in time.

With regard to the second point, the homogeneous nature of comuni classified as urban, we have constructed Table 3.1. This table shows the

TABLE 3.1

TOTAL AND CENTRAL CITY POPULATION, ELEVEN LARGEST COMUNI: 1901

Comune	Total population (000)	Population living in central city: Number (000)	Population living in central city: Percentage of total
Torino	336	283	84.2
Milano	491	464	94.5
Genova	235	159	67.7
Venezia	152	143	94.1
Bologna	152	145	95.4
Firenze	206	159	77.2
Roma	463	425	91.8
Napoli	564	493	87.4
Catania	149	92	61.7
Messina	150	124	82.7
Palermo	310	267	86.1
Total	3,208	2,754	85.8

SOURCE: G. MORTARA, Le popolazioni delle grandi città italiane, Biblioteca dell'Economista, Serie V, Vol. XIX, p. 509, 1908.

total population of comuni with more than 100,000 inhabitants and the population concentrated in the central city. In all but two of the comuni (Genova and Catania), the population concentrated in the central cities was more than three-fourths of the total population of the comune; moreover, the remaining part of the population was itself largely urban in character.

Urbanization has been more rapid in the North and in the Center than in the South. In 1871, large comuni (100,000 and more) accounted for 6.6 percent of the population in the North, 9.1 percent in the Center, and 7.6 percent in the South; a century later, the respective distribution was 29 percent, 39 percent, and 22 percent. Until 1921, Napoli was the largest Italian city; it was surpassed a decade later by Milano and Roma. The differential pattern of urbanization can be better seen from the classification adopted by ISTAT and based on six demographic, social, and economic parameters.[3] In 1961, 55 percent of the population in the North was classified as urban, against 51 percent in the Center, and only 34 percent in the South. Whatever criteria we may follow in the classification of the population, the South has experienced a slower rate of urbanization than the rest of the country.

3.1.2. Proceeding on the assumption that the size of the comune is directly correlated with the degree of urbanization, we have grouped the comuni in three broad classes:

Comuni with less than 30,000:	*mainly rural population*
Comuni with 30,000 to 100,000:	*semi-urban population*
Comuni with more than 100,000:	*mainly urban population*

A more detailed classification, although possible, would not be of great help, since we are trying to delineate major fertility differentials only in broad sectors of the population.

Consideration of the demographic characteristics of urban populations is complicated by certain special features of urban societies. These include:

(1) The existence of a large, fluctuating, and highly mobile population

(2) The demographic behavior of certain highly differentiated sectors of the urban population. Special groups include the institutional population, living in communities for religious, educational, military, sanitary, or penal purposes: this population is a larger fraction of the total population of cities than of the rest of the country. To the institutional population may be added domestic servants, paupers, prostitutes, etc., persons whose marital and reproductive life is largely affected by their profession or status. In Table 3.2 we have reported the fraction of the total population of the cities that consists of persons in these special categories at the 1901 census. The higher proportion of these spe-

[3] ISTAT, *Norme di classificazione dei comuni secondo le caratteristiche urbane e rurali,* Metodi e Norme, c (1963).

TABLE 3.2

SPECIAL "NONMARRIED" GROUPS AS PERCENTAGE OF TOTAL POPULATION, BY SEX, ELEVEN LARGEST COMUNI AND REST OF ITALY: 1901 CENSUS

Comune	Males	Females
Torino	11.0	12.8
Milano	6.2	11.2
Genova	6.9	13.2
Venezia	11.8	11.0
Bologna	11.0	10.8
Firenze	13.5	12.8
Roma	12.0	11.6
Napoli	7.2	9.3
Catania	5.2	5.9
Messina	7.5	5.9
Palermo	9.0	8.3
Total, 11 comuni	9.0	10.7
Rest of Italy	3.2	3.2

NOTE: Special "nonmarried" groups refer to domestic servants, priests and nuns, members of the armed services, inmates of hospitals and prisons, paupers, and prostitutes.

cial groups in the urban population (11 percent for females in the cities, compared with 3 percent in the rest of the country) has certainly contributed to different fertility and nuptiality in the cities, although a precise estimate of the effect would be difficult to construct.

(3) The influx of mothers from rural areas to deliver their children at a hospital or clinic in the city. When a double classification of births according to the place of residence of parents and place of birth of the baby is available, virtually unbiased fertility measures can be computed for the de jure population. In our analysis this has not been possible, because such double classification does not start until the late 1950s; thus, rates have been computed for the de facto population. The bias of the de facto calculation becomes very strong after World War II, when the practice of delivering the baby at home was rapidly abandoned. In 1958, the first year for which the double classification is available, the ratio of resident to all births was .882 in the 11 largest comuni.

Fertility rates computed for the de facto population would have probably been 12 percent higher than those computed for the de jure. In 1951 (the last year for which we have computed fertility rates for classes of comuni) the bias was probably lower; it must have been negligible for earlier times. This is proved by the fact that, while in 1958 about one out of three deliveries took place in institutions (hospitals and clinics), in 1951 the ratio was one of seven, and in 1932 it was only one out of twenty.

3.2 *Marriage Habits of Urban Populations*

3.2.1. Some of the elements cited in the preceding paragraphs, particularly the mobility and professional structure of the urban population and the presence of special occupational groups, affect the propensity to marriage in the cities. Table 3.3 reports the proportion married among women 15 to 49 years (M) for three classes of comuni in 1871, 1901, 1931, and 1951.

In 1871 and in 1901 the situation is, at the national level, almost identical; the highest proportion married can be found in the mainly rural population and the lowest in the mainly urban, while the semi-urban has intermediate values. The difference between the extremes is very strong: in 1871, a high of 57.3 percent and a low of 49.0 percent; in 1901, 57.6 percent against 48.8 percent. This inverse relationship between the size of the comuni and the propensity to marriage can be found in almost all the regions. The proportion married is below 50 percent in the urban population (except in Sicilia) and is often above 60 percent in the rural areas.

Primarily because of a fall in the proportion married in small comuni, there is no longer a large difference between rural and urban populations in 1931. It is interesting to note that the proportion married substantially increased in the large comuni of Torino, Genova, and Firenze, although no appreciable changes can be detected in the large comuni of other regions. This finding seems to lend further support to the theory that where effective control over marital fertility has been established, as in the large cities after 1901, the Malthusian means of fertility control, such as postponement or avoidance of marriage, are less essential. As a consequence, propensity to marriage, formerly checked by the prospect of immediate pregnancy and continuous childbearing, may tend to resume less restrictive patterns.

In 1951, the inverse relationship between propensity to marriage and

TABLE 3.3

PROPORTION FEMALES AGED 15-49 MARRIED, THREE CLASSES OF COMUNI, BY REGION: 1871 TO 1951

	1871				1901			
Region	Less than 30,000	30,000 to 100,000	More than 100,000	Total	Less than 30,000	30,000 to 100,000	More than 100,000	Total
Piemonte	56.4	58.5	48.8	55.8	54.6	54.0	44.8	53.4
Liguria	58.4	--	48.5	55.3	52.8	56.6	45.4	51.5
Lombardia	57.7	46.6	45.6	56.4	56.8	47.0	51.3	55.4
Trentino Alto Adige	--	--	--	--	--	--	--	--
Veneto	60.4	49.8	46.7	58.5	56.4	46.7	45.4	54.8
Venezia Giulia	--	--	--	--	--	--	--	--
Emilia	61.0	53.0	48.2	58.5	57.4	49.2	45.2	54.6
Toscana	58.7	50.4	49.3	56.6	58.0	51.3	44.8	55.5
Marche	52.1	52.2	--	52.1	55.8	54.0	--	55.7
Umbria	54.2	54.3	--	54.2	55.7	55.0	--	55.6
Lazio	59.4	--	48.7	56.2	54.9	--	48.5	52.2
Abruzzi	58.5	--	--	58.5	61.8	--	--	61.8
Campania	56.6	--	49.4	55.3	58.9	56.2	48.2	56.7
Puglia	56.9	52.4	--	56.5	60.5	60.8	--	60.6
Basilicata	58.6	--	--	58.6	63.6	--	--	63.6
Calabria	54.8	49.3	--	54.7	60.3	55.7	--	60.0
Sicilia	55.8	52.4	52.5	55.1	60.0	55.8	54.9	58.6
Sardegna	56.7	48.4	--	55.9	53.0	--	43.4	51.8
Italy	57.3	51.7	49.0	56.3	57.6	52.8	48.8	56.2
	1931				1951			
Piemonte	52.7	52.2	51.8	52.5	59.0	59.5	59.3	59.1
Liguria	49.6	49.4	49.4	49.5	56.0	58.6	57.5	56.9
Lombardia	51.5	52.9	49.1	51.1	55.9	54.6	54.7	55.5
Trentino Alto Adige	43.7	39.8	--	42.9	46.3	54.5	--	47.9
Veneto	49.3	46.6	44.6	48.5	52.7	51.5	52.3	52.6
Venezia Giulia	51.3	44.1	46.6	50.0	57.6	51.1	57.3	56.9
Emilia	53.8	49.7	46.8	52.0	58.4	57.2	56.5	57.8
Toscana	58.6	50.9	48.2	55.2	62.2	58.4	57.0	60.6
Marche	54.0	53.3	--	53.9	58.3	55.4	--	57.8
Umbria	59.5	--	55.7	58.0	61.9	62.1	--	62.0
Lazio	57.9	55.4	47.9	53.1	59.9	60.2	53.1	56.4
Abruzzi	58.3	49.2	--	57.3	57.2	51.4	--	56.5
Campania	53.9	52.9	45.8	51.7	51.9	50.2	49.6	51.2
Puglia	55.2	55.1	58.7	55.6	54.1	55.7	56.4	54.5
Basilicata	57.5	--	--	57.6	58.1	53.3	--	57.6
Calabria	55.5	51.0	50.0	54.9	55.4	51.5	48.8	54.6
Sicilia	57.5	56.8	51.0	56.0	57.5	60.7	53.8	56.9
Sardegna	50.6	44.6	41.7	49.2	51.4	45.8	46.1	50.4
Italy	53.8	51.9	48.7	52.5	56.3	55.9	54.5	55.9

NOTE: Boundaries for regions are those existing at time of each census.

urbanization had practically disappeared in the North and in the Center, while it still existed to some degree in the South. In the regions of the North and of the Center the proportion married had greatly increased in the three classes of comuni, but particularly in the large ones.

The reasons for the low propensity to marriage in the urban areas in 1871, 1901, and 1931 are complex and manifold. The major factors affecting the proportions married (M), are the same as those affecting I_m. These are the purely demographic factors of age and sex composition, but since the composition of the urban population was generally more favorable to marriage than the composition of the rural, this structural difference could hardly have been the source of lower *M* in the cities. The major elements determining *M* are the mean age at marriage, and the proportion remaining single.

3.2.2. To start with, the hypothesis that a shortage of males in the young age groups may have produced a "compulsory" lower propensity to marriage among women in the urban areas has to be rejected. In Table 3.4, we have reported the sex ratio for the 11 largest comuni in

TABLE 3.4

SEX RATIO OF POPULATION AGED 20-29, ELEVEN LARGEST COMUNI: 1871 AND 1901

Comune	1871	1901
Torino	99.1	84.2
Milano	87.6	94.2
Genova	96.8	90.8
Venezia	105.3	81.0
Bologna	89.3	106.9
Firenze	101.1	106.4
Roma	62.2	86.4
Napoli	98.2	97.4
Catania	98.9	106.1
Messina	99.2	88.8
Palermo	75.5	95.0

NOTE: The sex ratio refers to the number of females divided by the number of males, multiplied by 100.

1871 and 1901. A shortage of females was more common than a shortage of males, and in many cases it was very serious. The immigration of domestic servants (mainly females) was more than offset in the majority of cases by the large institutional population composed mainly of males.

In Table 3.5, data collected by Mortara show that the mean age at marriage was relatively high in the large cities. Age at marriage of brides was one to three years higher in the large cities than in the general population. Although some slight influence on age at marriage may be

TABLE 3.5

MEAN AGE AT MARRIAGE, BY SEX, SELECTED LARGE COMUNI: CIRCA 1900

Comune	Date	Mean age at marriage	
		Females	Males
Milano	1901-1904	26.0	29.7
Venezia	1903-1904	26.8	30.1
Bologna	1897-1900	28.0	31.10
Firenze	1905	27.2	30.3
Roma	1885	27.9	32.2
Napoli	1903-1905	27.6	30.9

SOURCE: G. MORTARA, Le popolazioni delle grandi città italiane, Biblioteca dell'Economista, Serie V, Vol. XIX, p. 564, 1908.

NOTE: Mean ages at marriage are expressed in years and months.

produced by the older age structure of the urban population, two factors probably account for most of the difference:

(1) The type of occupation prevailing in the cities calls for a higher degree of education and preparation. Male professionals, entrepreneurs, clerical workers, etc. have a higher age at marriage than males with other occupations. These occupational groups usually account for a larger share of the labor force in the cities than in the general populations.[4]

(2) The economic cost of marriage is much higher in urban, than in rural, society; this factor probably contributed to the lower frequency of marriage and to the higher mean age at marriage.

[4] E. Raseri, "Sulle variazioni dei quozienti di natività e sull'età media degli sposi secondo la condizione economica," in Atti della Società Romana di Antropologia v, 1897-1898, Roma, 1898, pp. 61-75. The differential age at marriage for the various professional groups is shown for the city of Rome in 1896. The highest mean age at marriage for grooms was that of army officers (33 years and 3 months), the lowest that of masons (25.6), against an average, for all professional groups, of 27.9. It is well known that the differentials are partly caused by the fact that certain professions (that of officer in the army, or of magistrate, or of entrepreneur) are entered at a relatively older age than other professions; however, given the close correlation between the age of grooms and the age of brides, differentials are reflected in the mean age at marriage of brides and, therefore, in fertility.

The mean age of brides has oscillated, for the entire country, between 23 and 25 years since the beginning of the century, but was 2 to 3 years higher, for instance, in Milano and Roma. See N. Federici, *Lezioni di Demografia*, Roma, 1965, p. 164. Interesting data on differential nuptiality are also reported by C. Gini, "Sulla nuzialità differenziale delle classi sociali," *Metron*, XI, no. 1 (1933): 111-115.

The proportion remaining single at the end of the reproductive period is the second main factor influencing the proportion married. In Table 3.6, we have reported the percentage of females aged 50-54 in the provinces containing the 11 largest comuni in 1871, 1901, 1931, and 1951, and compared this percentage with that of the rest of the population in each province.

TABLE 3.6

PERCENTAGE FEMALES AGED 50-54 SINGLE, BY COMUNE AND REST OF PROVINCE, SELECTED PROVINCES: 1871 TO 1951

	Comune				Rest of province			
Area	1871	1911	1931	1951	1871	1911	1931	1951
Torino	18.4	19.7	20.2	17.6	17.1	17.9	17.2	18.8
Milano	21.2	13.7	14.9	16.7	9.2	10.2	10.3	13.1
Genova	23.0	20.6	17.5	19.1	14.2	13.5	19.6	20.1
Venezia	19.3	21.5	20.1	20.0	5.9	7.6	7.5	11.8
Bologna	17.7	18.2	17.3	17.6	6.4	6.2	7.7	10.4
Firenze	18.1	16.9	11.8	18.0	8.5	7.1	6.9	9.0
Roma	22.3	24.7	15.2	18.3	8.9	6.0	7.5	7.6
Napoli	20.5	29.1	18.6	19.1	12.3	6.9	10.9	12.5
Catania	15.5	8.6	11.3	14.2	24.4	10.7	8.4	10.0
Messina	11.8	7.3	8.6	15.2	11.3	9.2	9.8	14.4
Palermo	19.6	14.3	15.0	18.5	10.0	7.9	8.6	14.0

Note: The comuni within the provinces are the eleven largest in Italy in 1901.

Excluding Catania and Messina, about 20 percent of the women who had reached the end of their reproductive period in 1871 and who lived in a large comune had never married. This proportion is almost twice as high as that recorded for the rest of the provincial population. A very similar pattern is also shown by the 1911 census. In the 1931 and 1951 censuses, the percentage remaining single in the cities stayed constant (although differences among the various comuni are less conspicuous) while in the rest of the provincial population it increased. The narrowing of differences between the comune and the rest of the province reflects the spread of urban growth into what were once largely rural areas. Such a large difference is one aspect of the deep structural peculiarities of the urban societies. Further analysis ought to explain whether the high proportion of women avoiding marriage was caused by a selective immigration to the cities of women whose status or profession was an obstacle to marriage, or by an actual lower propensity to marriage caused by the peculiar living conditions of the cities, or by a combination of the two factors.

A final illustration of the lower propensity to marriage in the large cities is provided by Table 3.7, drawn from the rich material of Mortara, concerning marriage rates around the 1871, 1881, and 1901 censuses.

TABLE 3.7

MARRIAGE RATES, BY COMUNE AND REST OF PROVINCE, SELECTED PROVINCES: 1871-1872 TO 1900-1901

	Comune			Rest of province		
Area	1871-1872	1881-1882	1900-1901	1871-1872	1881-1882	1900-1901
Torino	37	36	29	47	38	39
Milano	36	40	37	67	57	60
Genova	36	31	30	54	44	41
Venezia	27	27	26	60	52	53
Bologna	28	30	28	49	46	52
Firenze	40	36	29	54	54	53
Roma	22	41	33	21	48	48
Napoli	37	40	32	55	56	48
Catania	50	50	45	52	48	51
Messina	42	47	42	50	46	43
Palermo	36	40	39	63	68	55

SOURCE: G. MORTARA, Le popolazioni delle grandi città italiane, Biblioteca dell' Economista, Serie V, Vol. XIX, pp. 533 and 598, 1908.

NOTES: Marriage rate refers to the number of marriages per 1,000 unmarried women. The comuni within the provinces are the eleven largest in Italy in 1901.

Summing up, large cities, in comparison with the residual population of the provinces to which they belong, have (1) a lower frequency of marriage and (2) a lower proportion of fecund women who are currently married; this is due to (3) the substantially higher mean age at marriage and (4) the higher proportion of females who never get married.

3.3 *Urban-Rural Differential Fertility*

3.3.1. General and marital fertility rates (*GFR* and *MFR*) have been computed for three classes of comuni, by region; the data are from the censuses of 1871, 1901, 1931, and 1951. Absolute levels appear in

Tables 3.8 and 3.9 (see also Figure 3.1); Table 3.10 shows the percentage differences.

As early as 1871, marital fertility, as expressed by *MFR*, shows evidence of urban-rural differentials; the semi-urban population was 9.8 percent and the urban population was 15.1 percent below the rate for the mainly rural population. In most of the large cities of the Center and

TABLE 3.8

GENERAL FERTILITY RATE, THREE CLASSES OF COMUNI, BY REGION: 1871 TO 1951

	1871				1901			
Region	Less than 30,000	30,000 to 100,000	More than 100,000	Total	Less than 30,000	30,000 to 100,000	More than 100,000	Total
Piemonte	143.9	148.3	109.9	141.2	128.8	105.4	73.8	120.6
Liguria	142.0	--	115.6	137.4	116.7	123.1	89.4	110.8
Lombardia	152.8	127.1	103.9	148.5	157.6	107.6	94.3	145.6
Trentino Alto Adige	--	--	--	--	--	--	--	--
Veneto	161.9	128.9	107.8	156.7	168.2	118.1	97.2	159.0
Venezia Giulia	--	--	--	--	--	--	--	--
Emilia	146.2	129.6	106.9	141.1	156.7	119.9	81.5	142.4
Toscana	159.6	129.3	141.1	153.3	138.6	113.5	79.9	128.3
Marche	130.6	127.2	--	130.5	137.7	121.9	--	136.2
Umbria	136.8	124.1	--	135.6	128.6	114.3	--	126.5
Lazio	158.6	--	110.9	144.4	132.3	--	95.1	116.5
Abruzzi	142.8	--	--	142.8	133.9	--	--	133.9
Campania	144.8	--	140.6	144.1	131.6	140.6	109.9	127.8
Puglia	156.2	167.4	--	158.0	143.2	148.0	--	144.6
Basilicata	149.2	--	--	149.2	140.7	--	--	140.7
Calabria	144.3	167.3	--	144.8	132.3	135.8	--	132.5
Sicilia	162.8	144.8	133.5	157.4	148.2	127.4	122.9	141.4
Sardegna	149.8	132.9	--	148.1	131.0	--	110.9	128.4
Italy	150.4	135.5	123.7	147.3	143.0	123.1	98.0	135.9
	1931				1951			
Piemonte	63.4	52.5	43.8	58.6	42.2	57.5	34.3	41.9
Liguria	64.6	48.4	47.6	54.6	37.0	41.1	36.3	36.9
Lombardia	90.1	66.5	50.1	78.5	58.6	63.6	40.5	54.4
Trentino Alto Adige	91.1	60.4	--	84.3	72.4	70.2	--	72.0
Veneto	105.2	89.5	69.6	98.9	71.9	65.7	56.8	68.9
Venezia Giulia	98.4	59.5	47.5	74.6	51.7	65.6	34.4	48.9
Emilia	91.9	70.5	55.6	82.4	83.5	87.2	68.5	81.5
Toscana	78.8	70.1	49.9	72.1	77.2	90.7	71.4	78.8
Marche	103.3	78.7	--	99.2	63.7	59.7	--	63.1
Umbria	108.3	89.4	--	100.4	61.9	54.9	--	60.2
Lazio	116.0	93.8	78.8	96.8	78.7	76.5	54.6	66.0
Abruzzi	121.2	96.8	--	118.5	74.0	70.3	--	73.5
Campania	136.2	123.6	100.0	125.0	93.3	98.7	95.8	94.3
Puglia	136.1	127.0	141.1	132.6	99.8	109.0	102.4	101.4
Basilicata	143.3	--	--	143.4	99.8	111.0	--	100.9
Calabria	129.8	125.5	117.2	128.7	107.2	109.9	84.4	105.7
Sicilia	116.2	102.0	102.4	111.1	85.6	85.8	96.0	88.0
Sardegna	121.5	102.2	99.5	117.7	111.1	98.0	95.3	105.3
Italy	103.1	85.4	69.7	94.4	72.1	72.5	58.1	69.1

NOTES: The general fertility rate refers to live births per 1,000 women aged 15-49.
Boundaries for regions are those existing at time of each census.
1871 data computed from average of births in 1871-1872.

TABLE 3.9

MARITAL FERTILITY RATE, THREE CLASSES OF COMUNI, BY REGION: 1871 TO 1951

Region	1871				1901			
	Less than 30,000	30,000 to 100,000	More than 100,000	Total	Less than 30,000	30,000 to 100,000	More than 100,000	Total
Piemonte	248.1	221.0	188.2	242.5	231.5	183.4	143.5	219.3
Liguria	242.1	--	200.9	235.9	213.0	201.0	172.7	202.7
Lombardia	257.9	193.9	189.5	252.1	273.5	210.7	168.8	256.8
Trentino Alto Adige	--	--	--	--	--	--	--	--
Veneto	264.9	212.5	195.9	258.8	284.8	222.5	186.7	274.8
Venezia Giulia	--	--	--	--	--	--	--	--
Emilia	219.5	206.0	182.7	215.0	244.8	203.7	150.6	230.2
Toscana	247.3	222.0	203.6	240.4	224.3	204.0	148.8	214.9
Marche	215.1	205.2	--	214.6	224.7	200.5	--	223.4
Umbria	212.6	196.6	--	211.6	199.9	187.3	--	198.0
Lazio	246.4	--	198.7	234.1	189.7	--	161.5	178.6
Abruzzi	230.9	--	--	230.9	209.0	--	--	209.0
Campania	255.9	--	242.8	245.9	218.2	227.7	201.9	216.0
Puglia	262.6	299.7	--	265.2	230.4	232.0	--	230.8
Basilicata	247.8	--	--	247.8	221.4	--	--	215.0
Calabria	238.0	294.8	--	239.3	206.3	225.9	--	207.3
Sicilia	267.7	243.5	231.3	261.0	234.4	216.7	203.3	227.3
Sardegna	243.3	255.0	--	244.3	233.1	--	221.1	231.8
Italy	247.7	223.5	210.2	243.8	236.0	212.6	176.6	228.0
	1931				1951			
Piemonte	116.3	92.7	75.8	106.3	70.2	92.3	55.4	69.0
Liguria	124.4	90.4	88.2	103.2	64.1	66.0	59.8	62.0
Lombardia	170.1	114.7	87.2	146.6	103.5	110.3	58.6	95.4
Trentino Alto Adige	194.9	126.8	--	181.0	147.9	123.0	--	141.4
Veneto	201.4	167.5	140.6	191.0	131.7	120.8	102.4	125.9
Venezia Giulia	172.9	115.4	83.1	134.5	86.5	115.4	67.5	82.1
Emilia	155.2	124.8	89.2	141.0	85.3	87.2	68.5	81.5
Toscana	130.8	130.8	93.9	125.3	77.2	90.7	71.4	78.8
Marche	191.3	139.0	--	177.5	108.8	104.9	--	108.2
Umbria	172.5	149.1	--	163.1	97.7	85.5	--	94.8
Lazio	194.2	160.8	141.8	170.4	128.5	122.6	95.6	112.0
Abruzzi	202.4	181.4	--	200.4	126.7	128.3	--	126.9
Campania	247.0	226.3	197.0	233.1	176.0	183.7	182.1	178.0
Puglia	235.3	223.1	224.2	231.6	181.9	186.4	173.3	181.3
Basilicata	243.4	--	--	243.4	168.6	196.9	--	171.3
Calabria	222.3	218.6	217.2	221.8	186.4	189.3	162.2	185.0
Sicilia	196.5	174.6	187.4	191.3	146.0	136.2	168.4	150.0
Sardegna	231.9	210.0	211.1	228.7	210.2	200.7	189.5	207.4
Italy	184.4	153.4	128.6	170.5	125.1	122.9	100.0	119.6

NOTES: The marital fertility rate refers to live legitimate births per 1,000 married women aged 15-49.
Boundaries for regions are those existing at time of each census.
1871 data computed from average of births in 1871-1872.

the North, *MFR* was under 200 per thousand; the corresponding value of I_g must have been below .55, thus clearly showing evidence of the existence of neo-Malthusian control over fertility.

The differences between urban and rural fertility vary according to the region. The gap is very wide in Torino, Milano, and Venezia, where *MFR* is 24 to 27 percent below the corresponding value for the rural population. The same is true for Genova, Bologna, Firenze, and

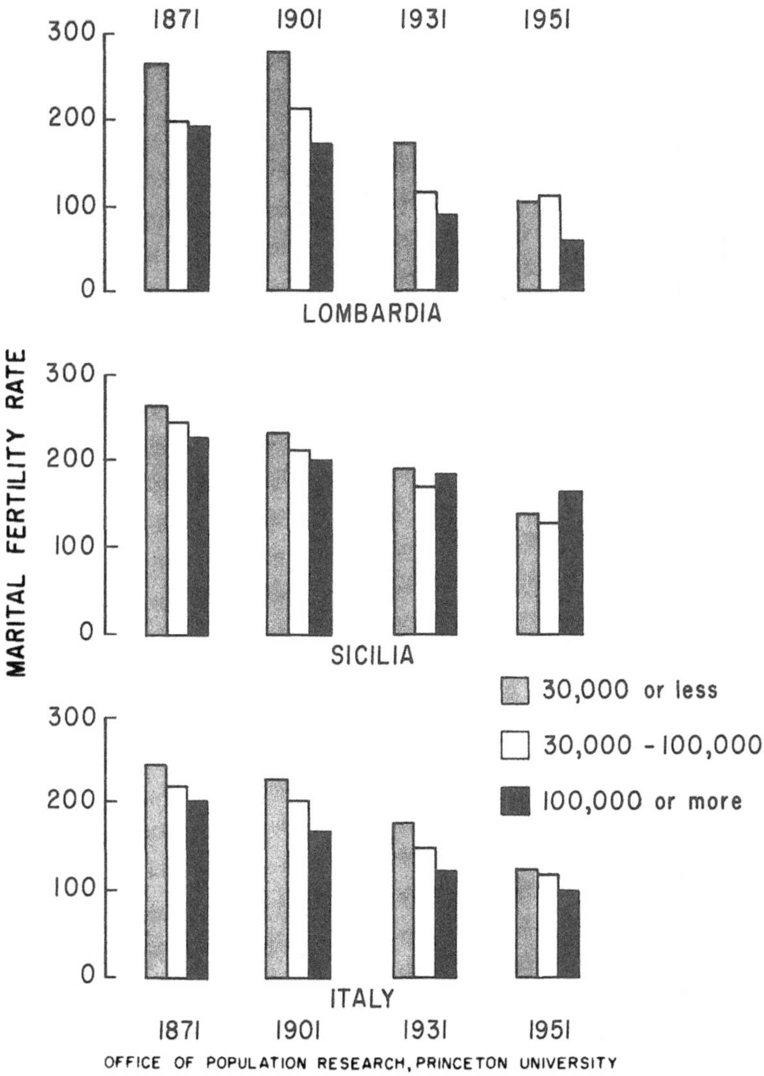

Figure 3.1 Marital Fertility Rate by Three Classes of Comuni, Lombardia, Sicilia, and Italy: 1871 to 1951

Roma, where it was 17 to 19 percent lower. Urban-rural differences were less sizeable in Napoli, Messina, and Palermo, varying from 5 to 14 percent.

While marital fertility was inversely correlated (lower in urban areas and higher in rural) with the size of the comuni in the Center and the

TABLE 3.10

PERCENTAGE DIFFERENCE IN MARITAL FERTILITY RATES AMONG THREE CLASSES OF COMUNI, BY REGION: 1871 TO 1951

	Population size of comuni											
	30,000-100,000 and less than 30,000				More than 100,000 and 30,000-100,000				More than 100,000 and less than 30,000			
Region	1871	1901	1931	1951	1871	1901	1931	1951	1871	1901	1931	1951
Piemonte	-10.9	-20.8	-20.3	+31.5	-14.8	-21.8	-18.2	-40.0	-24.1	-38.0	-34.8	-21.1
Liguria	--	- 5.6	-27.3	+ 3.0	--	-14.1	- 2.4	- 9.4	-17.0	-18.9	-29.1	- 6.6
Lombardia	-24.8	-23.0	-32.6	+ 6.5	- 2.3	-19.9	-24.0	-37.8	-26.5	-38.3	-48.7	-33.8
Trentino Alto Adige	--	--	-34.9	-16.8	--	--	--	--	--	--	--	--
Veneto	-21.8	-21.9	-16.8	- 8.3	- 7.8	-16.1	-16.1	-15.2	-26.0	-34.4	-30.2	-30.8
Venezia Giulia	--	--	-33.3	+33.4	--	--	-28.0	-50.2	--	--	-51.9	-33.5
Emilia	- 6.2	-16.8	-19.6	+ 2.2	-11.3	-26.1	-28.5	-21.5	-16.8	-38.5	-42.5	-19.7
Toscana	-10.2	- 9.1	- 0.5	+17.5	- 8.3	-27.1	-27.9	-21.3	-17.7	-33.7	-28.2	- 7.5
Marche	- 4.6	-10.8	-27.3	- 3.6	--	--	--	--	--	--	--	--
Umbria	- 7.5	- 6.3	-13.6	-12.5	--	--	--	--	--	--	--	--
Lazio	--	--	-17.2	- 4.6	--	--	-11.8	-22.0	-19.4	-14.9	-27.0	-25.6
Abruzzi	--	--	-10.4	+ 1.3	--	--	--	--	--	--	--	--
Campania	--	+ 4.4	- 8.4	+ 4.4	--	-11.3	-12.9	- 0.9	- 5.1	- 7.5	-20.2	+ 3.5
Puglia	+14.1	+ 0.7	- 5.0	+ 2.5	--	--	+ 0.5	- 7.0	--	--	- 4.7	- 4.7
Basilicata	--	--	--	+16.8	--	--	--	--	--	--	--	--
Calabria	+23.9	--	- 1.7	+ 1.6	--	--	- 0.6	-14.3	--	--	- 2.3	- 3.8
Sicilia	- 9.0	+ 6.6	-11.1	- 6.7	- 5.0	- 6.2	+ 7.3	+23.6	-13.6	-13.3	- 4.6	+15.3
Sardegna	+ 4.8	--	- 9.4	- 4.5	--	--	+ 0.5	- 5.6	--	- 5.1	- 9.0	- 9.8
Italy	- 9.8	- 9.9	-16.8	- 1.8	- 6.0	-16.9	-16.2	-18.6	-15.1	-25.2	-30.3	-20.1

North, there was no such relationship in Puglia, Calabria, and Sardegna. It is probable that while the diffusion of neo-Malthusian practices was well on its way in the large cities of Central and Northern Italy, the existence of such ideas was unknown in the South. As we have already pointed out, many large cities of the South lacked any urban characteristics; populations living in comuni of different size had similar social structures, and we do not expect different patterns of fertility in populations living in the same social environment.

We have pointed out that both *MFR* and the proportion married *M* hold an inverse relationship with the size of the comuni, and this fact tends to inflate the differences in the level of general fertility (and of the birth rate) between rural, semi-urban, and urban populations (see Table 3.8).

3.3.2. From 1871 to 1901, marital fertility experienced a dramatic decrease in the large cities of the North and of the Center, widening the gap between urban and rural patterns of demographic behavior. In Torino, Milano, Venezia, Bologna, and Firenze, the *MFR* was 34 to 39 percent below that of the rural population; Genova was 19 percent below (here, however, the rural population was also experiencing a decline in fertility); Roma, 15 percent; and Napoli, Catania, Messina, Palermo, and Cagliari, 5 to 13 percent below.

With regard to the semi-urban comuni, the prevailing marital fertility was well below that of the smaller comuni in Central and Northern Italy; no major differences can be found in Southern Italy (with the exception of Sicilia).

Between 1901 and 1931, marital fertility had continued to drop in each of the three classes of comuni in Northern and Central Italy (Veneto excluded); moreover, the gap between large and small comuni was even wider than before. In the comuni with over 100,000 inhabitants, the *MFR* was 22 to 52 percent below the corresponding levels observed in the mainly rural population. In the South, marital fertility had started to decline in the large cities, but the difference between urban and rural population was still limited. In many of the large comuni of Northern and Central Italy, the marital fertility rate had dropped below 100 births per thousand married women, while in the South it was generally over 200. In conclusion, by 1931, a neo-Malthusian decline had dramatically affected all regions, regardless of size or density, of the North and of the Center, while in the South, only the metropolitan population showed evidence of adopting neo-Malthusian controls of fertility.

Using three classes of comuni from one census to another to analyze changes in fertility is far from being precise. The share of total population and of the national territory for each class changed between 1871 and 1931. The steady process of urbanization shifted many small comuni to the larger categories; at the same time, middle-size comuni grew to large ones. As a consequence, the number of comuni with over 100,000 inhabitants increased from 9 in 1871 to 22 in 1931, and the number of comuni with 30,000 to 100,000 inhabitants grew from 36 to 110 during the same period. Eleven comuni, however, had populations exceeding 100,000 throughout the entire period; this allows greater comparability in the analyses of changes in marital fertility. In Table 3.11 and Figure 3.2 the rates for these comuni are shown for 1871,

TABLE 3.11

MARITAL FERTILITY RATE, ELEVEN LARGEST COMUNI: 1871, 1901, AND 1931

	Absolute level			Percentage change		
Comune	1871	1901	1931	1871-1901	1901-1931	1871-1931
Torino	188.2	143.5	75.8	-23.8	-47.1	-59.7
Milano	189.5	168.8	83.8	-10.9	-50.4	-55.8
Genova	200.9	172.7	85.5	-14.0	-50.5	-57.4
Venezia	195.9	186.7	142.7	- 4.7	-23.6	-27.2
Bologna	182.7	150.6	89.2	-17.6	-40.8	-51.0
Firenze	203.6	148.8	86.3	-26.9	-58.0	-57.6
Roma	198.7	161.5	141.8	-18.7	-12.2	-28.6
Napoli	242.8	201.9	197.0	-16.8	- 2.4	-18.9
Catania	257.9	189.9	179.2	-26.4	- 5.6	-30.5
Messina	219.1	197.2	169.4	-10.0	-14.1	-22.7
Palermo	236.9	213.3	201.7	-10.0	- 5.4	-14.9

NOTE: Marital fertility rate refers to legitimate live births per 1,000 married women aged 15-49.

1901, and 1931. In 60 years, marital fertility fell 50 to 60 percent in Torino, Milano, Genova, Bologna, and Firenze, and 15 to 30 percent in Venezia, Roma, Napoli, Catania, Messina, and Palermo.

As mentioned in Section 3.1.2, the analysis of marital fertility rates by urban-rural classification is complicated by the fact that rural women

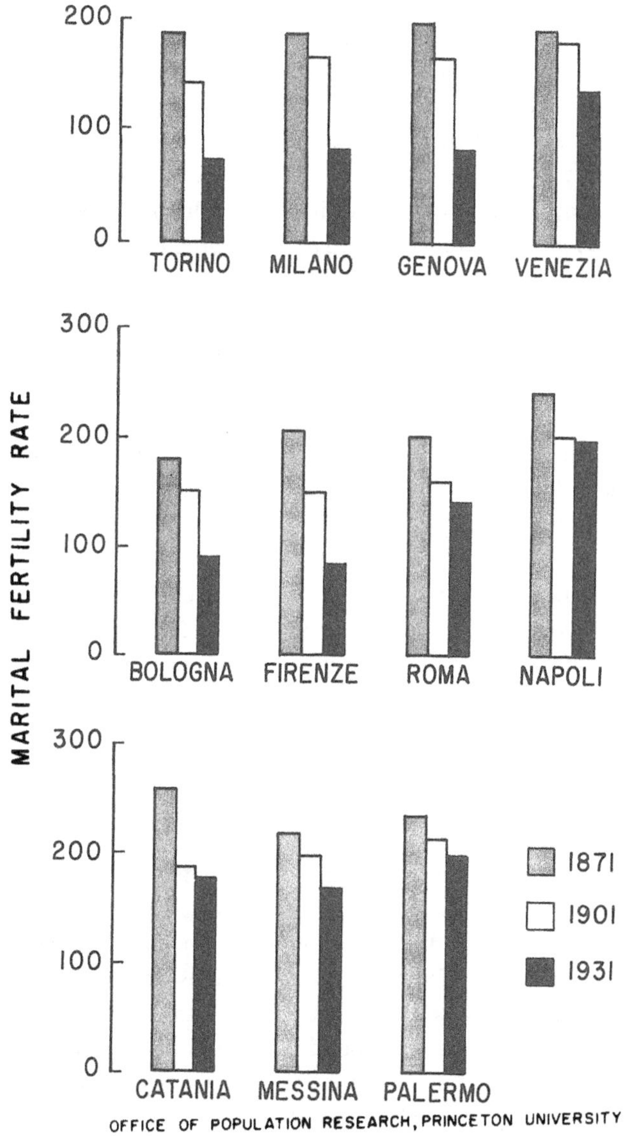

Figure 3.2 Marital Fertility Rate, Eleven Largest Comuni: 1871, 1901, and 1931

began to deliver children in city hospitals or clinics after World War II; women having children at home declined from 95 percent of total births in 1932, to 85 percent in 1951, and 67 percent in 1958. Therefore, urban fertility is probably overestimated, especially in the North and in the Center, while it is underestimated in the rural areas. The amount of distortion cannot be exactly measured, although it is our opinion that in 1951 it must have been modest, owing to the fact that the large majority of women still had their babies delivered at home.[5]

After 1931, marital fertility fell in all classes of comuni in the Center and the North; in some regions (Liguria, Emilia and Toscana, Marche and Umbria) urban-rural differentials were greatly reduced. Elsewhere in the Center and the North, the typical inverse relationship between size of the comune and *MFR* does not hold anymore; in Piemonte, Lombardia, Venezia, Giulia, the population of the comuni of intermediate size had the highest fertility. In the regions of the South, marital fertility decreased in all classes of comuni, but the decline took place at approximately the same rate in the rural as in the urban population. As a consequence, differentials are very modest indeed, and not always in the expected sense.

3.3.3. No allowance has yet been made for the effects of the unbalanced sex ratio of the married population on marital fertility. This unbalance was stronger in the rural areas than in other sectors of the population because of the differential impact of internal and external migration. Throughout Italy the ratio of married females to married males (either all ages, or women 15-49 per men 20-54) shows a strong shortage of men in comuni with less than 30,000 inhabitants. When marital fertility rates are corrected for this unbalance, the result tends to increase the gap separating rural, semi-urban, and urban fertility.

Large cities in Italy at all times have attracted a large number of illegitimate births, either because unmarried pregnant women came to the city to avoid censure from home communities or, perhaps even more important, because large cities in Italy often had charitable institutions where illegitimate children and foundlings could be placed.

Table 3.12 illustrates the rapid fall of illegitimacy by size of comune. In 1951, illegitimacy was only one-fifth of the 1871 level. Since the decline was similar in all three classes of comuni, differentials have remained unchanged over time. In 1871, as in 1951, the illegitimacy of

[5] This type of distortion could have been avoided in 1961, when the classification of births by place of residence of parents and place of occurrence of birth was available, but the combined age-sex-marital status distribution of the population has been published only for the provinces, with no breakdown by comune.

TABLE 3.12

ILLEGITIMATE FERTILITY RATE, BY CLASS OF COMUNE: 1871 TO 1951

	Actual levels				Relative levels (1871 set at 100)			
Class of comune	1871	1901	1931	1951	1871	1901	1931	1951
Less than 30,000	19.7	16.3	8.6	3.9	100	82.7	43.7	19.8
30,00 to 100,000	41.1	23.0	12.0	8.7	100	56.0	29.2	21.2
More than 100,000	39.2	23.0	13.8	8.0	100	58.7	35.2	20.4
Total	23.1	18.0	10.1	5.3	100	77.9	43.7	22.9

NOTE: Illegitimate fertility rate refers to the number of illegitimate births per 1,000 unmarried women aged 15-49.

the comuni with over 30,000 inhabitants was approximately twice the level of illegitimacy of the smaller comuni.

Summing up our discussion of differentials in urban-rural fertility, the following findings seem the most important:

(1) Fertility differentials by size of comuni were evident in the North and in the Center in 1871, and increased until 1931. Variability in the South (Sicilia excepted) was very modest. Over time fertility levels changed at approximately the same rate in the three classes of comuni.

(2) The inverse relationship between marital fertility and the propensity to marriage, on the one hand, and the size of the comuni, on the other, inflates the differentials in terms of birth rates and general fertility rates.

(3) Corrections for the sex unbalances produced by emigration tend to increase urban-rural differentials.

(4) A neo-Malthusian decline tended to spread in two directions: from the urban to the rural population, and from the Northwest to the South. As late as 1931, however, very little, if any, neo-Malthusian command over marital fertility is to be found in the rural population of the South.

3.4 *Other Sources for the Study of Urban Fertility*

3.4.1. The 1931 census special report on fertility provides us with further insight into urban-rural differentials.[6] Census data show the

[6] ISTAT, *Indagine sulla fecondità della donna.*

number of children ever born to married women (husband present) cross-classified by age and by place of residence (comuni over and under 100,000 inhabitants and individual data for comuni with more than 500,000 inhabitants—Roma, Milano, Napoli, Torino, and Genova).

It was possible to calculate the average number of children ever born for three cohorts with completed fertility (women aged 45-49, 50-59, and 60 and over at the 1931 census). The data show evidence of an increasing differential fertility (Table 3.13); women born before 1871 and

TABLE 3.13

MEAN NUMBER OF CHILDREN PER MARRIED WOMAN AGED 45-49, 50-59, AND 60 AND OVER, BY CLASS OF COMUNE: 1931 CENSUS

Class of comune	Mean number of children ever had by cohort			Percentage difference between cohorts		
	45-49	50-59	60+	45-49 and 50-59	50-59 and 60+	45-49 and 60+
Less than 100,000	5.48	5.78	5.98	- 5.2	- 3.3	- 8.4
More than 100,000	3.82	4.29	4.97	-11.0	-13.7	-23.1
More than 500,000:						
Roma	3.72	3.98	4.48	- 6.5	-11.2	-17.0
Milano	3.01	3.86	4.75	-22.0	-18.7	-36.6
Napoli	5.09	5.11	5.44	- 0.4	- 6.1	- 6.4
Torino	2.35	3.02	4.01	-22.2	-24.7	-41.4
Genova	3.13	3.71	4.56	-15.6	-20.4	-32.8
Italy	5.11	5.53	5.84	- 7.6	- 5.3	-12.5

NOTE: Data are for women with husband present.

living in comuni under 100,000 inhabitants had 20 percent more children than women of the same age living in the urban areas; the comparable figure for women born 1871–1881 was 35 percent more children and for those born in 1881–1886, 44 percent more. This increasing gap among cohorts in their reproductive behavior by urban-rural residence shows the steadiness of the neo-Malthusian decline in urban areas at the beginning of the century. Moreover, in the population living in comuni of over 100,000, the older cohort had 23 percent more children, on the average, than the younger cohort; the difference is only 8 percent in the comuni with under 100,000 inhabitants.

The difference in fertility levels between the older and the younger cohorts is particularly evident in cities with over 500,000 inhabitants, and amounts to over one-third in Milano, Torino, and Genova; however, in Napoli the difference is only 6 percent, and there is little evidence of change in fertility over time. Roma holds an intermediate position.

Although of a different nature from the current fertility measures, census data give full support to the findings outlined in the preceding pages, so that the hypothesis advanced at the beginning of this chapter can be fully accepted.

3.4.2. Around the turn of the century there was considerable interest among European scholars in the demography of urban areas. In Italy, statisticians, with the limited resources then available, attempted detailed classifications of births—by age of mother, sometimes by age of father, and by parity—in several cities. Table 3.14 summarizes data for seven cities: Milano, Cremona, Trieste, Udine, Venezia, Bologna, and Roma. The table also shows, for comparison, the age-specific fertility rates of

TABLE 3.14

AGE-SPECIFIC MARITAL FERTILITY, SELECTED CITIES, SARDEGNA, AND ITALY: LATE 19TH AND EARLY 20TH CENTURIES

Area	Date	15-19	20-24	25-29	30-34	35-39	40-44	45-49
Milano	1901	.490	.374	.247	.173	.121	.045	.003
Cremona	1866-1875	--	.363	.311	.246	.166	.063	.008
Trieste	1910-1911	.416	.382	.293	.218	.146	.057	.006
Udine	1872-1875	.605	.502	.393	.286	.190	.083	.007
Venezia	1903-1905	.302	.345	.305	.253	.194	.070	.005
Bologna	1898-1900	.319	.295	.251	.208	.156	.055	.003
Roma	1894-1896	.414	.372	.345	.252	.173	.066	.008
Sardegna	1931	.395	.419	.357	.298	.228	.106	.014
Italy	1931	.470	.333	.255	.193	.140	.066	.008

SOURCES: Roma: See G. MORTARA, Le popolazioni delle grandi città italiane, Biblioteca dell'Economista, Serie V, Vol. XIX, p. 622, 1908 (data drawn from Raseri, our correction). Cremona, Udine, Venice: E. RASERI, I nati in rapporto all'età dei genitori, In "Giornale della Società d'Igiene", nn. 19-20, Oct. 1897. Trieste: P. MEDANI, La fecondita legittima a Trieste dal 1900 al 1937, In "Atti III Riunione Soc. Ital. Econ. Dem. Stat.", Firenze, 1939. Milano: G. MORTARA, Le popolazioni delle grandi città italiane, Biblioteca dell'Economista, Serie V, Vol. XIX, p. 622, 1908.

NOTE: Age-specific marital fertility refers to the number of legitimate live births per 1,000 married women in each age group.

Italy and Sardegna in 1931, the first year for which these rates are available. Sardegna is included because it had the highest fertility among Italian regions in 1931 and was still largely unaffected by neo-Malthusian control.

The city of Udine (1872–1875) shows the highest fertility; and Milano (1901), the lowest; the difference is about 30 percent. Further information on urban fertility is presented in Table 3.15, which shows the

TABLE 3.15

HYPOTHETICAL NUMBER OF CHILDREN PER MARRIED WOMAN, BY AGE AT MARRIAGE, SELECTED CITIES, SARDEGNA, AND ITALY: LATE 19TH AND EARLY 20TH CENTURIES

		Actual levels		Relative levels (Sardegna, 1931, set at 100)	
Area	Date	Age at marriage 20	Age at marriage 25	Age at marriage 20	Age at marriage 25
Milano	1901	4.82	2.95	67.8	59.0
Cremona	1866-1875	5.78	3.97	81.3	79.4
Trieste	1910-1911	5.51	3.60	77.5	72.0
Udine	1872-1875	7.31	4.80	102.8	96.0
Venezia	1903-1905	5.86	4.14	82.4	82.8
Bologna	1898-1900	4.84	3.37	68.1	67.4
Roma	1894-1896	6.08	4.22	85.5	84.4
Sardegna	1931	7.11	5.00	100.0	100.0
Italy	1931	4.98	3.31	70.0	66.2

SOURCE: Based on data in Table 3.14.

period number of children per married woman getting married at age 20 and at age 25. The data were compiled by adding the age-specific marital fertility rates from 20 to 50 years and from 25 to 50 years. The hypothetical number of children per woman married at age 25 (a more realistic hypothesis) was 5.00 for Sardegna and 4.80 for Udine; the minimum was 2.95 in Milano. Using the fertility performance of Sardinian women in 1931 as a standard level for Italian fertility prior to neo-Malthusian control, Udine had approximately the same level and all others were below—ranging from Roma with a minimum of 16 percent difference to Milano with a maximum of 41 percent. This is a further piece of evidence that urban fertility, at least in the North and in the Center of the country, was already under extensive control at the turn of the century.

3.5 *Conclusion*

Data presented in this chapter have shown, beyond any reasonable doubt, that in the second part of the nineteenth century marital fertility in the urban areas north of Roma was below the levels of the adjacent rural population. Although drawing upon scarcer and less reliable material, it also appears that since the time of Napoleon, urban fertility has been lower than rural fertility. Furthermore, at least until the beginning of this century, the lower urban marital fertility was coupled with a much lower propensity to marriage as evidenced by a higher age at marriage and a higher proportion of women who never got married.

The low propensity to marriage in the urban areas—a typical Malthusian type of birth control—is reinforced by several obvious features of urban life. The occupational structure of the urban population and the higher economic cost of marriage tend both to raise the age at marriage and to reduce its frequency. Another factor of the low propensity is certainly the concentration, in the large cities, of those distinctive segments of the population that because of their profession or status never, or rarely, get married. Finally, selective immigration into the cities of unmarried people could be another element contributing to the lower proportions married, but we lack statistical evidence to support this hypothesis.

Reasons for lower marital fertility are more obscure. The most likely conclusion is, of course, that the urban population was more ready to accept new attitudes toward the family, and to implement these attitudes either by discovery of traditional methods of contraception or abortion, or by imitation of practices used by restricted sectors of the population (i.e., the nobility). We have no means to evaluate the possibility that other factors may have contributed to the lower fertility of the urban areas. One factor could be the high mobility and short-term residence of a large segment of the population. This could result in the periodical return of the mother into the community of origin for delivering babies or in the frequent, although temporary, separation of the couple because of the absence of one of the two spouses. Mobility could also be selective of infecund or subfecund couples, who would find it less difficult to move into the city than more fecund couples with larger families. Finally, de facto termination of marriages because of the physical separation of the couple could be more frequent in urban, than in rural, areas.

The available data do not allow the exploration of these hypotheses. Ad hoc techniques have yet to be developed for the historical analysis of the urban population; its mobility and complex interrelationship with the population of the surrounding territories make the traditional tools of analysis of limited use.

Another interesting finding is the increase in the propensity to marriage in some large cities in the North and Center in connection with the fall of fertility to very low levels. The hypothesis that traditional Malthusian control has been substituted by modern neo-Malthusian techniques has found new support.

Finally, a result of great sociological interest is the diverging situation in the South and in the rest of the country. In the South, the inverse relationship between size of the comune and marital fertility—so evident in the rest of the country—is obscured by contradictory regional patterns. Fertility falls at approximately the same rate in the urban areas and in the rural areas, and differentials according to the size of the comune, if they exist at all, are as small in 1871 as they are in 1951. In the Center and the North, marital fertility falls more rapidly in the urban areas until 1931; then there is an extraordinary acceleration of the fall in the rural areas. By 1951 the inverse relationship between fertility and urbanization is blurred in many regions. New uniform patterns of behavior have been established.

CHAPTER 4: The Geography of Fertility and Nuptiality Changes

4.1 *How Geography Can Help a Demographer*

4.1.1. This chapter is dedicated to the analysis of the association of fertility and nuptiality trends with the geographic characteristics of the country. Some introductory remarks are necessary to clarify our aims. In Chapters 2 and 3, the long-term trends in nuptiality and fertility were examined for the 18 regions retained in our analysis. A detailed and, as far as possible, varied battery of indicators was used in the analysis, providing a suitable frame for the interpretation of nuptiality and fertility changes during the last century. However, the average size of the regions, ranging from less than 1.5 million inhabitants in 1861 to 3.0 million in 1971, and the existence of regions with a very large population (Lombardia, in 1971, had 8.0 million inhabitants) makes them too large as units for an adequate territorial study.

Why do we need to take into consideration smaller demographic areas? One of the tools of social science is the use of comparison between segments of the population having in different degree the qualities or characteristics believed to influence the phenomenon under investigation. If populations were homogeneous with regard to such characteristics and qualities (or, more accurately, if distribution of such characteristics were similar within the various populations) territorial analysis would be meaningless. But no large population is composed of units with identical average characteristics, certainly not that of Italy, where at all times there has been a great variety in the social structure. A detailed territorial analysis is necessary, then, mainly for the following reasons:[1]

(1) It may clarify the mechanism of fertility decline, identifying environmental or geographic conditions that retard or facilitate the diffusion of lower fertility.

(2) Detailed territorial investigations extend the usefulness of the

[1] The following studies deal with the geography of demographic features of Italy. DIRSTAT, *Carte e diagrammi di demografia italiana*, Roma, 1878. E. Raseri, *Atlante di demografia e di geografia medica d'Italia*, Roma, 1906. ISTAT, *Atlante Statistico*, Roma, 1931. Ministero dell'interno, *Carta della natalità* (General fertility rates for 795 agrarian districts, 1935-1937), Roma, 1940. U. Giusti, *Caratteristiche ambientali italiane: agrarie, sociali e demografiche, 1815-1942*, Roma, 1943.

tools of statistical analysis when applied to the relation between indexes of fertility and quantitative measures of socioeconomic variables, such as literacy, occupational status, or urban-rural residence.

This second point will be analyzed at length in Chapter 5; the first point, in this chapter.

When discussing fertility trends, the term "diffusion" as applied to birth control or fertility decline is very often used. It is not our intention, in this chapter, to enter into an extended discussion of the nature of the decline in an effort to determine whether it was induced by "innovation" or by "diffusion." It is obvious that the word *diffusion* is rather gross and unprecise. The habit of controlling fertility is seen as a physical phenomenon, like the spreading of an epidemic in a population or the territorial spread of a new species of insects. It gives the idea, somehow, that a new attitude—like that of planning the timing, spacing, and number of children—involving a complex psychological change, can be contracted from another person through mere physical contact or vicinity.

To avoid a controversy over the interpretation of the decline of fertility as a result of diffusion or of innovation, we shall entertain the hypothesis that *part* of the mechanism of the decline was the spread of ideas, attitudes, or information through the population, and examine the most obvious implications of such a hypothesis. One evident implication is that a decline of fertility occurs more rapidly and more readily in populations with extensive communication with other populations where the decline has been initiated.

We shall, therefore, expect a more rapid diffusion of birth control wherever mobility is greater and contacts among populations is traditionally established: along the valleys, the coasts, or the plains, wherever communication is physically easier; among the more densely settled populations rather than among the more sparsely inhabited areas. On the other hand, in all areas of difficult access because of their peculiar conformation (mountain areas, alpine valleys, remote islands, etc.), the diffusion of birth control should, according to the hypothesis, take place later.

Geographic analysis also helps in examining the possible influence on diffusion of factors of a less physical nature. Communication (and imitation of behavior) occurs more readily among those with the same language or dialect and with common traditions and customs. The hypothesis of diffusion thus suggests that borders separating linguistic minorities or areas speaking different dialects, areas once politically associated, and areas sharing common political or religious attitudes are likely also to be borders separating populations that at a given moment have reduced fertility in different degrees. Cultural, political, and linguistic differences not only serve as barriers to intercommunication, but also may be linked to different degrees of acceptance of, or resistance to, new ideas and patterns of behavior.

Finally, when the analysis is made on a sufficiently detailed basis, it may be possible to pinpoint areas with an exceptionally early or an exceptionally late decline. The study of these extreme cases may be particularly useful and may give an indication of the factors at play in determining the less extreme instances of the behavior of the population.

4.1.2. Although it would be desirable to extend the analysis to smaller administrative units, this is often impossible because of the lack of adequate data. The computation of the battery of standardized indexes is possible for all censuses (with the exception of those of 1901 and 1921). Map 4.1 gives the names and locations of all the provinces. Their number increased from 59 in 1861 to 69 in 1871 (annexation of Veneto and Lazio) and to 92 in 1961. From 1881 to 1961 we have reconstructed a homogeneous series of indexes for 87 of the provinces in their present boundaries.[2] Their average size, ranging from 350,000 to almost 600,000 inhabitants in 1961, makes them more suitable than the regions for geographic and cross-sectional analysis. The province is, however, an administrative territory, created in many cases without much consideration for the geographic, ethnic, or social peculiarities of the various areas. Below the provincial level, the battery of indicators has been computed for 1881 and 1911 for 284 circondari, smaller administrative areas later abandoned, with an average population of about 100,000 inhabitants. For later dates, it is impossible to go below the provincial level unless we give up the computation of the standardized indexes. With reference to 1935–1937, general fertility rates have been computed for 795 agrarian areas formed by the *Istituto Centrale di Statistica* by subdividing the territory into areas having common geographic, and often also economic and social, characteristics.[3] An attempt to

[2] For the technical problems concerning the provincial series, see Appendix C.
[3] Ministero dell'interno, *Carta della natalità.*

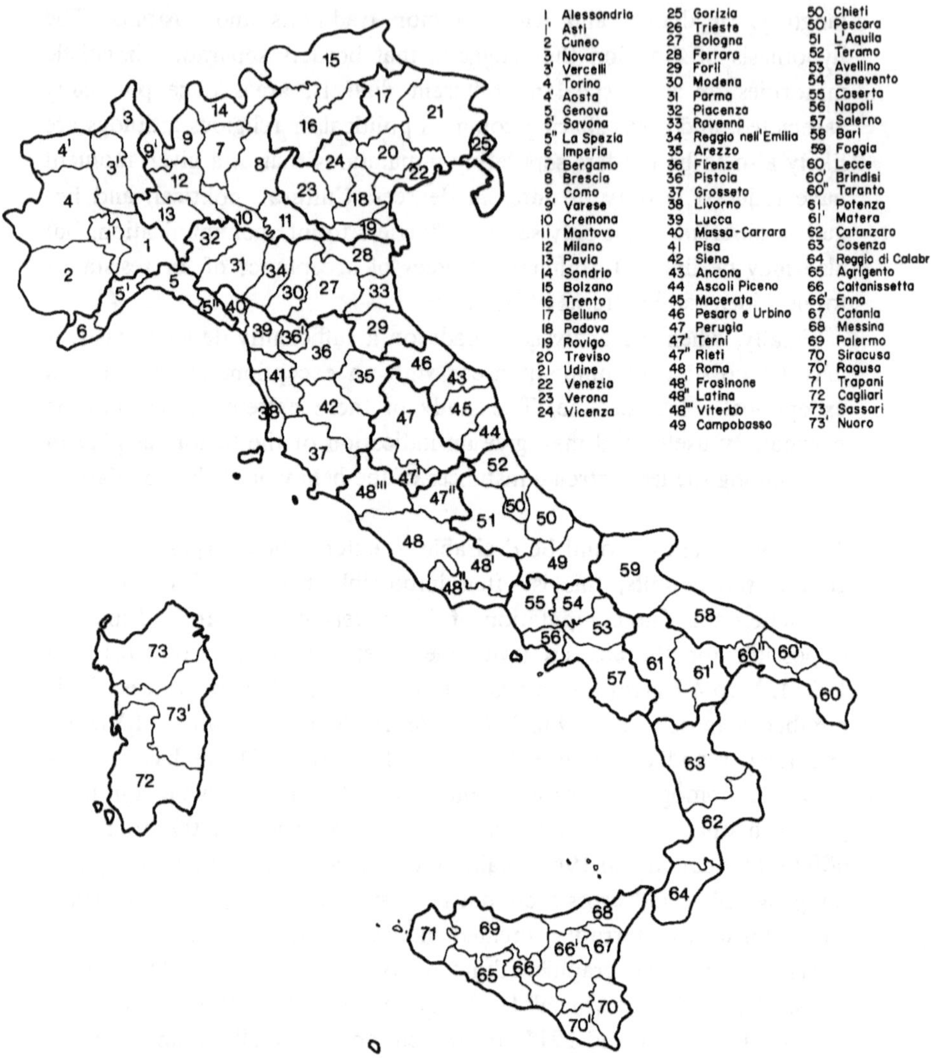

OFFICE OF POPULATION RESEARCH, PRINCETON UNIVERSITY

Map 4.1 Provinces of Italy

achieve an extreme degree of geographic detail by analyzing the birth rates of the 8,000 comuni would be of doubtful value given the different age structure and marital status of the communal populations, and the increasing habit of having the baby delivered outside the place of residence, not to speak of the difficulty of dealing with thousands of cases without losing sight of recognizable geographic patterns.

We have to recall, in general, that if the analysis of data for large areas has pitfalls, so does the multiplication of territorial areas analyzed. First, although territorial detail is useful for isolating segments of the population having approximately similar characteristics, it is always a very imperfect substitute for individual data that can be regrouped to present information about persons classified according to their individual characteristics (profession, education, income, etc.). This means that no matter how small it is, the population of the area considered will almost always comprise individuals who differ substantially in those characteristics we believe relevant for the interpretation of fertility differentials.

Second, certain disturbing factors become stronger as the demographic segments considered become smaller. In recent times, for instance, we have seen that an increasing proportion of women have their children delivered in hospitals and clinics, often far away from their place of residence. The smaller the territorial unit, the higher the risk that the birth of the child will take place outside the unit itself. In Chapter 2, we pointed out the bias introduced by emigration, which by altering the sex ratio of the married population generally produces an excess of married women over married men. In this case, measures of current fertility based on the female population underestimate the relevant level of marital fertility. Since the territorial incidence of emigration is very uneven, the smaller the size of the population considered, the higher the risk of an abnormal imbalance in the sex ratio. If we consider ratios (married women 15-49 per married men 20-54) varying between .95

TABLE 4.1

VARIABILITY IN SEX RATIO OF MARRIED POPULATION, DISTRIBUTION OF PROVINCES: 1861 TO 1931

Value of ratio	Distribution of provinces (percent)					
	1861	1871	1881	1911	1931	1951
Below normal (less than .95)	1.7	4.5	5.9	1.5	3.3	7.6
Normal (.95 - 1.05)	76.3	70.9	72.3	52.2	56.5	79.3
Above normal (more than 1.05)	22.0	24.6	21.8	46.3	40.2	13.1

NOTE: The sex ratio of the married population is defined as the ratio of married women 15-49 per 100 married males 20-54.

TABLE 4.2

MARITAL FERTILITY (I_g), BY PROVINCE: 1861 TO 1961

Province		1861	1871	1881	1911	1931	1936	1951	1961
1	Alessandria	.564	.575	.594	.480	.287	.242	.191	.219
1'	Asti	--	--	.631	.497	.299	.251	.207	.213
2	Cuneo	.696	.673	.690	.621	.439	.387	.290	.264
3	Novara	.658	.641	.662	.463	.291	.266	.225	.245
3'	Vercelli	--	--	.629	.384	.254	.228	.198	.204
4	Torino	.659	.643	.644	.433	.254	.231	.179	.224
4'	Aosta	--	--	--	--	.333	.280	.264	.232
5	Genova	.658	.627	.611	.474	.272	.246	.135	.220
5'	Savona	--	--	.620	.529	.322	.291	.191	.216
5"	La Spezia	--	--	.628	.537	.330	.293	.199	.226
6	Imperia	.657	.648	.609	.443	.321	.259	.195	.231
7	Bergamo	.711	.731	.743	.837	.669	.631	.453	.378
8	Brescia	.589	.619	.609	.745	.584	.545	.393	.346
9	Como	.710	.692	.735	.640	.422	.389	.317	.290
9'	Varese	--	--	.734	.570	.312	.300	.258	.294
10	Cremona	.655	.608	.611	.627	.427	.401	.310	.283
11	Mantova	--	.576	.558	.583	.354	.318	.254	.256
12	Milano	.693	.683	.671	.552	.326	.298	.221	.259
13	Pavia	.627	.616	.628	.491	.296	.259	.208	.221
14	Sondrio	.763	.760	.762	.719	.592	.539	.438	.405
15	Bolzano	--	--	--	--	.574	.517	.422	.449
16	Trento	--	--	--	--	.500	.476	.437	.391
17	Belluno	--	.778	.757	.724	.471	.426	.352	.321
18	Padova	--	.685	.623	.758	.597	.538	.392	.370
19	Rovigo	--	.675	.631	.713	.525	.474	.328	.310
20	Treviso	--	.713	.682	.823	.582	.549	.401	.368
21	Udine	--	.676	.668	.738	.439	.414	.296	.283
22	Venezia	--	.633	.598	.714	.542	.507	.341	.327
23	Verona	--	.630	.614	.665	.478	.459	.358	.335
24	Vicenza	--	715	.685	.747	.571	.545	.401	.386
25	Gorizia	--	--	--	--	.460	.404	.223	.253
26	Trieste	--	--	--	--	.270	.244	.159	.192
27	Bologna	.625	.597	.601	.585	.325	.282	.199	.209
28	Ferrara	.660	.589	.534	.633	.374	.333	.224	.224
29	Forli	.668	.569	.586	.673	.445	.413	.297	.283
30	Modena	.663	.616	.625	.689	.421	.361	.241	.245
31	Parma	.637	.612	.614	.656	.368	.330	.226	.230
32	Piacenza	.616	.577	.592	.676	.461	.399	.263	.254
33	Ravenna	.634	.569	.587	.550	.330	.300	.236	.247
34	Reggio nell'Emilia	.692	635	.623	.727	.404	.353	.243	.228
35	Arezzo	.753	.667	.669	.642	.429	.381	.264	.245
36	Firenze	.758	.679	.622	.509	.299	.274	.214	.233
36'	Pistoia	--	--	.691	.597	.340	.307	.219	.227
37	Grosseto	.710	.661	.644	.550	.341	.306	.224	.213
38	Livorno	.657	.545	.527	.454	.306	.279	.199	.226
39	Lucca	.738	.680	.664	.583	.383	.357	.371	.279
40	Massa-Carrara	.720	.694	.651	.637	.439	.380	.269	.255
41	Pisa	.727	.647	.625	.511	.315	.286	.215	.226
42	Siena	.693	.628	.602	.518	.319	.280	.202	.194

Province		1861	1871	1881	1911	1931	1936	1951	1961
43	Ancona	.700	.624	.650	.628	.433	.390	.278	.258
44	Ascoli Piceno	.679	.653	.704	.681	.522	.484	.329	.290
45	Macerata	.676	.626	.662	.681	.482	.461	.296	.256
46	Pesaro e Urbino	.672	.584	.633	.629	.475	.427	.297	.279
47	Perugia	.627	.600	.594	.630	.452	.401	.265	.245
47'	Terni	--	--	.604	.583	.403	.363	.235	.225
47"	Rieti	--	--	.597	.634	.523	.462	.332	.285
48	Roma	--	.610	.513	.541	.430	.380	.289	.323
48'	Frosinone	--	--	.599	.617	.590	.529	.383	.324
48"	Latina	--	--	.601	.614	.590	.551	.399	.355
48"'	Viterbo	--	--	.606	.587	.444	.400	.286	.262
49	Campobasso	.665	.649	.634	.567	.540	.498	.365	.334
50	Chieti	.665	.617	.615	.562	.526	.488	.344	.279
50'	Pescara	--	--	.642	.625	.575	.523	.355	.326
51	L'Aquila	.679	.652	.671	.594	.544	.480	.367	.323
52	Teramo	.668	.633	.682	.670	.623	.569	.376	.328
53	Avellino	.690	.766	.762	.672	.663	.610	.448	.405
54	Benevento	.655	.665	.672	.642	.619	.580	.417	.390
55	Caserta	.680	.656	.659	.684	--	--	.508	.492
56	Napoli	.717	.678	.666	.657	.641	.601	.528	.543
57	Salerno	.669	.594	.630	.694	.666	.605	.474	.437
58	Bari	.775	.744	.740	.704	.645	.607	.514	.491
59	Foggia	.725	.669	.693	.650	.620	.608	.513	.485
60	Lecce	.717	.670	.714	.762	.690	.640	.506	.464
60'	Brindisi	--	--	.718	.733	.624	.595	.472	.443
60"	Taranto	--	--	.711	.699	.616	.606	.464	.421
61	Potenza	.678	.645	.634	.645	.615	.589	.471	.423
61'	Matera	--	--	.669	.662	.646	.592	.482	.428
62	Catanzaro	.642	.646	.611	.578	.598	.577	.520	.496
63	Cosenza	.638	.619	.602	.583	.587	.552	.475	.434
64	Reggio di Calabria	.639	.658	.618	.675	.601	.571	.492	.457
65	Agrigento	.718	.717	.671	.657	.588	.543	.424	.401
66	Caltanissetta	.711	.712	.706	.699	.619	.568	.469	.482
66'	Enna	--	--	.667	.570	.537	.526	.437	.400
67	Catania	.719	.695	.654	.553	.499	.462	.416	.436
68	Messina	.684	.619	.657	.615	.518	.464	.390	.375
69	Palermo	.685	.716	.685	.629	.578	.526	.462	.451
70	Siracusa	.692	.712	.665	.535	.443	.431	.359	.366
70'	Ragusa	--	--	.693	.604	.459	.433	.326	.333
71	Trapani	.761	.715	.745	.615	.500	.483	.391	.389
72	Cagliari	.625	.620	.625	.698	.656	.630	.603	.554
73	Sassari	.671	.649	.669	.676	.638	.607	.531	.513
73'	Nuoro	--	--	.673	.657	.710	.677	.634	.577

and 1.05 as normal, and as below normal and above normal the ratios falling respectively below and above such limits, Table 4.1 can be obtained. From unification to 1931, in a high proportion of all provinces, ranging from over one-fifth to almost one-half, an abnormal prevalence of married fertile women over married fertile males can be observed and, consequently, a lesser probability of women to procreate. When the unbalanced sex composition is induced by seasonal or temporary emigra-

tion, the annual probability of conception for each married woman whose husband is absent will be reduced but not nullified. When the sex composition is affected by permanent emigration of males, the probability of legitimate pregnancies for married women whose husbands have left is zero. Corrections like those proposed in Section 2.5.3 will lead, in the first case, to an overstatement of actual marital fertility, while, in the second case, the correct value will be close to the truth. But, almost everywhere in the areas of emigration, streams of emigrants leaving for the season or for short periods coexisted, although in varying measure, with those leaving permanently or for long periods. It is therefore risky to attempt a correction for small areas when the characteristics of emigration are not exactly known, as is frequently the case. In the Alpine areas, for instance, a substantial excess of married females can be found almost everywhere until 1921, owing mainly to seasonal emigration that coincided with the date of the census; in Belluno and Udine, for instance, the ratio rose to the exceptional levels of 1.55 and 1.44 in 1911. The growing transoceanic and permanent emigration at the end of the century deeply affected the demographic equilibrium of the South, and the 1911 census showed a substantial surplus of married females (more than 10 percent) in all the provinces of Abruzzi, Campania (with the exception of Napoli), Basilicata, and Calabria.

4.2 *The Geography of Birth Control, 1861 to 1961*

4.2.1. Table 4.2 lists I_g by province from 1861 to 1961 and Maps 4.2 to 4.9 present the same data in graphic form. These data constitute the basic information for our analysis of the geography of fertility.

The first three censuses (1861, 1871, and 1881) comprise a period of high fertility, when birth control was still limited to small sectors of the population. Variations in fertility from one census to the other are therefore predominantly caused by short-term fluctuations. In any case, the geography of fertility does not show great variations during that period; and the areas of high fertility remain approximately the same: the provinces of northern Lombardia (particularly Sondrio, Bergamo, and Como) and Veneto (Belluno, Treviso, and Vicenza); the provinces of Puglia; a province of central Campania, on the Apennines (Avellino); and the provinces of Trapani and Caltanissetta in Sicilia. Most of the provinces of Toscana had a relatively high fertility in 1861, but then experienced a continuous, although initially slow, decline.

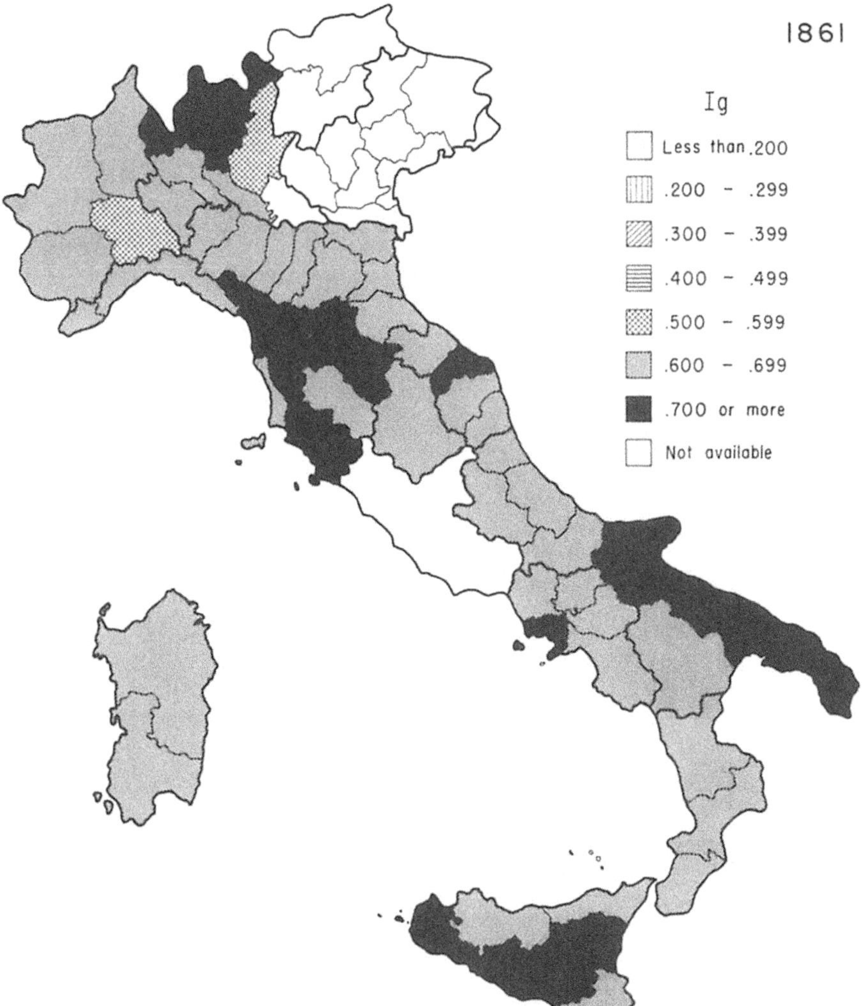

Map 4.2 Marital Fertility (I_g), by Province: 1861

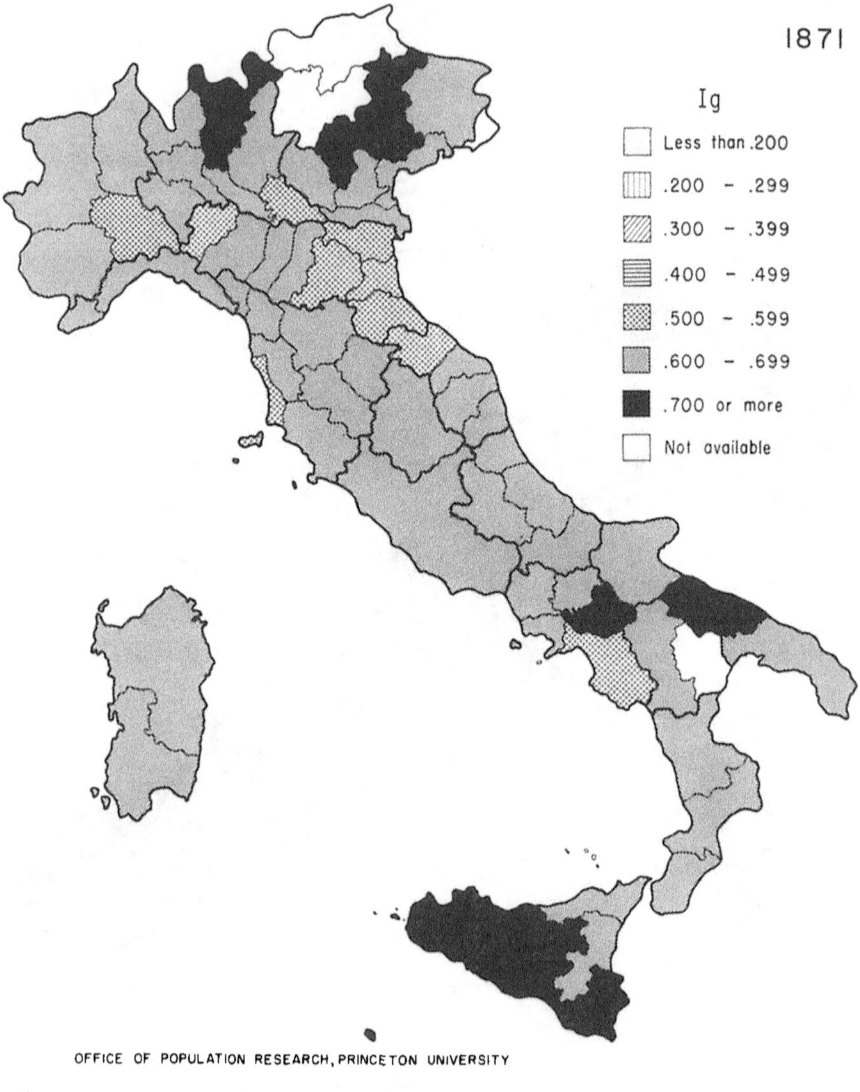

Map 4.3 Marital Fertility (I_g), by Province: 1871

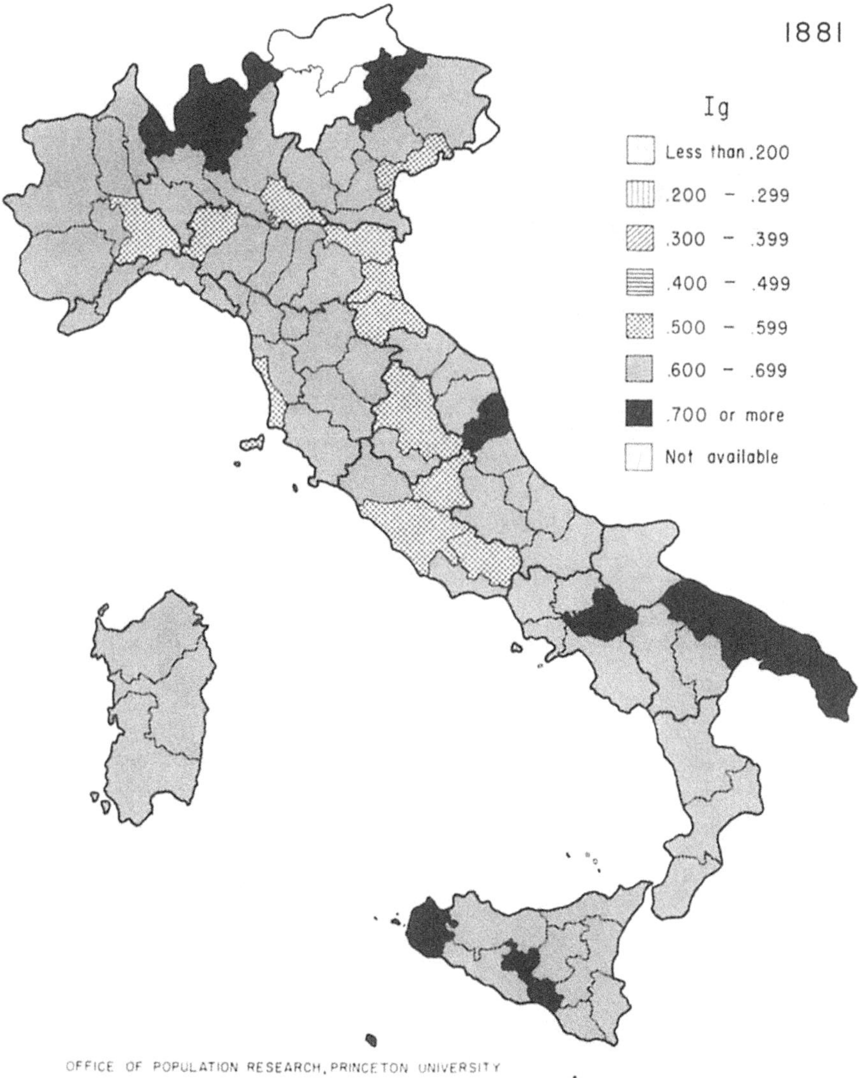

Map 4.4 Marital Fertility (I_g), by Province: 1881

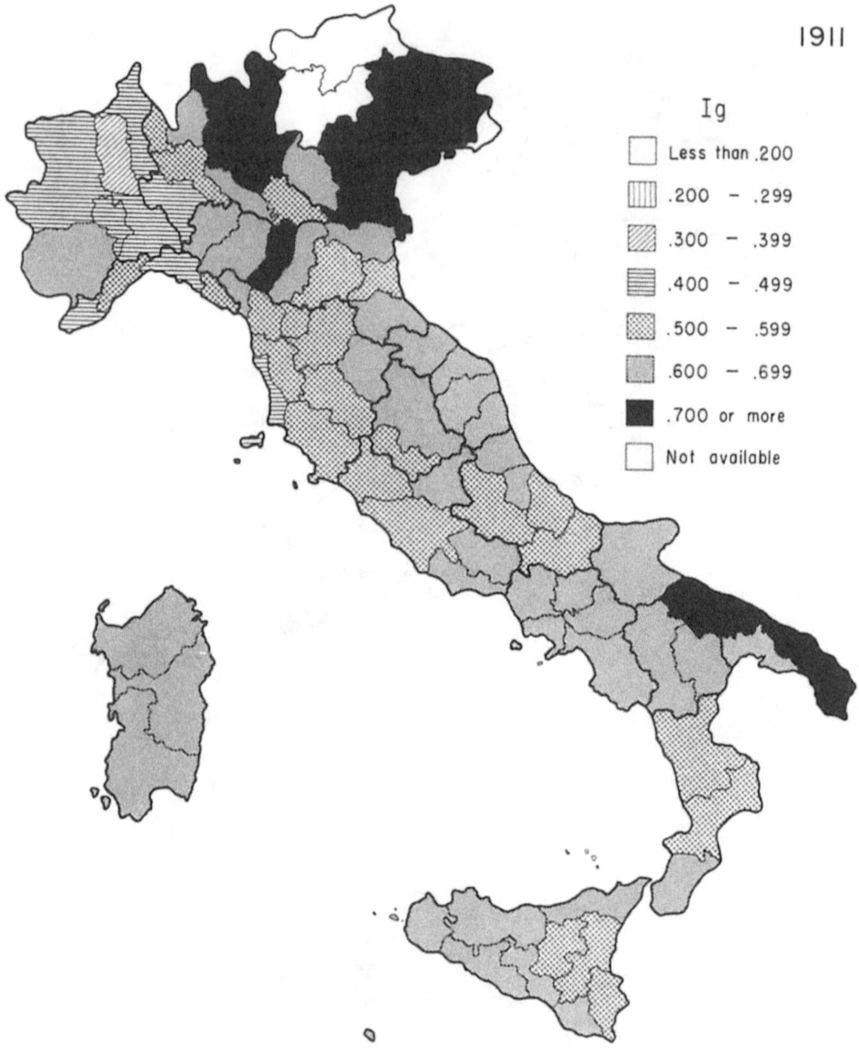

Map 4.5 Marital Fertility (I_g), by Province: 1911

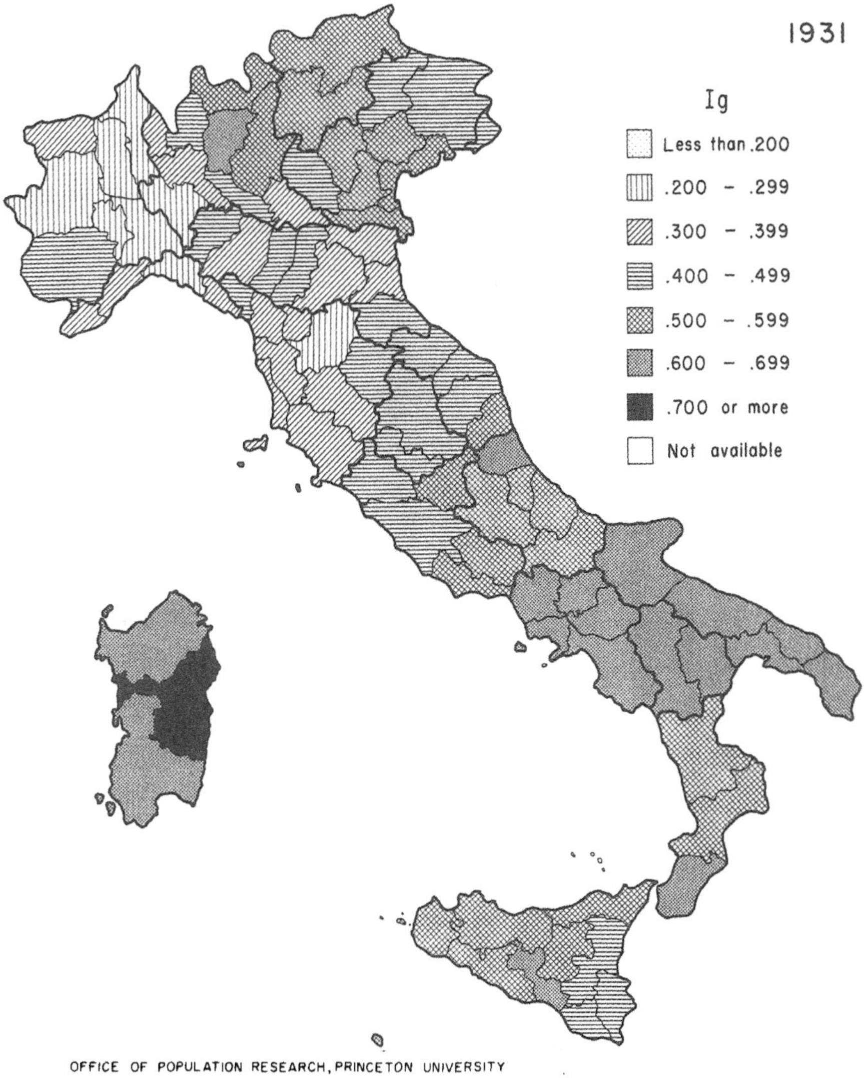

Map 4.6 Marital Fertility (I_g), by Province: 1931

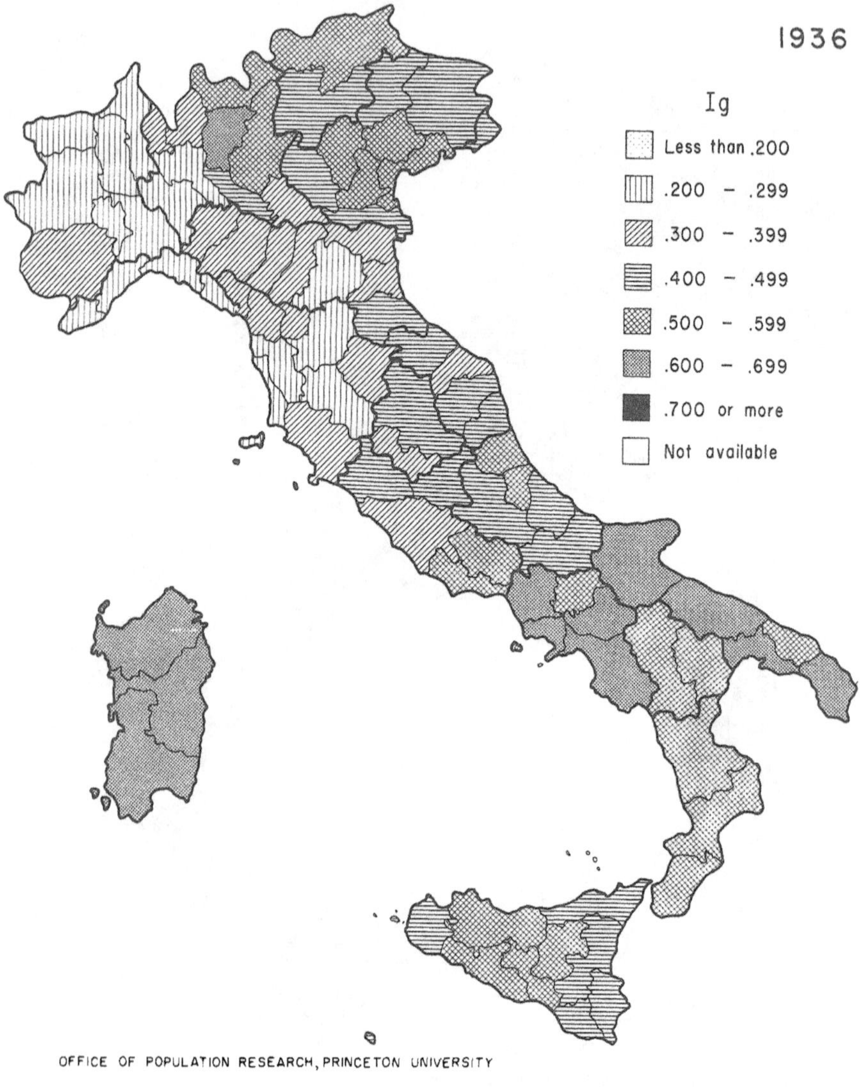

Map 4.7 Marital Fertility (I_g), by Province: 1936

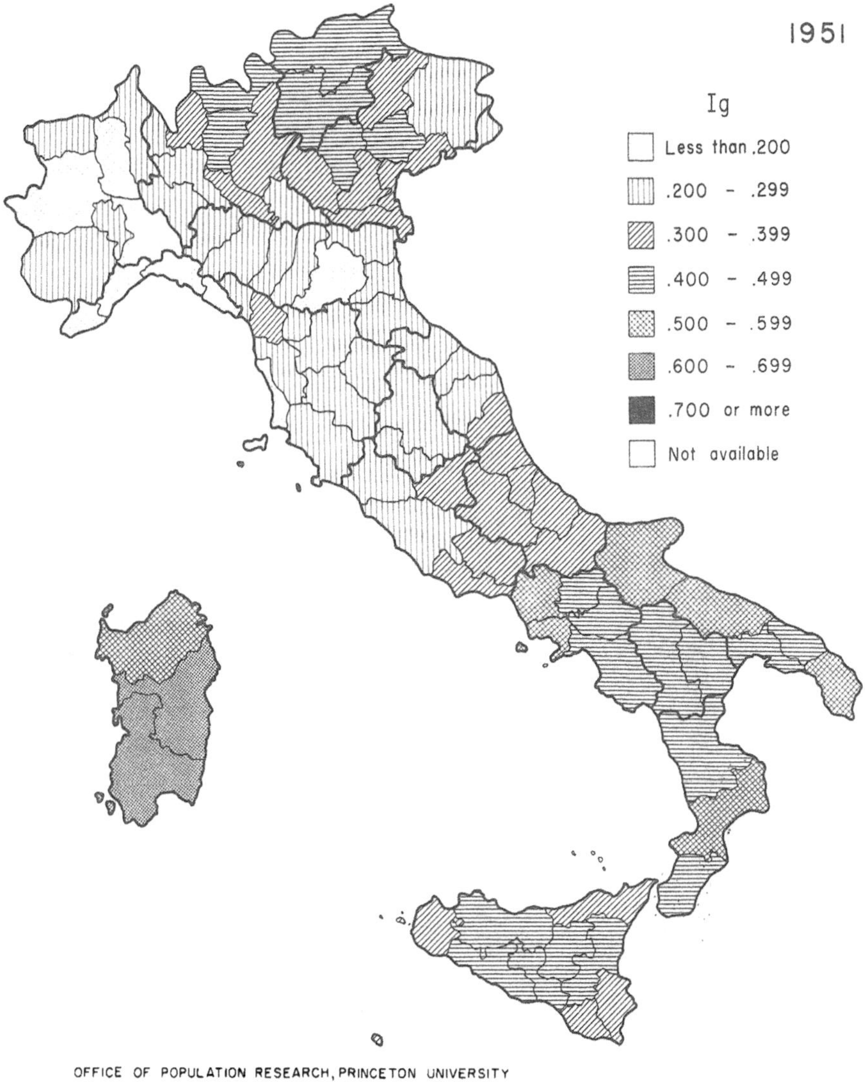

Map 4.8 Marital Fertility (I_g), by Province: 1951

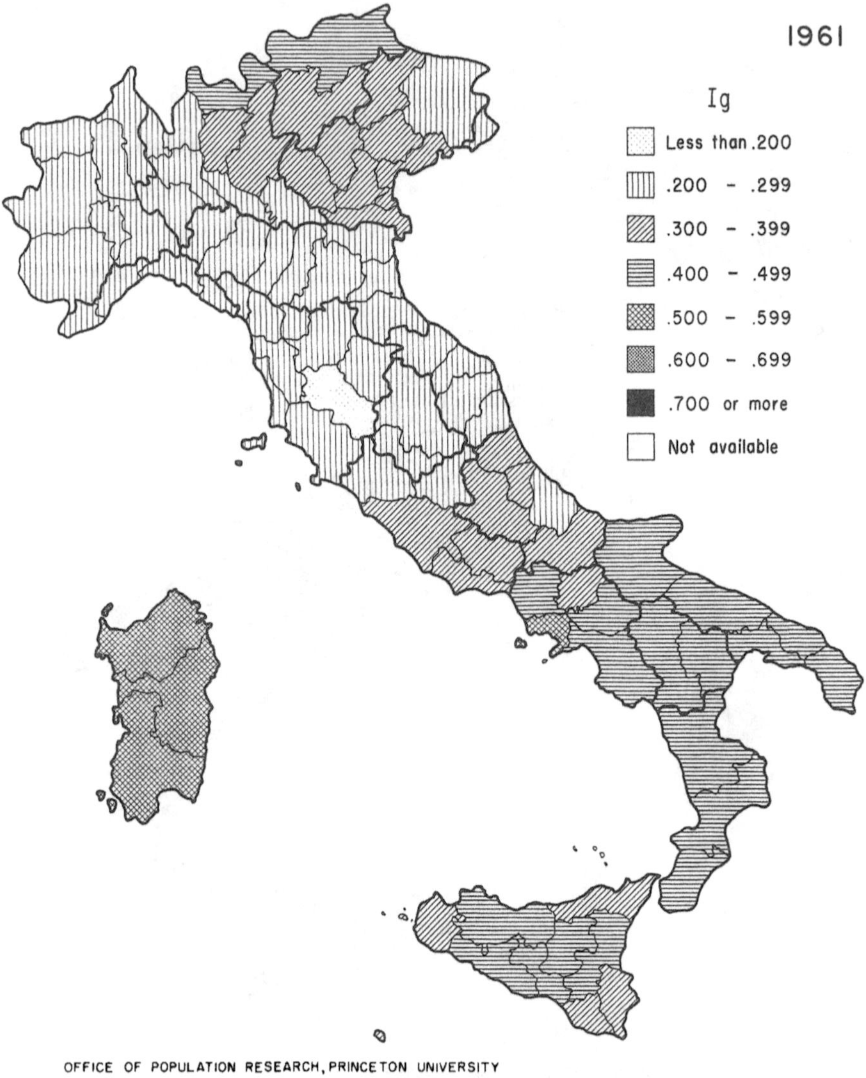

Map 4.9 Marital Fertility (I_g), by Province: 1961

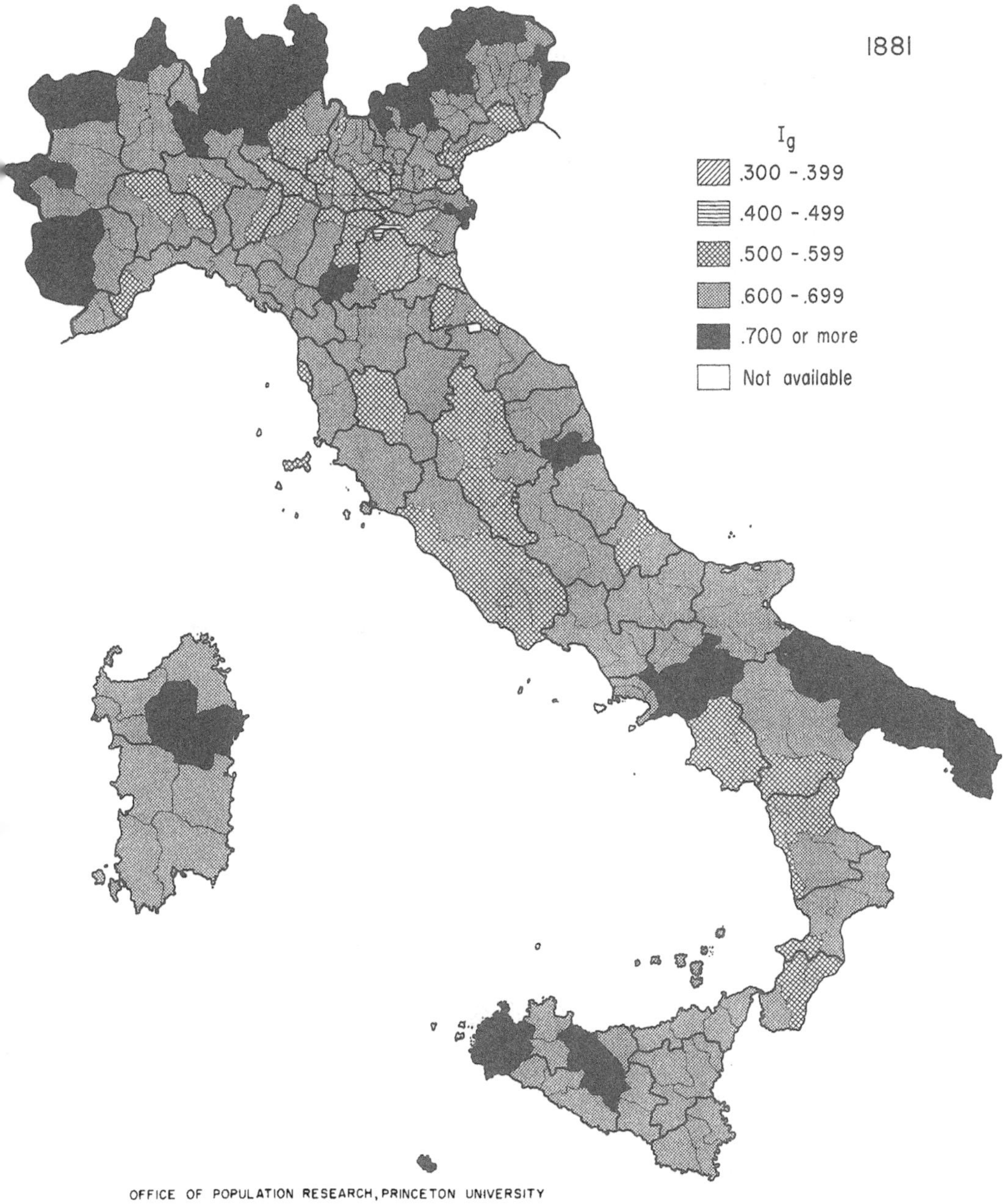

Map 4.10 Marital Fertility (I_g), by Circondario: 1881

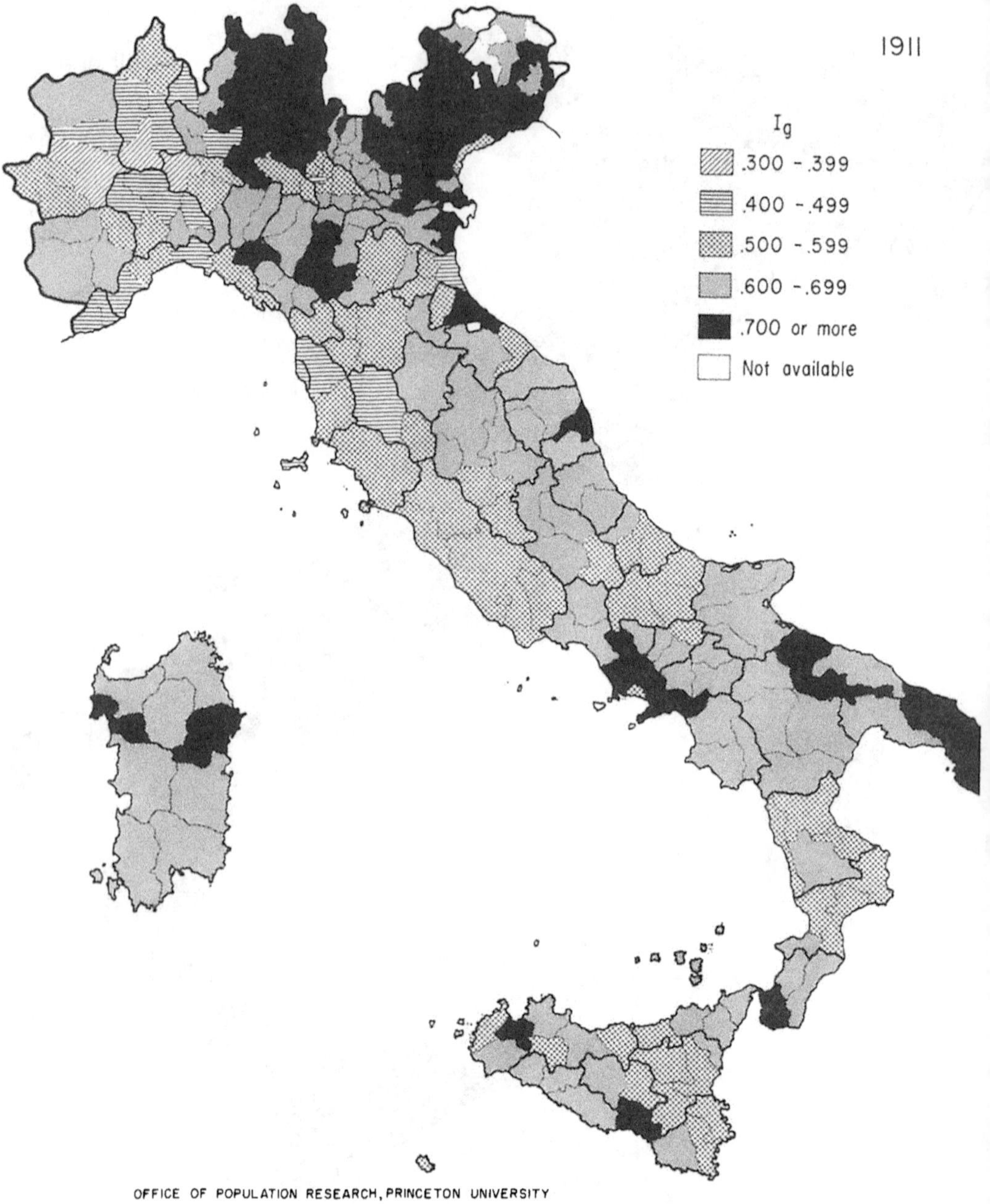

Map 4.11 Marital Fertility (I_g), by Circondario: 1911

Map 4.10, representing I_g in 284 circondari in 1881, gives a much more precise idea of the geography of fertility. For instance: the whole range of Alpine circondari forming the Italian border from the west (Cuneo, Piemonte) to the east (S. Pietro Natisone, Veneto) had a relatively high I_g, above .700. We will see that this high fertility was coupled with a very low propensity to marriage (measured by I_m) and constituted a particular type of Alpine high fertility. If we exclude some sporadic instances in Emilia and in the Marche, the four other areas of high fertility are in the South. The first comprises five circondari (the whole province of Avellino, Nola, and Salerno), mostly constituted by the mountainous and inaccessible areas of the Apennines, but also stretching down to the sea. The second comprises seven circondari, covering two-thirds of Puglia (the whole provinces of Bari and Lecce). The third comprises five circondari in the provinces of Trapani, Palermo, and Caltanissetta, constituting an almost continuous area in western Sicilia. A fourth minor spot of high fertility involves two circondari of northern Sardegna.

The existence of low fertility areas is less easy to identify. In 1881 illegitimacy reaches a maximum, in large part because of the introduction of civil marriage, which distorted the significance of measures of legitimate fertility. Therefore, the relatively low level of I_g (less than .600) in the provinces once belonging to the Papacy (Romagna, Umbria, Lazio) is probably artificial (see Section 2.5.1). However, moderate fertility prevails in many circondari lying on both sides of the Po River, from west (Casale-Monferrato, Piemonte) to east (Massa S., Veneto). In fact, I_g seems to fall gradually, passing from the Alpine areas to the Po valley. It is also important to note the existence of a few areas of low fertility along the coast of Liguria and Toscana, the starting point of a further rapid decline that came to cover a larger area. Another area of relatively moderate fertility comprises six contiguous circondari in Campania, Basilicata, and Calabria. However, this area will show an almost constant fertility until the 1930s.

4.2.2. The censuses of 1911, 1931, and 1936 testify to the acceleration of the fertility decline in the North and in the Center. In 1911, the distortion caused by high illegitimacy is much lower, but the mass emigration from the South and from many other areas introduces another bias that cannot be properly eliminated.

The trend, as illustrated in Map 4.11, is generally clear. The areas of high fertility (above .700) are still approximately the same as in 1881: in Lombardia, all the circondari in the provinces of Sondrio, Bergamo, and Brescia, plus three other adjoining circondari, have relatively high fertility; the same can be said for almost all of Veneto, which had many circondari above .800 and two above .900. Five other circondari of Emilia, either lying on the Apennines or along the Adriatic coast complete the enumeration of the high fertility areas in the North. Of the areas of high fertility existing in the South in 1881, the one covering central and southern Puglia is still there, with unchanged boundaries and levels of fertility; the other, in Campania, has somewhat changed its boundaries; the third zone, in Sicilia, is now reduced to only two circondari. But the most interesting feature is the extension of the area of low fertility in the North and in the Center. Three circondari on the left bank of the Po, have fallen below the .400 mark: going eastward, Torino and Vercelli (Piemonte) and Mortara (Lombardia). North of this area in five contiguous circondari fertility has dropped below .500, as it has, to the south, in four other adjoining circondari. This large area coincides with the western portion of the Po valley and includes the largest part of Piemonte, with over two million inhabitants. Another area of relatively low fertility is developing along the Tyrrhenian coast, in seven circondari in Liguria and Toscana.

Map 4.12, representing changes in I_g, 1881–1911, at the provincial level, gives a clear-cut picture. Declines in I_g ranging from 10 to over 30 percent cover a vast area, almost contiguous, including all the provinces of Piemonte (excluding Cuneo) and of Liguria, four provinces of western Lombardia and seven of the nine provinces of Toscana. In a large area of seven million inhabitants, fertility control has made substantial progress. Three other provinces of Abruzzi and Campania show falls in I_g above 10 percent, but we know that emigration played an important role in affecting our period measures. Emigration, on the other hand, was only partially responsible for the fall of fertility in Sicilia, particularly in the eastern portion of the island. This was the only area of the South to experience a precocious decline of fertility.

Changes above or below the 1881 level within a 10 percent limit cover most of the rest of the country and are due to varying factors, a description of which would be unsatisfactory and beyond the scope of this chapter.

4.2.3. From 1911 to 1931, legitimate fertility for Italy as a whole declined by almost one-fourth. The area of relatively low fertility (below

.500) described in 1911 embraced the largest part of the Center and the North by 1931: all provinces of Piemonte (with the exception of Cuneo), Liguria, and Toscana (except Arezzo and Massa); three provinces of western Lombardia and Mantova; and four provinces of Emilia. In a total of 25 provinces, accounting for 12 million people, or three-tenths of the total population, I_g is below .400, and in 8 of the 25 provinces (mainly in Piemonte) it is below .300.

Fertility above .500, and therefore possibly still close to pre-Malthusian levels, can be found in the three provinces of eastern Lombardia (Bergamo, Brescia, and Sondrio), in the mainly German-speaking province of Bolzano (Trentino), and in five provinces of lower Veneto. The area is still a large one, practically contiguous and covering most of Northeastern Italy. Three other provinces—Ascoli (Marche), Frosinone, and Rieti (Lazio)—have an I_g above .500 in the Center, but their contiguity with the large area of high fertility of the continental South explains the exception. Sicilia is the only region of the South where relatively controlled fertility prevails in four of the nine provinces. In 1936, with a national I_g reduced by a further 8 percent, I_g fell below .400 in all other provinces of the North and of the Center.

Map 4.13 represents the percent change in provincial I_g, 1911–1931. The Center and the North, with the sole exceptions of the provinces of Rieti (Lazio) and Sondrio (Lombardia) had undergone a reduction of I_g of 20 percent or more; in practically all the western section of the North and of the Center the decline exceeded 30 percent. A mild decline of less than 10 percent occurred in the South, with some areas registering a mild increase; only in Sicilia did the decline exceed 10 percent (in six of the nine provinces).

4.2.4. The year 1951 marked the breakthrough of low fertility in the South. Abruzzi and a large portion of Sicilia fell in the category of very low or strongly controlled fertility (I_g below .400). This category embraced all the Center and the North, with the exception of six provinces of Lombardia, Trentino, and Veneto, once the hard-core area of high fertility. In ten provinces of Piemonte, Liguria, Emilia, V. Giulia, and Toscana, I_g fell below .200. This corresponds, on the average, to a period, hypothetical family size of 1.6 children or less per couple, a family size that gives a clear idea of the degree of neo-Malthusianism permeating the largest part of the country. Moderately high fertility (above .500) is limited in 1951 to six provinces in the South (in Campania, Puglia, and Calabria) and to Sardegna. Map 4.14 represents the

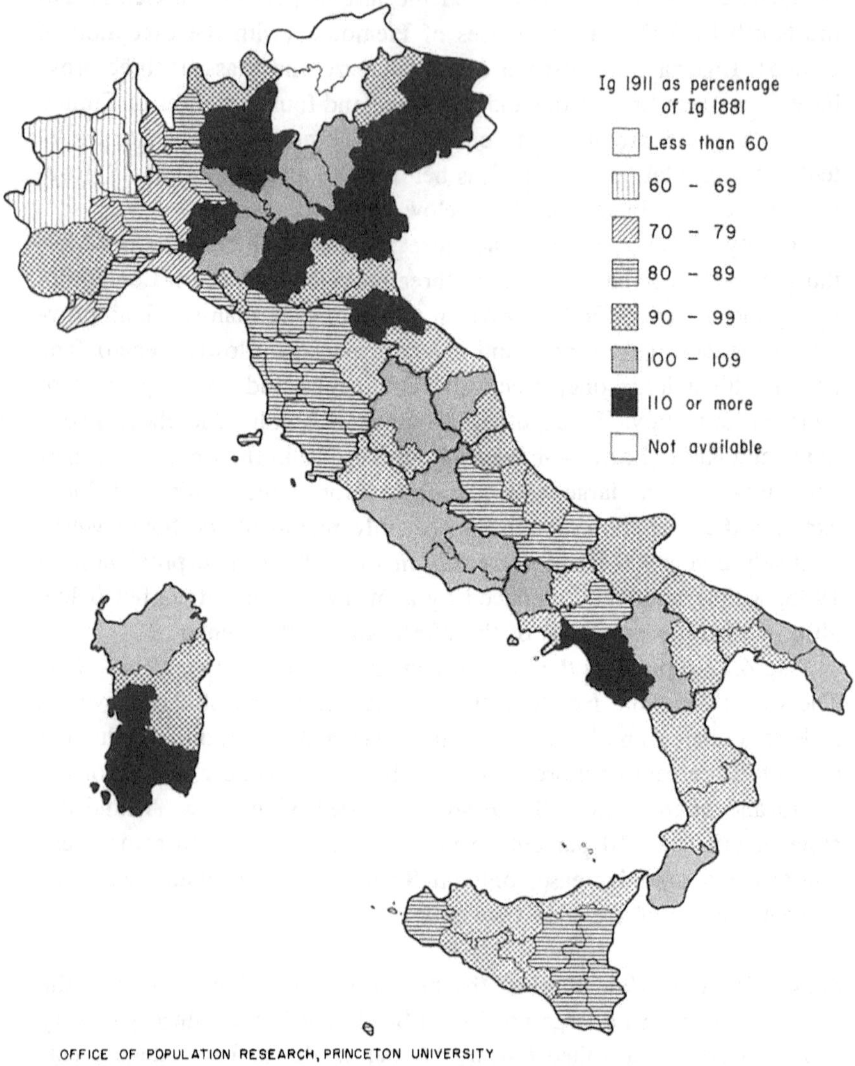

Map 4.12 Change in Marital Fertility (I_g), by Province: 1911 as Percentage of 1881

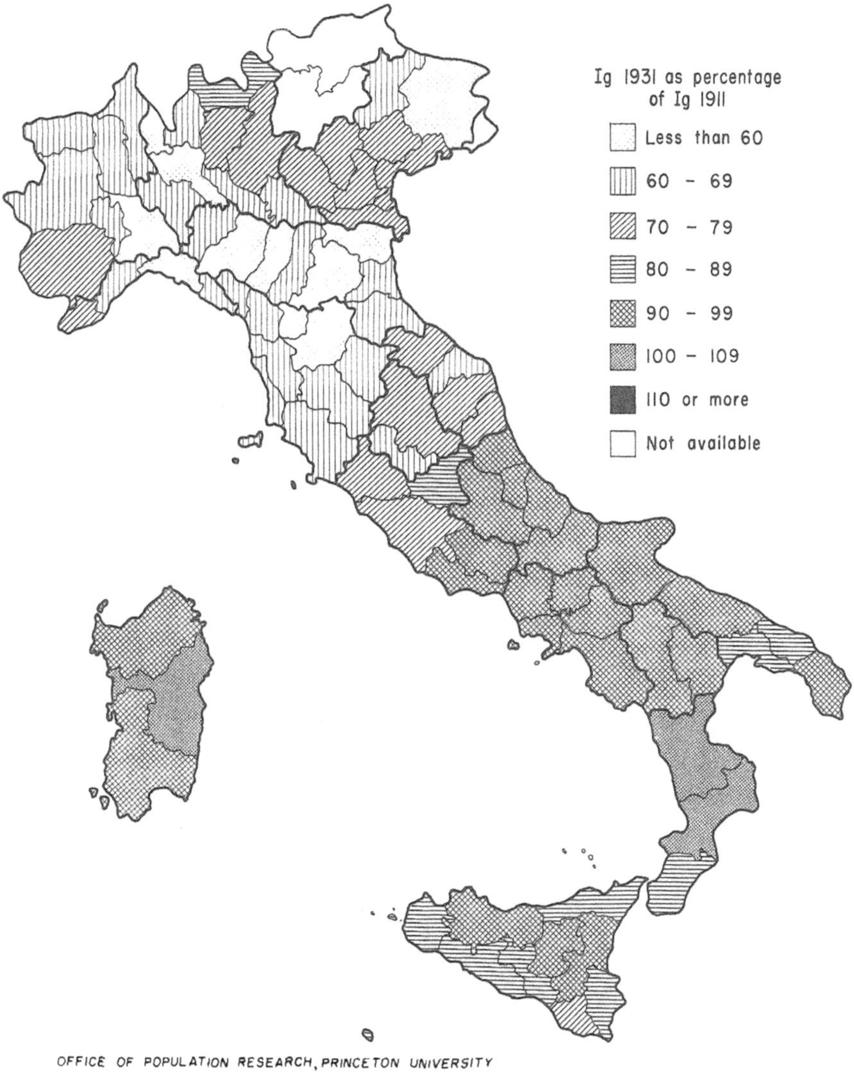

Map 4.13 Change in Marital Fertility (I_g), by Province: 1931 as Percentage of 1911

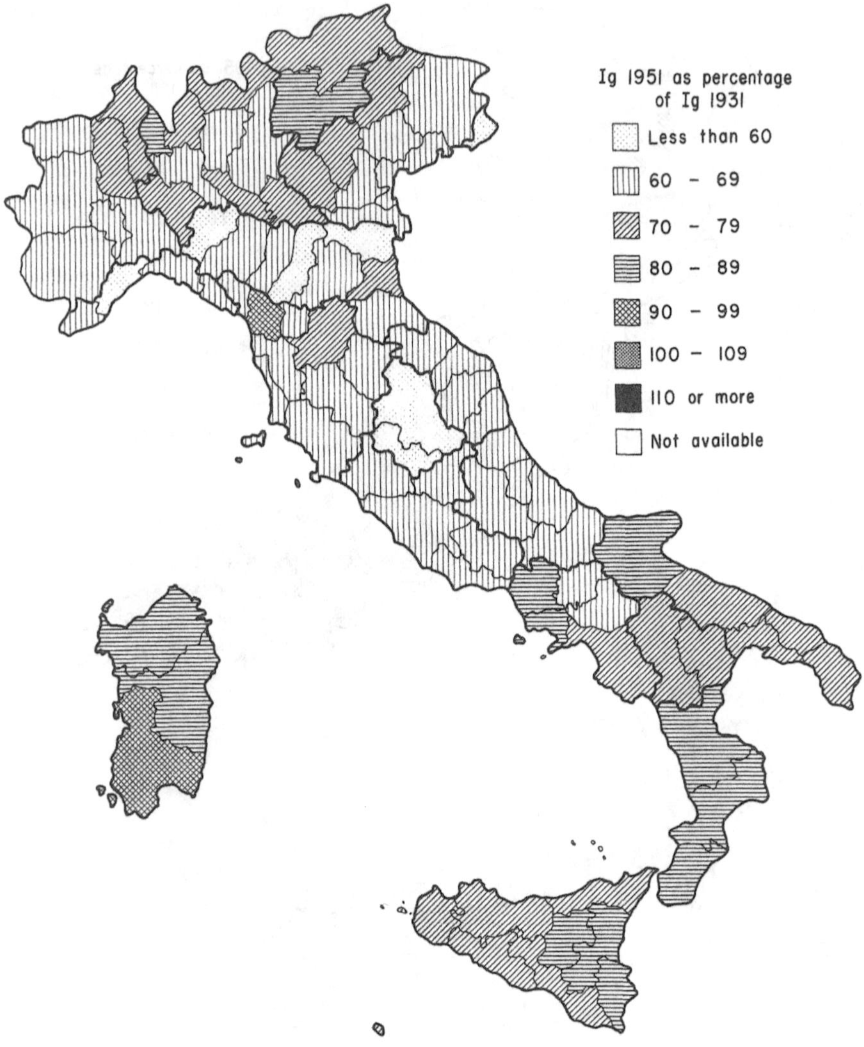

Map 4.14 Change in Marital Fertility (I_g), by Province: 1951 as Percentage of 1931

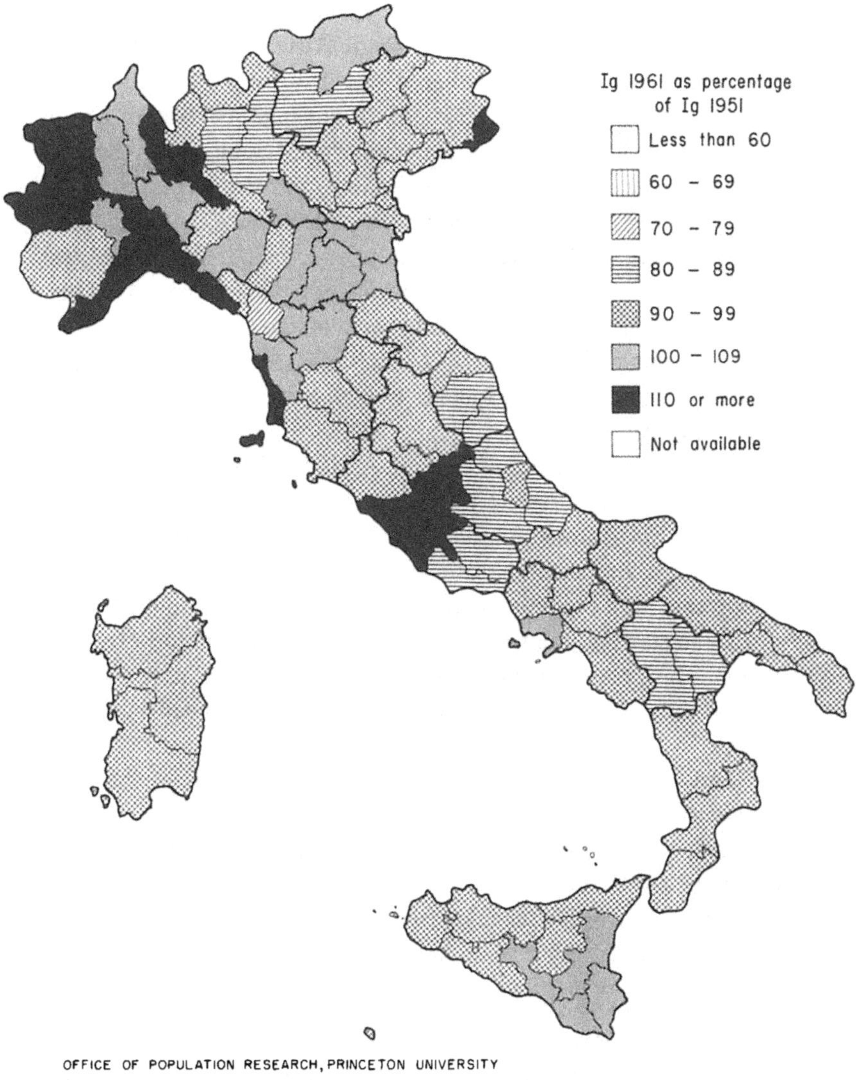

Map 4.15 Change in Marital Fertility (I_g), by Province: 1961 as Percentage of 1951

fall of I_g, 1931–1951, and shows that I_g not only declined in all provinces of the country, but also did so by more than 10 percent in all but two provinces. A decline of more than 30 percent took place in all but two provinces of Piemonte and Toscana; all but one province of Lazio and Emilia; all of Liguria, V. Giulia, Umbria, Marche, and Abruzzi, and ten other provinces in Lombardia, Veneto, and Campania.

In 1961 very low fertility (I_g below .400) finally broke through into the hard-core area of Northeastern Italy; marital fertility remained above .400 in only two provinces, Sondrio and the German-speaking Bolzano. In the continental South, only one of the six provinces that had moderately high fertility in 1951 did so in 1961: the highly urbanized, metropolitan Napoli. Moderately high fertility still prevailed in Sardegna, however.

Map 4.15, representing the change of I_g, 1951–1961, shows a new fact: a recovery of legitimate fertility in most of the provinces of Piemonte, Liguria, Lombardia, Emilia, and Toscana; these provinces had experienced, since the beginning of the century, a precocious and rapid decline. Together with the persistent, although mild, decline in the South, this trend is the starting point of a new process of equalization of fertility behavior. The process of differentiation between the South and the rest of the country, initiated at the turn of the century, ended by 1961.

4.2.5. Is there any lesson we can derive from the analysis of the geographic patterns of fertility decline? Some of the usual interpretations are reinforced; others are neither proved nor disproved; others can at least be rejected for Italy.

Conclusions that readily emerge from a consideration of the geographic patterns of fertility decline are as follows:

(1) In the North and Center, the fertility decline seems to have proceeded with a classic process of diffusion; from the west portion of the Po valley in Piemonte it moved eastward, and southward along the coast of Liguria, Toscana, and, later, Lazio.

(2) In areas of predominantly high fertility, or of predominantly low fertility, it is rare, if not impossible, to find isolated instances of low or high fertility. The decline may lag behind, or precede, that of the remaining area by a few years, but the lag is never very long.

(3) During the process of fertility decline the areas of high fertility are always very large; this is true not only in the South but also

in the North, where the hard-core area of Lombardia, Trentino, and Veneto embraces quite a large population.

(4) The hypothesis that the diffusion process might be accelerated—or delayed—by natural, geographic obstacles, cannot be proved. The Po valley is certainly an area where mobility has always been easier than elsewhere in Italy, but high fertility persisted in the 1930s in Veneto's eastern portion of the valley, while the decline arrived earlier in the more mountainous and less accessible areas of the same region. On the other hand, inaccessible Abruzzi controlled fertility much earlier than the lower provinces of Lazio and the coastal ones of Campania with their much easier communications and closer contacts with the rest of the country. The province of Napoli, practically one large metropolitan area, is the province with the highest legitimate fertility in the continental South in 1961. Of the two islands, Sicilia and Sardegna, the first underwent a substantial decline of fertility at the end of the last century, over 50 years before Sardegna.

Our opinion is that geographic location is only one among the many factors at play in determining the level of fertility in the various areas of the country. In relatively homogeneous populations diffusion of fertility control may be delayed by natural obstacles; this may be the case, for instance, with the populations of the Apennines between Toscana and Emilia. Other cases might be easily discovered if detailed maps (such as the 1936 one for the 795 agrarian districts for general fertility) were available. Nothing more can be said if we stick to scientific evidence. Moreover, it is obvious that geographic location is a qualitative concept that can be defined only approximately. Finally, a natural obstacle may not remain forever; when a bridge is laid across a river, a tunnel excavated in a mountain, or a road built through a mountain chain, the isolation of a certain area may come to an end. Our impression is that any attempt to construct an index of the degree of isolation on the basis of the available data would be vain.

4.3 *The Geography of the Propensity to Marriage, 1861 to 1961*

The geographical variation of nuptiality—as described by the weighted proportion of married females aged 15-49 (I_m)—is less informative for our purposes than the variation of I_g. In fact, I_m is not a suitable measure for analyzing variations in nuptiality over time or space, except when interest in nuptiality is limited to the contribution of marital

TABLE 4.3

PROPORTION MARRIED (I_m), BY PROVINCE: 1861 TO 1961

Province		1861	1871	1881	1911	1931	1936	1951	1961
1	Alessandria	.686	.668	.649	.558	.532	.528	.558	.609
1'	Asti	--	--	.663	.610	.600	.598	.590	.641
2	Cuneo	.545	.573	.566	.517	.493	.514	.528	.576
3	Novara	.541	.557	.533	.526	.517	.549	.573	.619
3'	Vercelli	--	--	.550	.475	.510	.548	.580	.625
4	Torino	.496	.514	.556	.470	.506	.527	.574	.633
4'	Aosta	--	--	--	--	.502	.541	.595	.626
5	Genova	.554	.569	.504	.474	.455	.459	.523	.576
5'	Savona	--	--	.549	.505	.478	.500	.554	.598
5"	La Spezia	--	--	.604	.530	.528	.545	.574	.618
6	Imperia	.505	.521	.509	.488	.500	.521	.560	.625
7	Bergamo	.530	.548	.537	.533	.472	.474	.492	.548
8	Brescia	.555	.567	.541	.513	.490	.503	.516	.564
9	Como	.516	.504	.514	.513	.465	.497	.500	.547
9'	Varese	--	--	.569	.556	.487	.488	.542	.587
10	Cremona	.595	.617	.563	.536	.506	.529	.533	.575
11	Mantova	--	.655	.609	.554	.540	.566	.594	.635
12	Milano	.562	.561	.570	.552	.497	.496	.526	.578
13	Pavia	.640	.634	.614	.536	.517	.531	.547	.604
14	Sondrio	.487	.499	.475	.481	.484	.500	.515	.578
15	Bolzano	--	--	--	--	.373	.388	.440	.498
16	Trento	--	--	--	--	.421	.424	.467	.518
17	Belluno	--	.541	.502	.576	.489	.495	.549	.569
18	Padova	--	.621	.575	.519	.468	.475	.482	.554
19	Rovigo	--	.674	.613	.563	.534	.555	.545	.614
20	Treviso	--	.620	.556	.520	.452	.465	.495	.558
21	Udine	--	.543	.506	.548	.466	.499	.563	.588
22	Venezia	--	.558	.521	.506	.479	.496	.526	.583
23	Verona	--	.573	.550	.500	.465	.465	.499	.558
24	Vicenza	--	.594	.564	.433	.449	.457	.491	.537
25	Gorizia	--	--	--	--	.443	.460	.530	.579
26	Trieste	--	--	--	--	.463	.508	.544	.588
27	Bologna	.594	.562	.501	.504	.502	.510	.552	.618
28	Ferrara	.606	.637	.561	.538	.509	.547	.591	.661
29	Forli	.612	.577	.515	.544	.544	.558	.574	.617
30	Modena	.618	.602	.554	.566	.528	.544	.575	.643
31	Parma	.563	.575	.537	.541	.489	.505	.555	.604
32	Piacenza	.627	.620	.579	.554	.447	.443	.477	.548
33	Ravenna	.566	.521	.465	.503	.529	.540	.559	.640
34	Reggio nell'Emilia	.593	.595	.553	.576	.509	.529	.572	.630
35	Arezzo	.528	.547	.517	.553	.580	.586	.600	.648
36	Firenze	.550	.565	.526	.504	.504	.506	.546	.597
36'	Pistoia	--	--	.557	.544	.528	.553	.596	.628
37	Grosseto	.628	.620	.499	.612	.624	.630	.659	.677
38	Livorno	.504	.506	.462	.532	.551	.547	.622	.641
39	Lucca	.514	.537	.499	.490	.484	.497	.389	.580
40	Massa-Carrara	.524	.582	.532	.556	.544	.561	.577	.623
41	Pisa	.575	.578	.543	.572	.556	.566	.599	.636
42	Siena	.594	.585	.555	.600	.596	.598	.621	.660

Province		1861	1871	1881	1911	1931	1936	1951	1961
43	Ancona	.547	.527	.510	.550	.530	.531	.567	.613
44	Ascoli Piceno	.500	.434	.433	.505	.501	.504	.533	.611
45	Macerata	.530	.487	.471	.523	.517	.517	.567	.629
46	Pesaro e Urbino	.584	.535	.512	.569	.576	.591	.603	.635
47	Perugia	.550	.529	.476	.442	.573	.581	.607	.647
47'	Terni	--	--	.488	.536	.569	.568	.615	.641
47"	Rieti	--	--	.522	.561	.541	.560	.571	.617
48	Roma	--	.575	.501	.473	.501	.486	.515	.563
48'	Frosinone	--	--	.525	.613	.566	.578	.588	.652
48"	Latina	--	--	.513	.553	.565	.615	.600	.639
48"'	Viterbo	--	--	.494	.514	.564	.564	.608	.642
49	Campobasso	.624	.621	.627	.623	.604	.617	.586	.631
50	Chieti	.586	.618	.621	.593	.582	.590	.576	.617
50'	Pescara	--	--	.564	.543	.534	.540	.525	.582
51	L'Aquila	.532	.548	.547	.565	.561	.557	.536	.585
52	Teramo	.490	.518	.496	.497	.497	.518	.518	.598
53	Avellino	.567	.551	.600	.558	.563	.574	.522	.586
54	Benevento	.557	.594	.595	.556	.542	.551	.509	.573
55	Caserta	.533	.554	.530	.522	--	--	.490	.542
56	Napoli	.526	.537	.520	.488	.479	.462	.480	.514
57	Salerno	.543	.588	.554	.542	.528	.525	.499	.565
58	Bari	.558	.593	.592	.564	.535	.527	.532	.549
59	Foggia	.566	.586	.605	.579	.574	.576	.560	.575
60	Lecce	.530	.560	.549	.527	.516	.505	.480	.518
60'	Brindisi	--	--	.581	.562	.517	.504	.524	.572
60"	Taranto	--	--	.608	.571	.560	.552	.556	.565
61	Potenza	.584	.608	.627	.623	.606	.614	.572	.623
61'	Matera	--	--	.652	.644	.600	.611	.563	.607
62	Catanzaro	.560	.573	.575	.586	.560	.562	.563	.603
63	Cosenza	.542	.577	.554	.581	.568	.567	.545	.592
64	Reggio di Calabria	.534	.545	.543	.575	.520	.520	.519	.558
65	Agrigento	.624	.605	.612	.627	.590	.594	.568	.593
66	Caltanissetta	.629	.618	.619	.651	.608	.604	.574	.602
66'	Enna	--	--	.620	.630	.600	.639	.609	.626
67	Catania	.565	.535	.531	.573	.584	.582	.569	.615
68	Messina	.537	.540	.519	.535	.514	.504	.507	.552
69	Palermo	.572	.561	.578	.523	.509	.503	.529	.560
70	Siracusa	.621	.567	.575	.604	.613	.613	.624	.652
70'	Ragusa	--	--	.562	.554	.585	.605	.623	.662
71	Trapani	.617	.565	.548	.521	.496	.505	.545	.579
72	Cagliari	.565	.562	.534	.468	.479	.484	.502	.502
73	Sassari	584	.591	.560	.497	.459	.464	.478	.486
73'	Nuoro	--	--	.513	.501	.448	.447	.441	.449

status to overall fertility. In an analysis of the factors affecting differences in nuptiality, it is necessary to consider separately age at marriage, the proportion remaining single, and widowhood and divorce. The same I_m can characterize two populations, one having relatively early marriage but a high incidence of permanent celibacy and widowhood, the other having relatively late, but more nearly universal, marriage. Similarly, a relatively level trend in I_m may conceal extensive changes in marriage habits. The usefulness of I_m is not in differentiating populations with different marriage customs but in providing a measure of marriage that is the complement of the measure of marital fertility in the determination of overall fertility. Its usefulness in Italy for this purpose is limited by the rather narrow range of its variation both historically and geographically. Table 4.3 and Maps 4.16-4.29 give in full detail the modifications undergone by I_m through the century-long period considered.

Map 4.24, I_m by circondario in 1881, reveals a much greater range of variation than the maps of I_m by province. There is an area of high nuptiality (I_m above .600) along the Po valley, particularly in the provinces of Asti, Alessandria, Pavia, and, in the eastern portion of the valley, in the provinces of Mantova, Verona, and Rovigo. I_m declines passing from the Po valley to the Alpine areas; many circondari (nine) mainly Alpine, from the west (Aosta, Piemonte) to the east (Tolmezzo, Veneto) have an I_m below .450 and, in some instances, below .400. The variability in the North is very high, I_m being as low as .379 in Varallo (Piemonte) and as high as .700 in Casale-Monferrato, less than 40 miles south of Varallo.

A second area of relatively low I_m can be found among the circondari once belonging to the Papacy, particularly those in the provinces of Forlí and Ravenna (Emilia), Macerata and Ascoli (Marche), all of Umbria, and part of Lazio (Roma, Viterbo). In this area of low fertility the effects—both direct and indirect—of the introduction of civil marriage, should be recognized. In the South and in Sicilia—excluding the north of Abruzzi and Campania—propensity to marriage is generally above the national mean.

Map 4.25, I_m by circondario in 1911, has little resemblance to Map 4.24. While the Alpine circondari continued to have a lower propensity to marriage than elsewhere in the North, the area of high I_m in the Po valley cannot be identified anymore. In the Center, patches of relatively low nuptiality (Umbria, Marche, Lazio) remained, but overall I_m increased in the 30-year period. Throughout the South, nuptiality remained relatively high.

From 1911 to 1931, I_m declined almost everywhere; national I_m reached an all-time low (excluding 1921, heavily affected by the consequences of the war). I_m increased in only 23 provinces, mainly in the North and Center. While areas of substantial decline were scattered everywhere, they were most often found in Lombardia, Emilia, Veneto, and Sardegna.

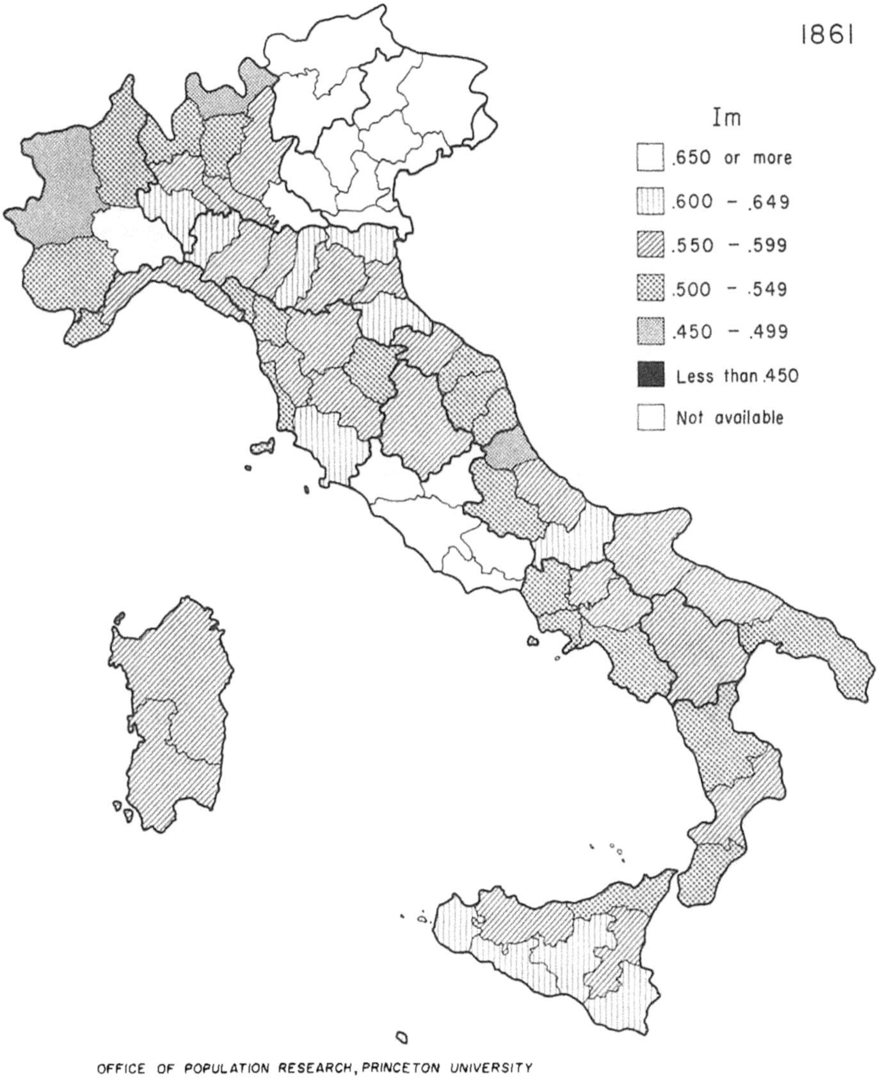

Map 4.16 Proportion Married (I_m), by Province: 1861

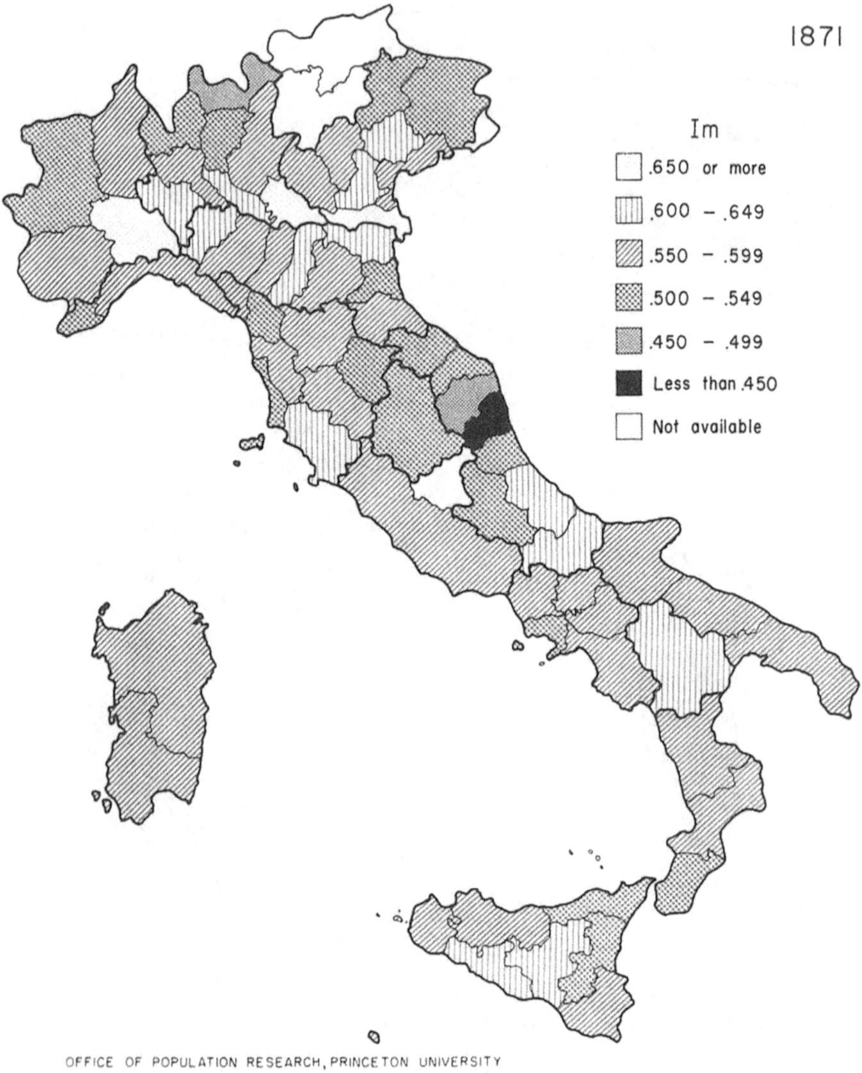

Map 4.17 Proportion Married (I_m), by Province: 1871

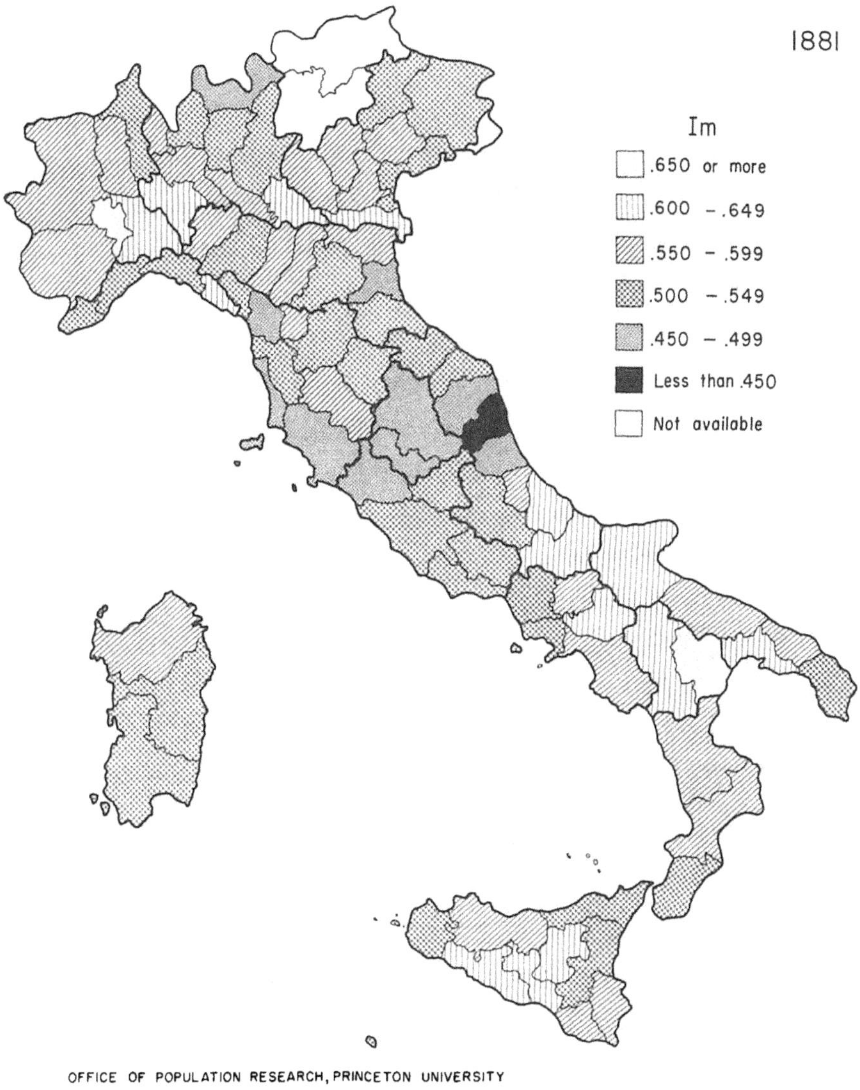

Map 4.18 Proportion Married (I_m), by Province: 1881

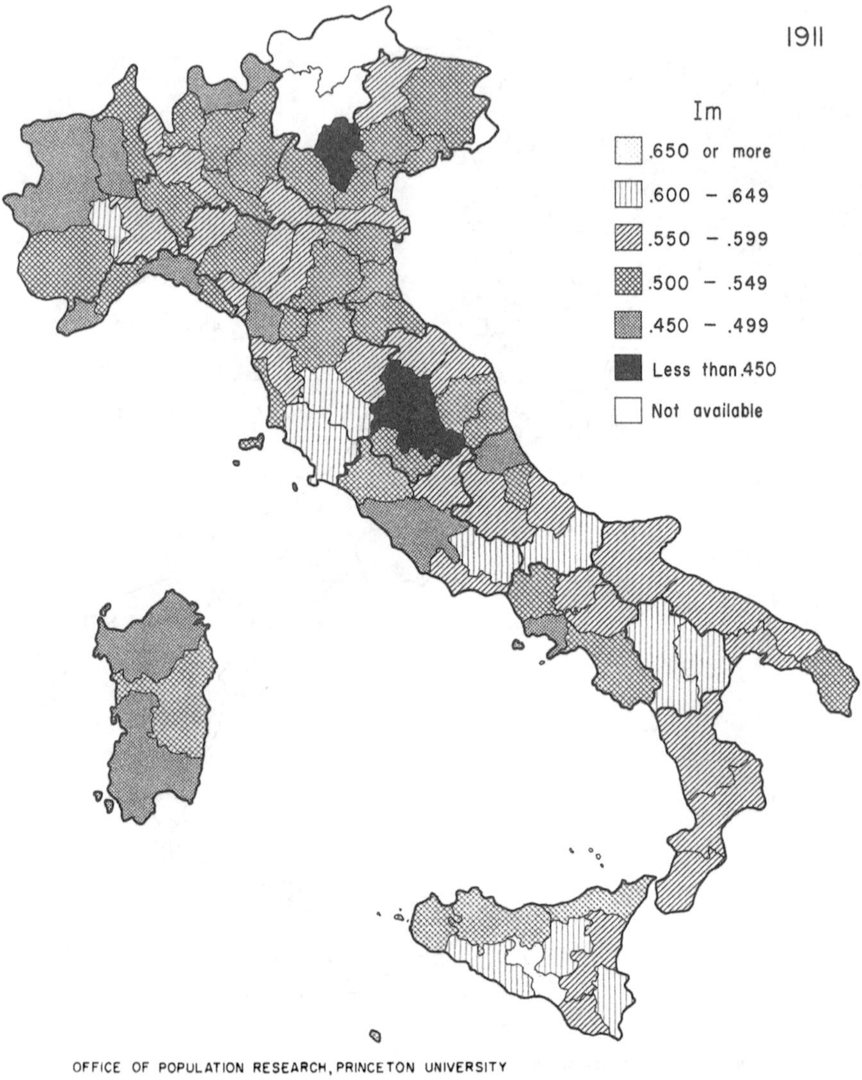

Map 4.19 Proportion Married (I_m), by Province: 1911

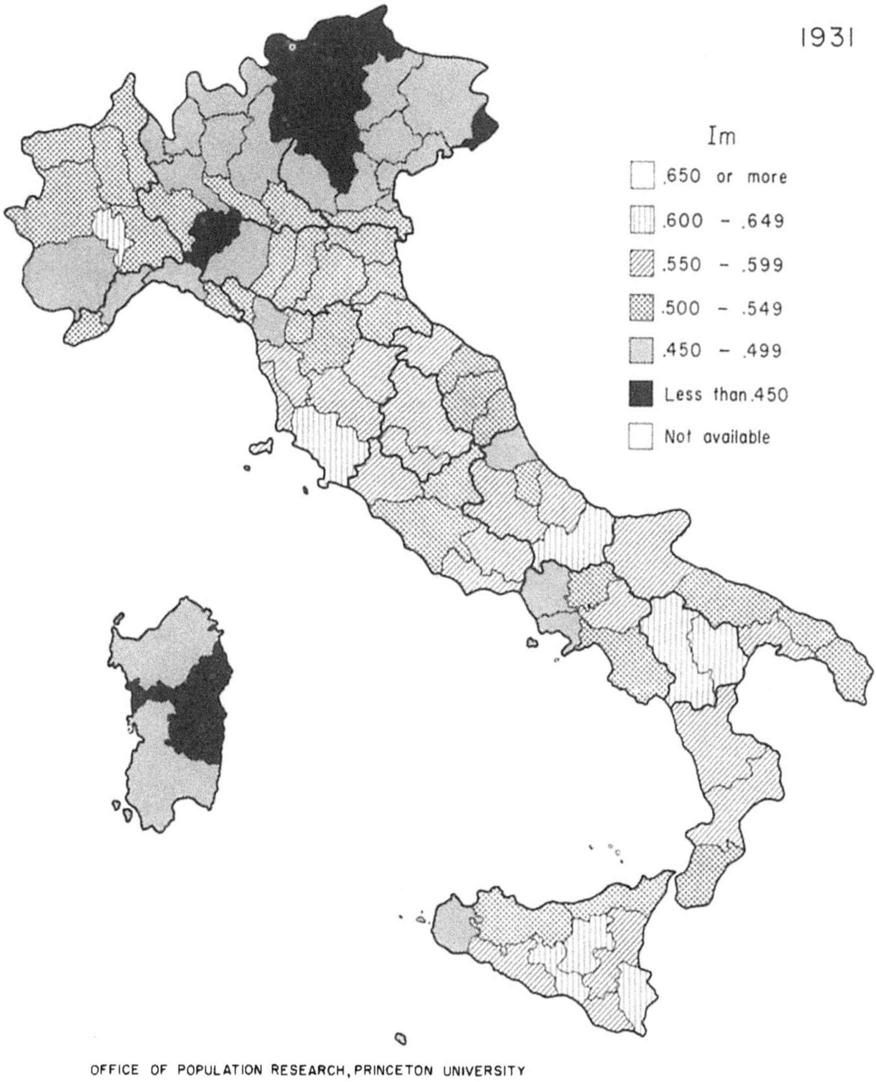

Map 4.20 Proportion Married (I_m), by Province: 1931

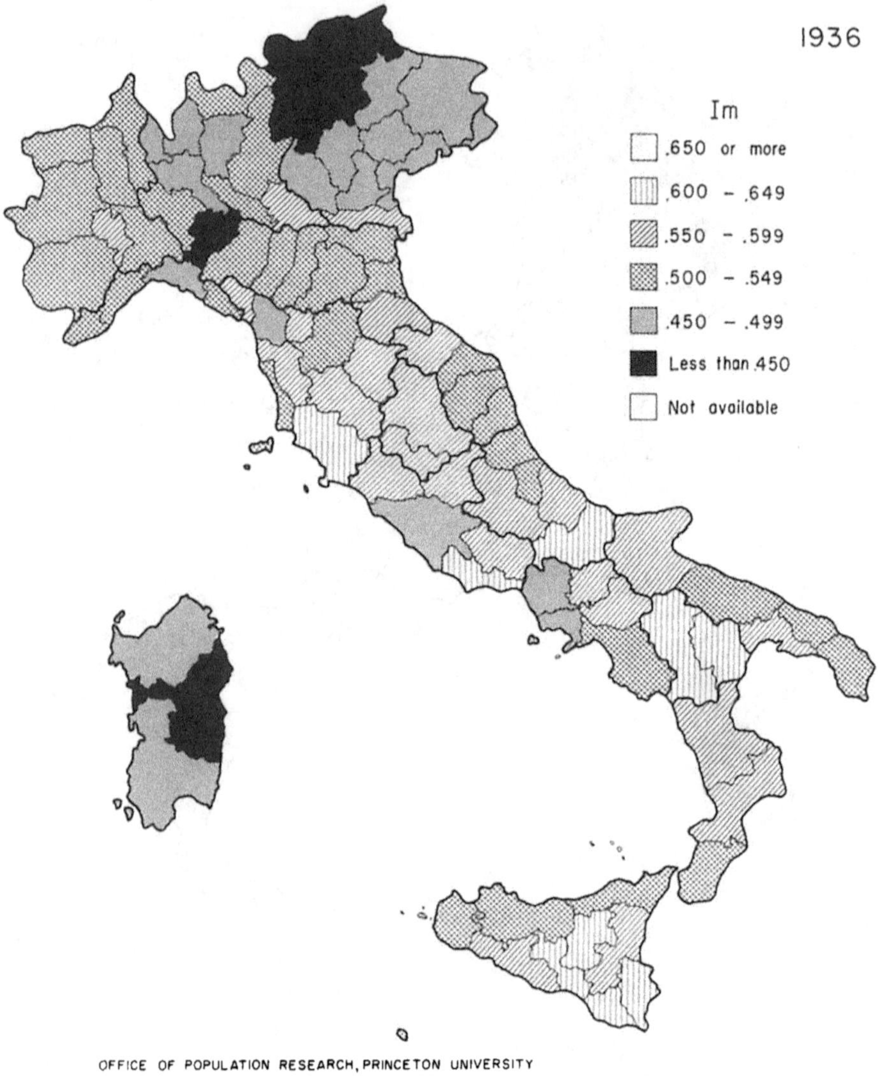

Map 4.21 Proportion Married (I_m), by Province: 1936

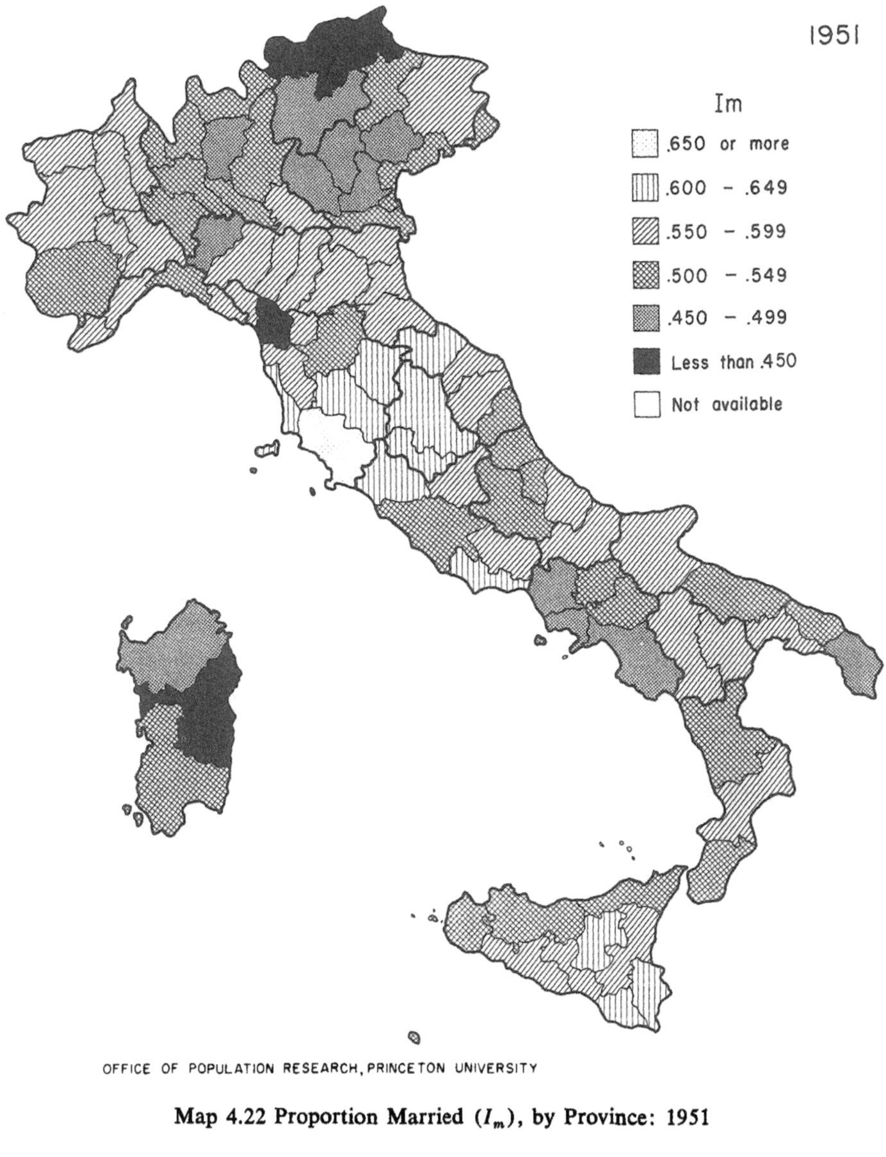

Map 4.22 Proportion Married (I_m), by Province: 1951

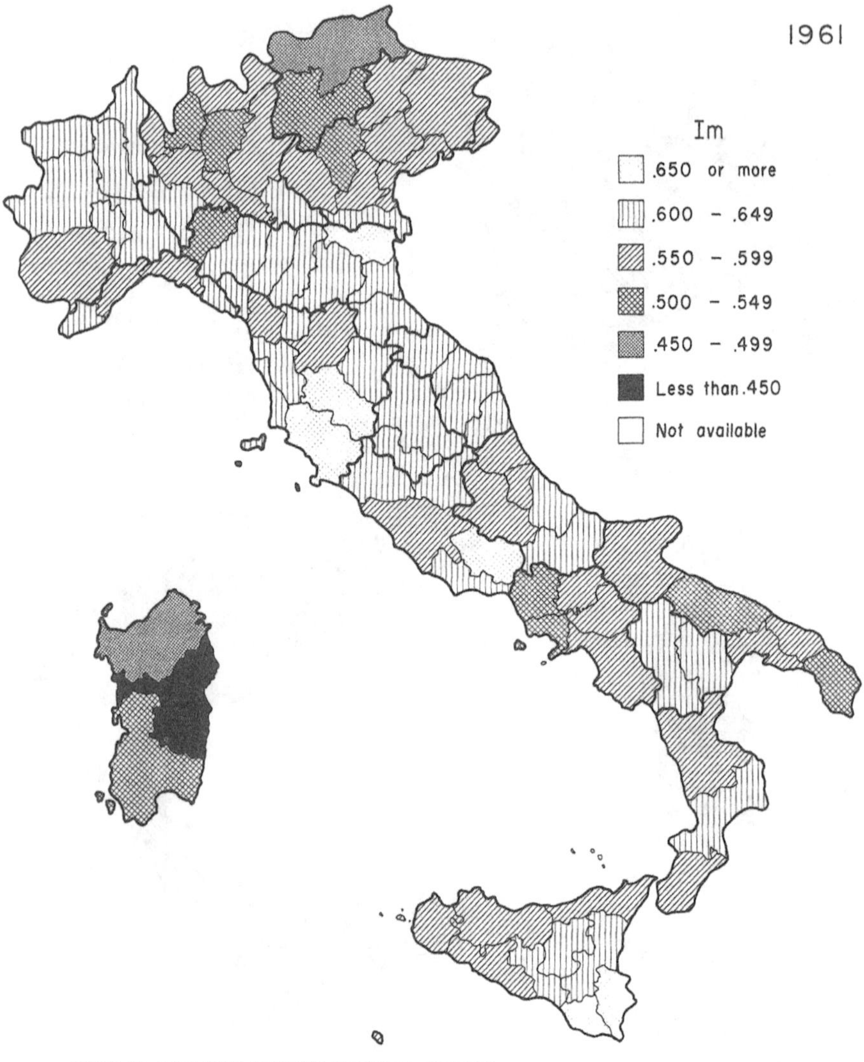

Map 4.23 Proportion Married (I_m), by Province: 1961

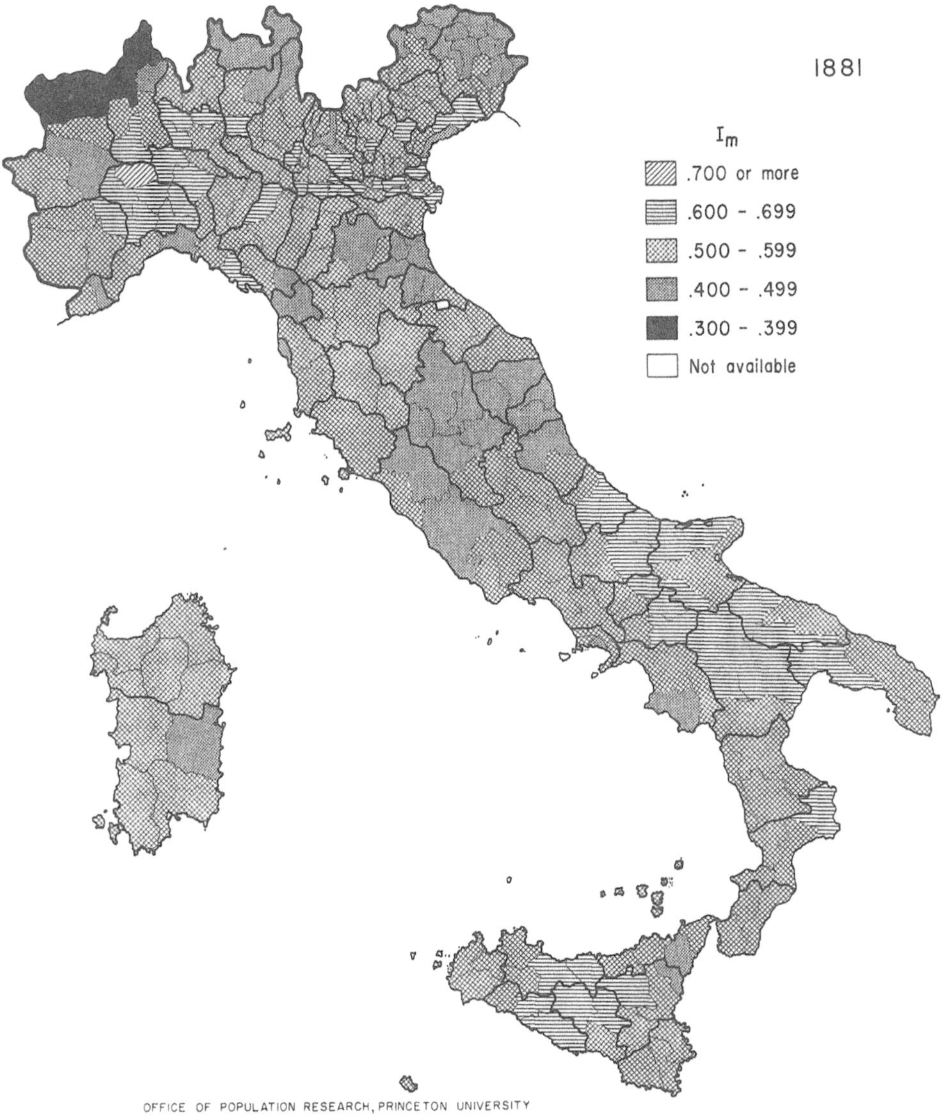

Map 4.24 Proportion Married (I_m), by Circondario: 1881

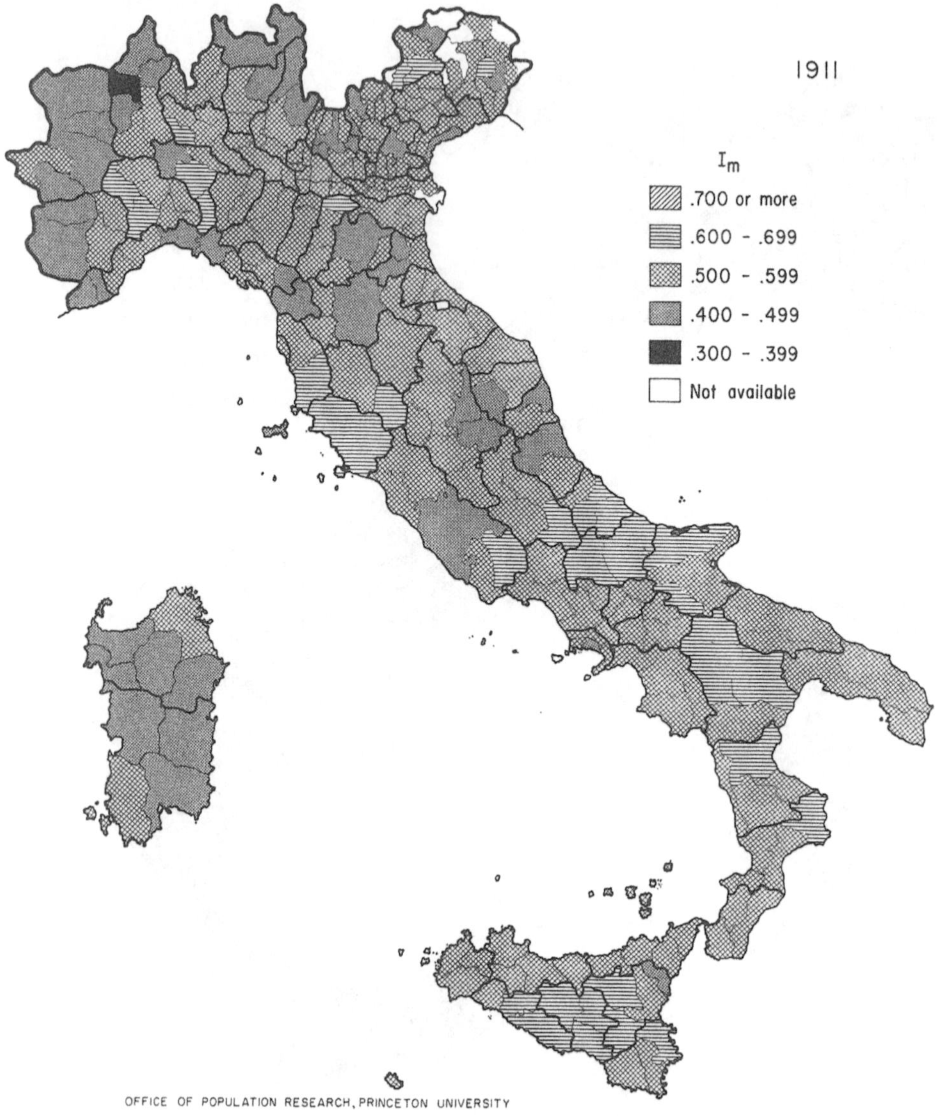

Map 4.25 Proportion Married (I_m), by Circondario: 1911

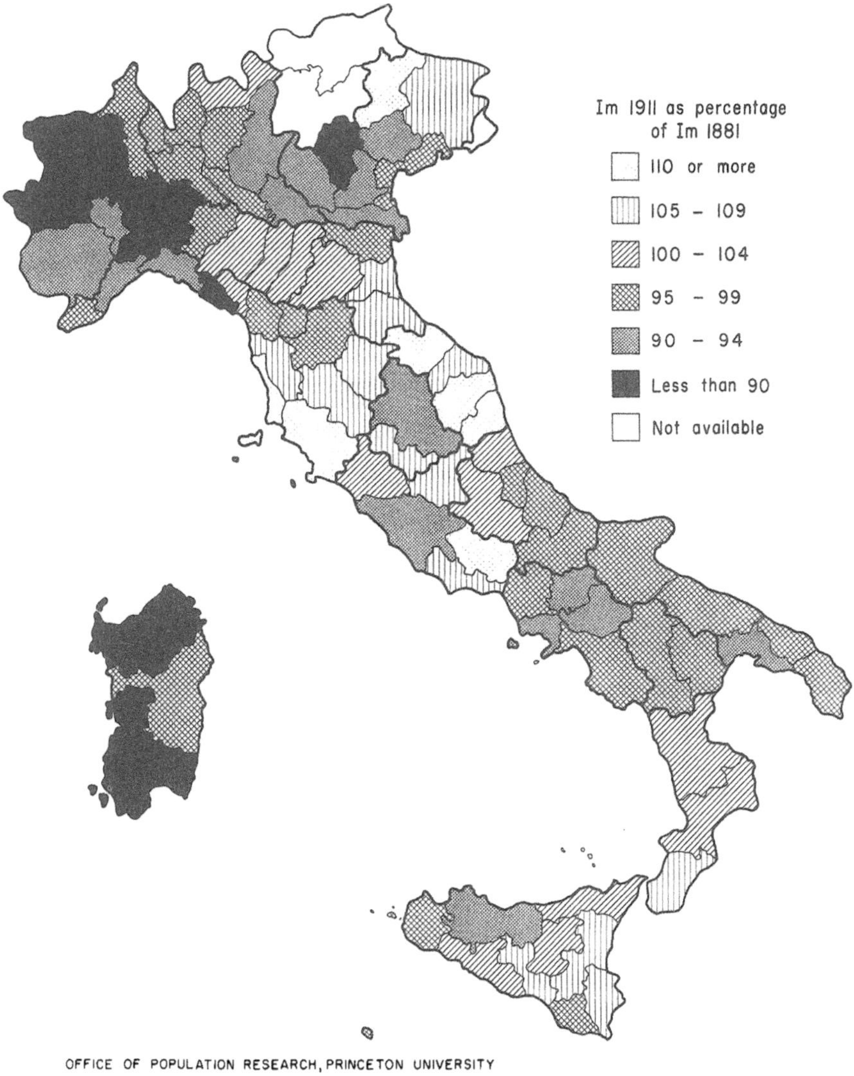

Map 4.26 Change in Proportion Married (I_m), by Province: 1911 as Percentage of 1881

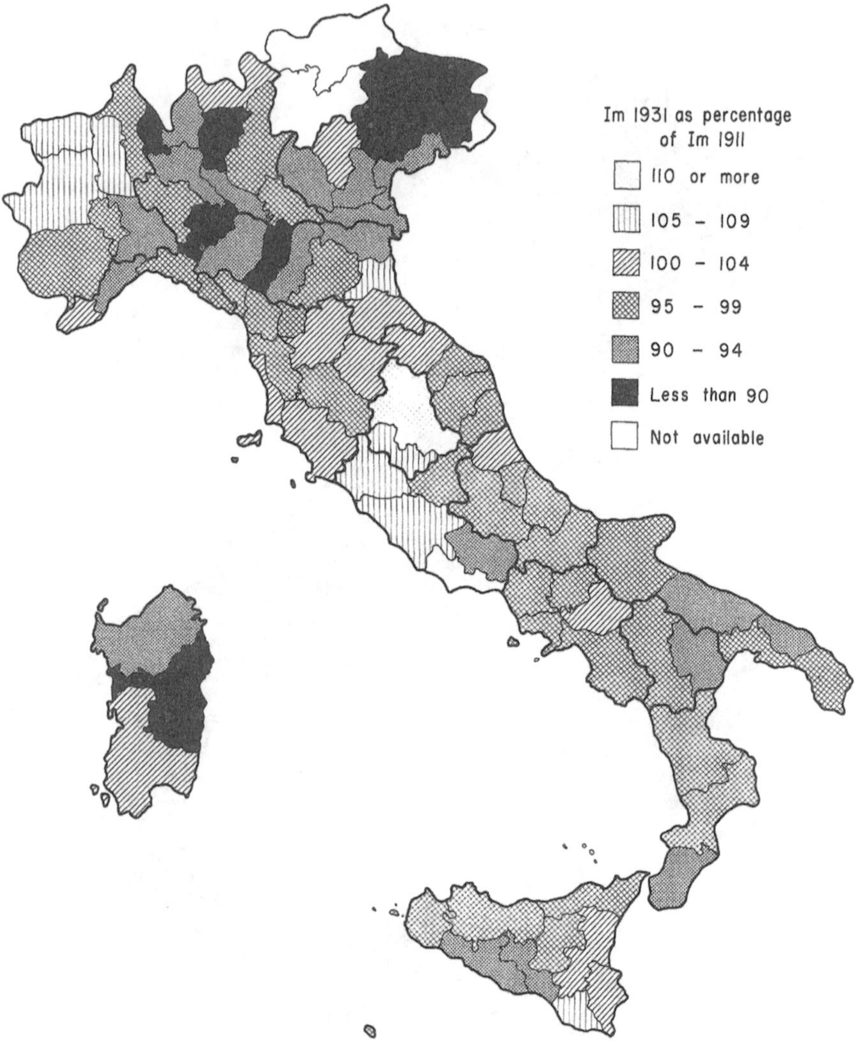

OFFICE OF POPULATION RESEARCH, PRINCETON UNIVERSITY

Map 4.27 Change in Proportion Married (I_m), by Province: 1931 as Percentage of 1911

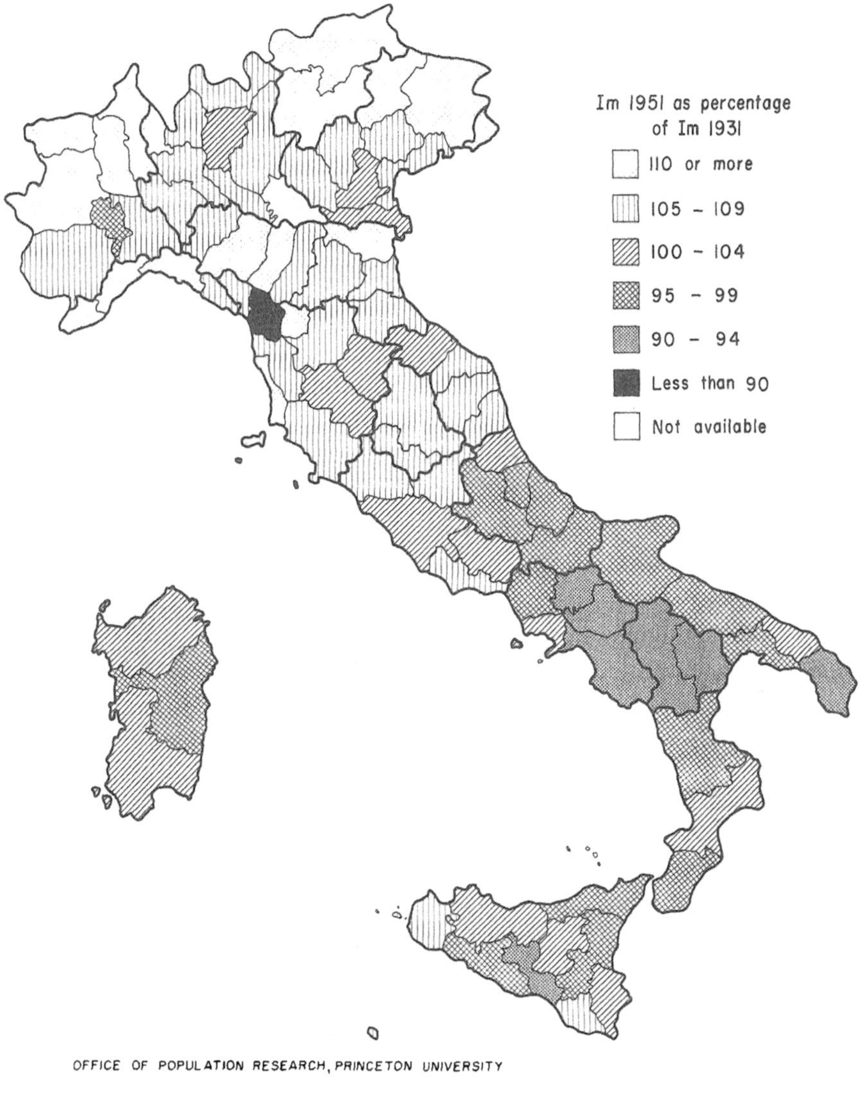

Map 4.28 Change in Proportion Married (I_m), by Province: 1951 as Percentage of 1931

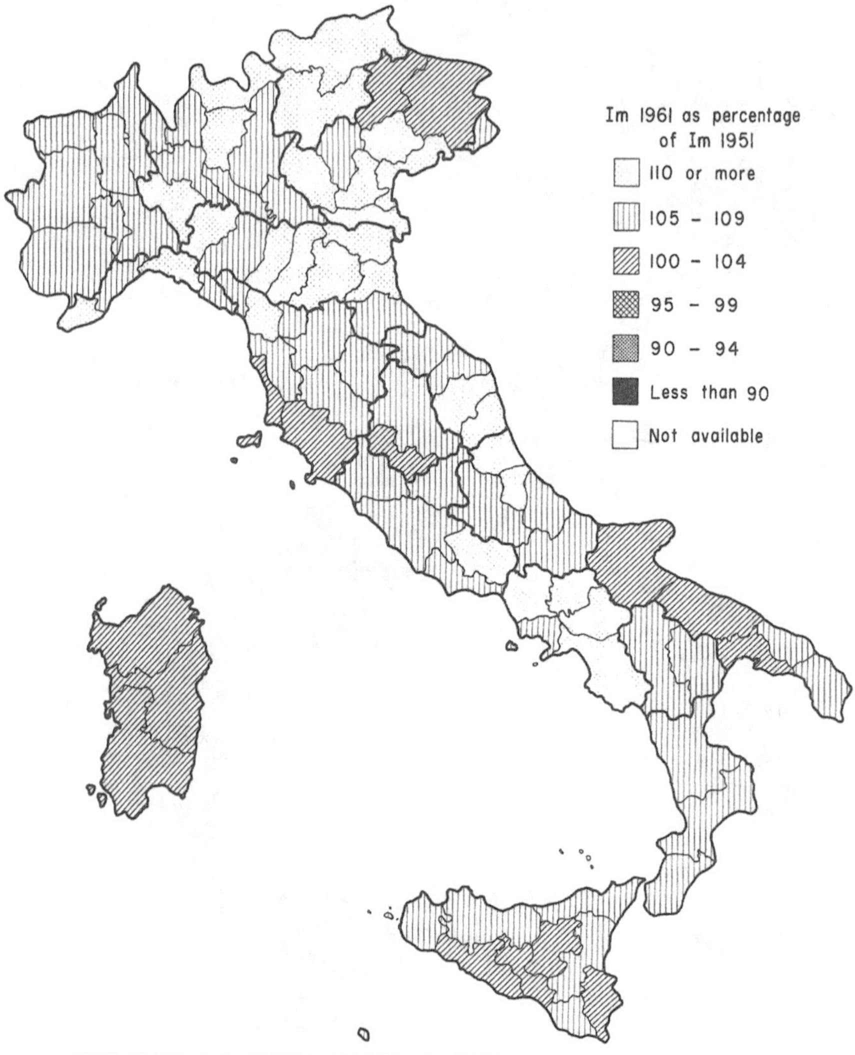

Map 4.29 Change in Proportion Married (I_m), by Province: 1961 as Percentage of 1951

From 1931 to 1951, two distinctive patterns of change in I_m are evident: a substantial increase occurred in the North and the Center (with the sole exception of the province of Latina), and a further substantial decrease in the continental South.

During the last decade (1951 to 1961) I_m increased in all provinces, without exception. In 28 provinces, of which 18 are in the North, the increase exceeded 10 percent.

In Chapter 5, the association between the decline of I_g and the increase in I_m—already noted in examining urban-rural differentials—will be measured and interpreted in the light of multivariate analysis. We may here anticipate that the inverse association is generally maintained even when other variables are introduced, supporting the theory that Malthusian control of fertility through the reduction of nuptiality is often released when neo-Malthusian forms of control are introduced.

4.4 *Variability and Variation of Fertility*

4.4.1. The analysis of variability and variation of legitimate fertility and, to a lesser extent, of nuptiality may help to summarize some of the rather impressionistic findings of the preceding paragraphs.

In Table 4.4 we have reported the distribution of the provinces according to the level of I_g, 1861 to 1961. Until 1881, about two-thirds of the provinces had an I_g between .600 and .700; the mean and the median values fell from .678–.677 in 1861 to .649–.646 in 1871 and .643–.648 in 1881. A legitimate fertility around two-thirds of the fertility of the Hutterite women is not only the average, but also the normal or typical value of legitimate fertility in pre-Malthusian times. In 1911 less than one-half of the provinces were in the .600–.700 range, and the distribution of the provinces, from 1911 on, shifted toward lower values of I_g, with increasing variability. In 1951, provinces with premodern fertility (I_g above .600) coexisted with provinces where the average couple gave birth to 1.6 children or less (I_g below .200).

Table 4.5 shows the distribution of the circondari according to the level of I_g in different broad geographic areas, 1881 and 1911. The circondari having levels of legitimate fertility below the typical premodern level increased in the Islands, remained unchanged in the continental South, and decreased in the Northeast. In the Center and Northwest—but not in the Islands—the fall of fertility was accompanied by an increase in dispersion.

Finally, Table 4.6 gives the distribution (within the same geographic areas) of the 795 agrarian zones according to their general fertility in 1936. In the Northwest, Northeast, and Center, areas where fertility is in full transition, the entire range of fertility values is represented. In the South and in the Islands the distribution shows not only higher fertility, but also much lower dispersion, which, generally speaking, tends to be a function of the rapidity of the transition.

4.4.2. The fertility decline began, for the Italian population as a whole, in the early 1890s. Although marital fertility had already declined in a number of provinces, the extent of the decrease did not affect the general national level. As an obvious consequence of differential territorial trends, provincial variability of legitimate fertility greatly increased after the beginning of the century. In Table 4.7 values of the standard deviation (σ) and of the coefficient of variability (defined as standard deviation divided by the mean value multiplied by 100) of provincial I_g are shown from 1861 to 1961, for the North and Center, the South and Islands, and all Italy. For Italy, relative provincial dispersion is between 6 and 8 percent of the mean value from 1861 to 1881, testifying to the homogeneity of behavior of regional populations before that date. During this century, variability rapidly increased from about one-seventh in 1911 to one-fourth in 1931 and one-third in 1951. In the last 10 years, however, variability decreased because of the recovery of fertility in the North and Center and the further decline in the South. On the other hand, increasing dispersion was a consequence of differentiation of the demographic behavior of the various subpopulations, and of the loss of demographic homogeneity based upon a pattern of relatively high premodern fertility.

The trend of relative variability in the South compared to the rest of the country is especially interesting. In the South, relative dispersion remained between 5 and 8 percent from 1861 to 1911, increased slightly to 10 and 11 percent in 1931 and 1936, and then increased to 16 and 17 percent in 1951 and 1961. The trend in the North and Center is quite different: relative dispersion, very low from 1861 to 1881 at 6 to 8 percent, increased rapidly to 17 percent in 1911 and 27 percent in 1936 and 1951; it fell in the last two decades to 21 percent. This means that even for approximately equal levels of average fertility, relative dispersion of legitimate fertility in the South was much lower than in the rest of the country. This happens because in the areas with an early decline in fertility, neo-Malthusian attitudes had spread at an uneven pace

TABLE 4.4

DISTRIBUTION OF PROVINCES BY LEVEL OF MARITAL FERTILITY (I_g): 1861 TO 1961

Level of I_g	1861	1871	1881	1911	1931	1936	1951	1961
	Actual number of provinces							
Less than .200	--	--	--	--	--	--	10	2
.200 - .300	--	--	--	--	8	18	30	43
.300 - .400	--	--	--	1	17	17	23	23
.400 - .500	--	--	--	8	23	22	20	20
.500 - .600	2	10	12	24	23	23	7	4
.600 - .700	39	47	62	40	17	10	2	--
More than .700	18	12	13	14	1	--	--	--
Total	59	69	87	87	89	90	92	92
Median	.678	.649	.643	.630	.478	.432	.337	.315
Mean	.677	.646	.648	.616	.471	.434	.344	.338
	Percentage distribution of provinces							
Less than .200	--	--	--	--	--	--	10.9	2.2
.200 - .300	--	--	--	--	9.00	20.0	32.6	46.7
.300 - .400	--	--	--	1.1	19.10	18.9	25.0	25.0
.400 - .500	--	--	--	9.2	25.84	24.4	21.7	21.7
.500 - .600	3.4	14.5	13.8	27.6	25.84	25.6	7.6	4.4
.600 - .700	66.1	68.1	71.3	46.0	19.10	11.1	2.2	--
More than .700	30.5	17.4	14.9	16.1	1.12	--	--	--
Total	100.0	100.0	100.0	100.0	100.0	100.0	100.0	100.0

because of deep economic and social differences among the various sectors of the population. The greater acceptance of new attitudes in the more educated, urbanized, and affluent classes caused increasing differential fertility between urban and rural populations, and between provinces in a given region. On the other hand, in the South, where the population is perhaps more homogeneous in its socioeconomic characteristics, and certainly culturally less differentiated, acceptance of neo-Malthusian attitudes was relatively slow and late, and did not generate pronounced fertility differentials.

4.4.3. Analysis of variance is a useful way of examining the sources of variation in the provincial levels of marital fertility (I_g). We may assume that provincial fertility is affected by patterns of behavior shared by the regions, as well as by peculiar factors—known and unknown—characterizing the provincial population. The total variance of I_g by province can be subdivided into two components: the mean square variance "between," and the mean square variance "within," regions. If it is assumed that the fertility level of each province is determined only by

TABLE 4.5

DISTRIBUTION OF CIRCONDARI BY LEVEL OF MARITAL FERTILITY (I_g), BY GEOGRAPHICAL AREA: 1881 AND 1911

	Actual number of circondari											
	1881						1911					
Level of I_g	North-west	North-east	Center	South	Islands	Italy	North-west	North-east	Center	South	Islands	Italy
Less than .400	--	--	--	--	--	--	3	--	--	--	--	3
.400 - .500	--	1	--	--	--	1	15	1	4	--	--	20
.500 - .600	20	26	11	16	--	73	20	5	15	14	10	64
.600 - .700	28	50	22	28	23	151	13	28	14	20	19	104
More than .700	15	22	1	12	10	60	12	56	1	12	4	85
Total	63	98	34	56	33	285	63	90	34	56	33	276
	Percentage distribution of circondari											
Less than .400	--	--	--	--	--	--	4.8	--	--	--	--	1.1
.400 - .500	--	1.0	--	--	--	0.4	23.8	1.1	11.8	--	--	7.3
.500 - .600	31.7	26.5	32.4	28.6	--	25.6	31.7	5.6	44.1	25.0	30.3	23.2
.600 - .700	44.5	51.0	64.7	50.0	69.7	53.0	20.6	31.1	41.2	53.6	57.6	37.6
More than .700	23.8	22.5	2.9	21.4	30.3	21.0	19.1	62.2	2.9	21.4	12.1	30.8
Total	100.0	100.0	100.0	100.0	100.0	100.0	100.0	100.0	100.0	100.0	100.0	100.0

TABLE 4.6

DISTRIBUTION OF AGRARIAN DISTRICTS BY LEVEL OF GENERAL FERTILITY RATE, BY GEOGRAPHICAL AREA: 1935-1937

General fertility rate	Northwest	Northeast	Center	South	Islands	Italy
	Actual number of districts					
Less than 60	49	4	2	--	--	55
60 - 80	58	26	37	--	--	121
80 - 100	39	56	46	5	7	153
100 - 120	20	36	42	29	27	154
120 - 140	11	22	18	76	29	156
140 - 160	6	6	7	72	21	112
More than 160	2	1	2	30	9	44
Total	185	151	154	212	93	795
	Percentage distribution of districts					
Less than 60	26.5	2.6	1.3	--	--	6.9
60 - 80	31.4	17.2	24.0	--	--	15.2
80 - 100	21.1	37.1	29.9	2.4	7.5	19.2
100 - 120	10.8	23.8	27.3	13.7	29.0	19.4
120 - 140	5.9	14.6	11.7	35.8	31.2	19.6
140 - 160	3.2	4.0	4.5	34.0	22.6	14.1
More than 160	1.1	0.7	1.3	14.1	9.7	5.6
Total	100.0	100.0	100.0	100.0	100.0	100.0

NOTE: The general fertility rate refers to live births per 1,000 women aged 15-44.

the peculiarities of its own social and economic structure and is independent of the fact that it belongs to one or another region, "between" and "within" region mean square variances may be considered like two measures of the same universe, and, therefore, after allowance has been made for the number of degrees of freedom, should not show significant differences. The hypothesis can be tested by means of the *F* test, *F* being the ratio of the "between" to the "within" mean square variance. The larger the departure of *F* from unity, the smaller the probability that the two mean square variances can be thought of as measures of the same universe.

The computations shown in Tables 4.8 and 4.9 lead to the following conclusions. The *F* test shows that the null hypothesis (no significant difference between the two estimates of variance) becomes increasingly improbable with the passage of time, and must always be rejected at a .01 percent probability level, with the only exception being 1871. The values of *F* sharply increase during the period, growing from a minimum of 1.9 in 1871 to a minimum of 33.5 in 1961. In other terms, from 1861

TABLE 4.7

TERRITORIAL VARIABILITY IN MARITAL FERTILITY (I_g), BY PROVINCES IN NORTH AND CENTER, SOUTH, AND ALL ITALY: 1861 TO 1961

Area	Measure	1861	1871	1881	1911	1931	1936	1951	1961
North and Center	Number	34	44	53	53	60	61	58	58
	Mean	.676	.642	.635	.609	.415	.377	.276	.270
	Standard deviation	.046	.051	.053	.101	.101	.102	.075	.058
	Coefficient of variation	6.7	8.0	8.3	16.7	24.3	27.0	27.2	21.5
South	Number	25	25	34	34	32	33	34	34
	Mean	.687	.669	.666	.641	.593	.555	.450	.422
	Standard deviation	.036	.055	.041	.053	.064	.061	.072	.072
	Coefficient of variation	5.3	8.2	6.2	8.3	10.7	10.9	16.0	17.2
Italy	Number	59	69	87	87	92	94	92	92
	Mean	.680	.652	.647	.622	.477	.439	.340	.326
	Standard deviation	.042	.054	.051	.087	.123	.124	.112	.097
	Coefficient of variation	6.2	8.3	7.9	14.0	25.8	28.1	32.9	29.8

TABLE 4.8

ANALYSIS OF VARIANCE IN MARITAL FERTILITY (I_g) BETWEEN REGIONS AND PROVINCES: 1861 TO 1961

Analysis	Measure	1861	1871	1881	1911	1931	1936	1951	1961
Between regions	Sum of squares	53,112.65	71,498.28	103,213.72	408,220.18	1,043,060.31	1,083,479.37	993,768.67	771,060.45
	Degrees of freedom	13	15	15	15	17	17	17	17
	Mean square variance	4,085.59	4,766.55	6,880.91	27,214.68	61,356.49	63,734.08	58,456.98	45,356.50
Within region	Sum of squares	52,607.52	131,922.79	124,119.89	256,202.05	355,159.30	350,472.50	993,768.67	771,060.45
	Degrees of freedom	45	53	71	71	74	76	74	74
	Mean square variance	1,169.06	2,489.11	1,748.17	3,608.48	4,799.45	4,611.48	2,292.95	1,355.06
Total variation	Sum of squares	105,720.17	203,421.07	227,333.61	664,422.23	1,398,219.61	1,433,951.87	1,163,447.18	871,334.55
	Degrees of freedom	58	68	86	86	91	93	91	91
	F	3.495	1.914	3.936	7.541	12.784	13.821	25.494	33.472

NOTE: F significant at .01 level except for 1871, when it is significant at the .1 level.

through 1881, only one-third to one-half of the total variation among provinces arose from differences among regions, but from 1911 on "between" region variation accounted for over two-thirds of the total. Of course, the changing interrelations of "between" and "within" region variation are strictly connected with the diverging patterns of provincial (and regional) dispersion examined earlier.

TABLE 4.9

ANALYSIS OF VARIANCE IN MARITAL FERTILITY (I_g) BETWEEN REGIONS AND CIRCONDARI: 1881 AND 1911

Analysis	Measure	1881	1911
Between regions	Sum of squares	237,942.99	1,481,988.16
	Degrees of freedom	15	15
	Mean square variance	15,862.87	--
Within region	Sum of squares	937,784.93	1,399,829.88
	Degrees of freedom	268	260
	Mean square variance	3,499.20	--
Total variation	Sum of squares	1,175,727.91	2,881,818.04
	Degrees of freedom	283	275
	F	2.593	18,351

NOTE: F significant at .01 level.

4.5 *Conclusion*

The geographic analysis of fertility trends is insufficient, by itself, to provide a satisfactory interpretation of the factors of territorial trends and differentials. Data by region, province, or circondario are poor substitutes for individual data, since each area contains—although in different degrees—those many characteristics that are believed to have an impact on the behavior of the population. It is almost impossible to find a completely rural province or circondario, whose fertility could be usefully compared with that of another province or circondario completely urban. There is no province or circondario whose population is completely literate or illiterate.

We may also say that, although regions differ widely as far as their social structure and culture are concerned, there are no well-defined qualitative factors separating one region from the other. The identity of the various regions is evident enough, but it relies on the varying combinations of many factors and never on one alone. Ethnic origin, language, and religion do not provide any clear-cut dividing line between one group and another, as happens in many populations of Europe. The analysis of variance, however, has shown that regions have had a significant impact over the level of provincial fertility since the earliest times.

The geographic analysis stresses once again the distinctive patterns of fertility decline in the South. The decline is late and slow, and territorial variability is relatively unimportant. The lower level of social and economic achievement is not, however, the only distinctive pattern of the South. Regions of this area formed a state prior to unification, and their structure was at least partly shaped by common political and administrative ties. Dialects spoken in the South may be grouped in the same family, and the linguistic border with the rest of Italy closely follows the administrative boundaries. The cultural unity of the South therefore stands out clearly, but, as we will see in the next chapter, it cannot be defined by the classic socioeconomic indicators.

The gradual erosion of high fertility in the North and Center of the country seems to follow some of the typical patterns of diffusion. The diffusion of birth control starts from the cities and extends to the rural areas, and proceeds along a Northwest-Northeast and a Northwest-South direction.

Natural obstacles do, sometimes, delay the decline. But a number of instances exist in which barely accessible areas showed an earlier decline than areas with easy communications and high mobility. It is very difficult to give an exact definition of the "natural obstacle," whose characteristics vary from one zone to another with the passing of time and with the progress of techniques in the field of communications.

Consideration of geographic location is only one of many ways of examining the environment and the culture of each population. We are sure that the illustration of territorial trends and differentials attempted in this chapter has added insight to our knowledge. The same can be said of the analysis of variability and of variation. We are also convinced, however, that it would be unwise to lean upon this descriptive outline for drawing hypotheses as to the factors of fertility decline without, or before, giving consideration to the quantitative analysis of the social or economic factors that, among the many others influencing fertility, can be measured.

CHAPTER 5: Factors Involved in Italy's Fertility Decline

5.1 *Problems of Method*

In our monograph on Portugal, we encountered the many difficulties social scientists face in dealing with the determinants of a complex phenomenon such as the secular decline of fertility.[1] The difficulties are certainly not less in Italy, where the object of the analysis is the fall of fertility in the 90 or so provinces of the country, or, in other words, the differential experience of the populations of the various provinces in exercising control of their marital fertility. The questions to be answered are essentially two. The first asks why provincial populations show different levels of fertility at certain dates and what factors may account for the differences in the level of marital fertility at these dates. The second question concerns the differential rapidity of the decline: why has fertility, from one date to the other, declined more rapidly in some provinces and less rapidly, or not at all, or even increased, in others? What are the factors, of a social or economic nature, whose action has presumably affected differential trends of fertility?

There are essentially three limitations. First, we deal with aggregate data. The varying unit, in the study of the interrelationships between fertility and one or more quantitative, generally socioeconomic, variables, is the population of a given area, instead of the individual couple. Therefore the independent variables that demographers are forced to correlate with fertility are the social, economic, and educational characteristics of the population of each area, which have to be measured through the use of percentages, ratios, or rates. It is tempting, although not logically justifiable, to extend to individuals the relationships found between the "average" characteristics of each area and the corresponding level of fertility. For example, if the level of fertility in each area is positively correlated with the average level of illiteracy of the population, we are led to extend this correlation to individuals and assume that the higher the level of fertility, the lower the level of education, although there are many examples that show the fallacy of such analogical procedure.

The second grave, although unavoidable, limitation is that many fac-

[1] Livi-Bacci, *A Century of Portuguese Fertility*, p. 101.

tors are likely to be involved in a fertility decline—social, economic, cultural, religious, psychological, physiological, biological, etc.—but only a few have been recorded in the available statistics. More precisely, the degree of control over fertility is a matter of a complex personal choice, involving the whole personality of the individual and his manifold relationships with his spouse, his relatives, and his society. The available indicators can at best describe some aspects of the living conditions of the population as a whole, conditions that presumably influence to some degree the behavior of the individuals. The factual indicators employed in the statistical analysis are far from the complex behavior that we want to explain.

But, even assuming that an adequate battery of indicators are available, there is a third limitation. It is likely, in fact, that the impact of each factor affecting fertility will change according to the stage of demographic development. For example, education may play a very important role in determining the level of fertility at the beginning of the process of fertility decline because it facilitates the diffusion of birth-control knowledge; but education may be irrelevant when fertility has already reached a moderate level, at which time other factors previously of little consequence may take on importance. This fact may obscure the meaning of territorial, cross-sectional correlation analysis, and lead to mistaken conclusions.

In spite of the three limitations just mentioned, the method of analogy is often the only one open to demographers when they study historically the interrelations linking fertility to other variables; in spite of its shortcomings, this is the method we will follow in this chapter. Multiple regression, multiple and partial correlation, and the analysis of covariance are the statistical tools employed for determining the impact of the various factors on provincial fertility differentials and trends.

5.2 *Choice of the Variables*

5.2.1. As was said before, the limitations of the available data restrict the range of the indicators that may be employed in cross-sectional analysis. But before even choosing indicators, we must select the dates and the periods on which to base our study. The censuses prior to 1881 offer little choice of indicators, not to mention their often suspect reliability. Moreover, 1881 is the first census for which we were able to compute I_g in the provinces according to their present boundaries to ensure comparability with later censuses. Finally, in 1881 birth control was only in its initial stage of diffusion in a score of provinces, and the fertility levels of the Italian population were still high and premodern. In addition to 1881, we have also selected 1911, 1931, 1951, and 1961. In 1911, fertility had already dropped considerably in many areas of the North and the Center; the decline was already well under way. It must be borne in mind that 1911 levels of marital fertility were partly distorted by very heavy out-migration, particularly from the Southern regions. In 1931, some regions of the North and of the Center had fallen below replacement; yet in some areas of the South and of the Islands premodern levels of marital fertility still prevailed. In 1951 fertility had reached its historical minimum for the nation as a whole, and the decline was well on its way in the South. In 1961, fertility had recovered in many areas of the North and of the Center, while the decline continued in the South. The five dates coincide with significant periods in the history of Italian fertility: 1881 and 1951 correspond with the beginning and the end of the transition; 1911 and 1931 are two intermediate phases of the decline before and after the great shock of World War I; 1961 opens a new phase in the equalization of territorial fertility levels.

The dependent variable, I_g, has been correlated with levels of independent variables at each of five selected dates. This is the first step of the cross-sectional analysis, or the "static" step. In the second step, "dynamic" relationships have been tested by correlating changes in I_g (1881–1911, 1911–1931, 1931–1951, and 1951–1961) with changes in the various indicators used in the analysis.

5.2.2. Six indicators, comparable through time and available at the five dates selected, are the independent variables:

(1) *Proportion married* (I_m). The underlying hypothesis is that, at least in the initial phase of the decline, the lower is I_m, the higher is I_g. One reason to expect a negative correlation is that when a certain family size is envisaged, late marriage (generally corresponding to a low I_m) requires a higher "utilization" within marriage of the fecundity of the woman at the later age of child-bearing, say between 30 and 45 years. On the other hand, early marriage (high I_m), calls for a lower utilization of fecundity during married life, if the same family size is to be attained. In other words, control of marriage may act as a substitute for fertility control. This hypothesis is very controversial; van de

Walle[2] has shown with reference to Belgium and The Netherlands that the age at first marriage started to decline (and I_m to increase) before the onset of fertility decline. However, other factors, mainly associated with the selectivity of marriage, point to negative correlation between the propensity to marriage and marital fertility.

(2) *Infant mortality* (deaths under age 1 per 1,000 live births). A positive correlation is expected with I_g. The death of a newborn child requires replacement if a given family size is to be achieved. A reduction of infant mortality increases the number of surviving children and creates pressure for control.

(3) *Ruralization* (percentage of the labor force engaged in agriculture) and

(4) *Industrialization* (percentage of the labor force engaged in industry). We assume that ruralization is associated with a lower standard of living, and also with a traditional and conservative value-system, and hence, with higher fertility. Industrialization is, on the contrary, seen as a symptom of dynamism and of social change, and thus we expect it to lead to a decline in fertility.

(5) *Male illiteracy* (percentage of illiterates, unable to read or write, among males aged 20 to 39 years). The hypothesis of a direct relationship with fertility is obvious. Illiteracy is also a good indicator of socioeconomic status, since it is an essentially permanent characteristic of the individual, at least after a certain age, unlike income, profession, or place of residence, which may change through a person's lifetime.

(6) *Urbanization* (percentage of the population living in the capital city of each province). An inverse correlation with fertility is expected. Our definition of the urban population is only a very imperfect approximation, since we have considered as "urban" only the population living in the comune of the capital city of each province (the province has the same name as the capital city). To this definition apply most of the restrictive considerations examined in Chapter 3.

In Table 5.1 we have summarized the indicators used in the analysis, the method of their computation, and the expected relationship with marital fertility.

[2] E. van de Walle, *Marriage and Marital Fertility*, *Daedalus*, Spring 1969 (issue dedicated to *Historical Population Studies*), p. 497.

TABLE 5.1

SOCIO-ECONOMIC VARIABLES USED IN CORRELATION AND COVARIANCE ANALYSIS

Variable	Method of computation	Expected relationship with I_g
Marital fertility (I_g)	See paragraph 2.2.1.	--
Proportion married (I_m)	See paragraph 2.2.1.	Negative
Infant mortality	Deaths under one year of age per 1000 live births	Positive
Ruralization	Percentage of the labor force engaged in agriculture	Positive
Industrialization	Percentage of the labor force engaged in industry	Negative
Male illiteracy	Percentage of illiterate males 20-39 over total number of males 20-39	Positive
Urbanization	Percentage of the provincial population in the province's capital city	Negative

5.2.3. Before examining the results of the correlation analysis, it is interesting to have an idea of the levels and trends of the different indicators. Limitations of space make it impossible to report all the indicators for the more than 90 provinces. We have reported, in Table 5.2, only the mean provincial value of each indicator, for the North and the Center, the South and the Islands, and Italy as a whole.

This is not the place for speculation and interpretation of social, economic, and cultural differentiation of the two areas throughout the 80-year period considered. This is the complex job of sociologists and historians, and we will leave the task to them. It is helpful to note a few facts, however. Differences between the two areas are not very evident in 1881, but they rapidly increase in 1911 and after. According to the census data, the South and the Islands in 1881 had a higher industrialization and a lower ruralization than the North and Center; however, industrialization in the North and Center increased drastically in 1911, and decreased slightly in the South and the Islands. This fact is partly due to a genuine crisis in the industrial sector of the South, which had grown under the protective policy of the Regno delle Due Sicilie before unification; thereafter the South fell behind the North. In addition the 1881 census probably overestimated the industrial labor force by in-

TABLE 5.2

MEAN VALUE AND STANDARD DEVIATION OF SELECTED SOCIO-ECONOMIC VARIABLES, NORTH AND CENTER, SOUTH AND ISLANDS, AND ALL ITALY: 1881 TO 1961

		Mean value			Standard deviation		
Variable	Date	North and Center	South and Islands	All Italy	North and Center	South and Islands	All Italy
Marital fertility (I_g)	1881	634.9	666.3	647.1	53.4	42.1	51.4
	1911	609.3	641.1	621.7	102.5	54.2	87.9
	1931	415.1	592.9	476.9	101.6	64.6	124.0
	1951	275.9	450.4	340.4	75.8	73.0	112.7
	1961	270.9	422.0	327.4	59.3	73.9	98.0
Proportion married (I_m)	1881	536.3	569.1	549.1	46.2	40.4	46.7
	1911	529.3	563.2	542.6	38.4	46.7	44.8
	1931	504.4	546.8	519.1	46.2	46.3	50.2
	1951	550.9	541.5	547.5	48.4	44.0	46.8
	1961	597.0	580.1	590.7	55.0	48.3	53.0
Infant mortality	1881	223.5	234.3	227.4	34.9	32.9	34.4
	1911	143.4	155.0	147.9	23.5	24.9	24.6
	1931	94.3	134.8	108.4	25.1	25.3	31.7
	1951	48.3	82.8	61.1	9.6	15.7	20.7
	1961	30.6	48.0	37.1	6.2	8.4	11.0
Ruralization	1881	52.5	46.7	50.3	11.1	10.2	11.1
	1911	56.5	65.0	59.8	14.4	12.8	14.3
	1931	47.8	59.6	51.9	15.9	11.2	15.4
	1951	40.8	57.5	47.0	17.4	14.1	18.1
	1961	27.5	45.2	34.1	13.9	9.8	15.1
Industrialization	1881	20.4	23.7	21.7	6.8	7.5	7.2
	1911	29.9	23.0	27.2	10.8	7.3	10.1
	1931	30.0	21.6	27.1	11.1	5.8	10.4
	1951	33.6	20.8	28.9	12.7	6.0	12.4
	1961	41.8	30.6	37.6	11.4	5.1	11.0
Male illiteracy	1881	39.8	68.3	50.9	14.7	5.2	18.4
	1911	17.5	45.6	28.4	11.2	10.3	17.5
	1931	6.0	29.0	14.0	4.5	8.3	12.6
	1951	2.1	14.8	6.8	1.5	5.2	7.0
	1961	1.2	8.7	4.0	0.6	3.7	4.3
Urbanization	1881	20.7	15.6	18.7	13.8	13.1	13.7
	1911	24.6	19.0	22.4	17.5	16.5	17.3
	1931	28.9	22.1	26.5	18.5	16.2	18.0
	1951	31.7	26.3	29.7	18.7	18.1	18.5
	1961	35.3	29.4	33.1	18.7	18.4	18.7

cluding a large number of women working at home, particularly in the South.[3] The reader should also remember that the values of Table 5.2 are unweighted means of the provincial levels; this tends to penalize the North and the Center, where the large industrial agglomerations of Milano, Torino, and Genova were located.

[3] For an interpretation of historical census statistics on labor force, see O. Vitali, *Aspetti dello sviluppo economico italiano alla luce della ricostruzione della popolazione attiva,* Roma, 1970, pp. 33ff.

The gap in illiteracy between the South and the Islands, and the rest of the country was very conspicuous; the mean provincial proportion was, in 1881, 68 percent against 40 percent. One can, however, easily follow the increasing distance between the two areas during our century. As is proved by illiteracy, the gap existed and was substantial at the end of the last century, although the indicators are not detailed or flexible enough to show it. On the other hand, the take-off of the economy, especially in the North, has made the gap more visible during this century; the South and the Islands lagged behind, tied to their mainly rural economic and cultural life.

One last remark: the variability of the indicators is sensibly lower in the South and the Islands than in the rest of the country, with the sole exception of urbanization. This is shown by the coefficient of variation reported in Table 5.3.

TABLE 5.3

COEFFICIENT OF VARIATION, SELECTED SOCIO-ECONOMIC VARIABLES, NORTH AND CENTER, SOUTH AND ISLANDS: 1911, 1931, AND 1951

Variable	North and Center			South and Islands		
	1911	1931	1951	1911	1931	1951
Infant mortality	16.4	26.6	20.0	16.1	18.8	19.0
Ruralization	25.5	33.3	42.6	19.7	18.8	24.5
Industrialization	36.1	37.0	37.8	31.7	26.9	28.8
Male illiteracy	64.0	75.0	71.4	22.6	28.6	35.1
Urbanization	71.1	64.0	59.0	86.8	73.3	62.6

Note: Coefficient of variation is compiled from data reported in Table 5.2 and is defined as standard deviation divided by mean value and multiplied by 100.

The provinces of the South and of the Islands have a much more homogeneous social and economic structure than the provinces of the rest of the country.

5.3 *Multiple and Partial Correlation Analysis*

5.3.1. In the correlation analysis we have retained the six variables indicated in Section 5.2.2, two regional areas—the North and the Center on one side, the South and the Islands on the other (from now on referred to as North and South)—plus the entire country, and five dates: 1881, 1911, 1931, 1951, and 1961.

Originally, we planned to use other indicators, such as the female participation in the labor force and female illiteracy, the hygienic characteristics of households, the structural characteristics of the families, and the proportion of the population declaring, at the 1911 census, not to be affiliated with the Catholic church. Subsequently, we reduced the variables to six for the following reasons: (1) the variable could not be computed for all five dates; (2) it had a very high correlation with another variable; (3) it had a low correlation with the dependent variables. That the elimination of some variables does not greatly affect the correlation analysis is proved by the fact that the multiple correlation coefficients between the socioeconomic variables and fertility in all Italian provinces falls from .601 to .567 in 1911, when the number of variables is reduced from 10 to 6; from .900 to .842 in 1931 and from .935 to .911 in 1951 (reduction of the variables from 11 to 6).

There are also several reasons for retaining only two major geographic areas instead of a larger number. As mentioned before, the small number of provinces (87 in 1881, 92 in 1961) cannot be subdivided into too many groups without making the whole procedure meaningless (too many variables and too few cases). Also, there is the difficulty of regionalization, given the particular shape and conformation of the country. While the region South (islands included) can be easily identified, having common economic, social, historical, and even linguistic and climatic characteristics, the regionalization of the rest of the country is particularly difficult, and solutions may involve rather arbitrary decisions if an excessive fragmentation is to be avoided (as in our case, given the nature of the basic unit, the province). We have thought it preferable to pool together all provinces of the Center and of the North, which, as seen in Tables 5.2 and 5.3 have a much more variable structure than the provinces of the South, but at least share the common characteristic of being "other than South."

Once the six explanatory variables were chosen, and the two groups of provinces, the "static" and "dynamic" correlation analysis was done for the two territorial subdivisions and for Italy—the "static" by correlating at each date the provincial levels of I_g with the provincial levels of the indicators; the "dynamic" by correlating the percent changes of I_g over each period (1881–1911, 1911–1931, 1931–1951, and 1951–1961) with the corresponding percent changes of the indicators.

5.3.2. Tables 5.4 and 5.6 report the zero-order correlation coefficients for the "static" and "dynamic" analysis, while Tables 5.5 and 5.7 report the corresponding partial and multiple coefficients. We will forget, for the moment, the zero-order coefficients, since we are more interested in interpreting the impact of the various variables on I_g on a multiple basis.

The coefficient of multiple correlation (R) is a measure of the degree of association between marital fertility and the six independent variables simultaneously considered. It tells us, in the static case, how good an estimate of the provincial marital fertility based on the knowledge of the provincial levels of the six indicators would be, or, in other words, to what extent the level of marital fertility depends on the varying socioeconomic conditions of the provincial populations as measured by all six indicators considered together.

The multiple R^2, in the static analysis, is relatively moderate in 1881 and 1911. With the exception of the North in 1881 ($R^2 = .561$), the explained variance is between 22 and 40 percent. The predictive power of the variables is quite modest. Moreover, for the two territorial subdivisions, R^2 is lower in 1911 than in 1881. This fact can be explained, at least partially, by the disturbing action of mass emigration before World War I. The low multiple correlation is partly a consequence of the rather homogeneous distribution of the provinces according to marital fertility. Fertility was still largely uncontrolled and the generally small provincial differentials were largely produced by random and unknown factors. The weakness of the multiple association duly reflects this fact.

After 1911, multiple R^2 increases, reaching a maximum in 1951 for the North and Italy, and in 1961 for the South; around 80 percent of the variance of I_g is explained by taking the six variables simultaneously into account. Up to 1951, R^2 is larger for the North than for the South; the situation is reversed in 1961. This fact, too, is consistent with expectations. Up to the 1930s, much of the Southern population practiced birth control to a very limited extent, if at all. And, again, when fertility is largely uncontrolled, we do not expect to find an association with the traditional socioeconomic indicators. The association increases when the propensity to control family size grows in the population.

The fall in R in the North (from .882 in 1951 to .627 in 1961) marked the end of the fall in I_g as the practice of birth control spread through the population. In many populations at an advanced stage of demographic development, the traditional inverse relationship between

TABLE 5.4

MARITAL FERTILITY (I_g), ZERO ORDER "STATIC" CORRELATIONS WITH SELECTED SOCIO-ECONOMIC VARIABLES, NORTH AND CENTER, SOUTH AND ISLANDS, AND ALL ITALY: 1881 TO 1961

Geographical area	Variable	1881	1911	1931	1951	1961
North and Center	Proportion married (I_m)	-.077	(.053)	-.327	-.623	-.456
	Infant mortality	(-.261)	.454	.507	.569	.385
	Ruralization	.403	.381	.331	.146	(-.106)
	Industrialization	(.083)	-.350	-.293	-.007	(.140)
	Male illiteracy	(-.392)	.141	.109	.031	(-.228)
	Urbanization	-.525	-.330	-.286	-.462	-.347
South and Islands	Proportion married (I_m)	(.209)	-.330	-.463	-.623	-.740
	Infant mortality	(-.255)	.033	(-.169)	.115	.312
	Ruralization	(-.214)	(-.129)	.052	(-.029)	(-.189)
	Industrialization	(.075)	(.147)	-.014	(.144)	(.027)
	Male illiteracy	.020	.174	(-.201)	.251	.308
	Urbanization	(.395)	-.008	-.351	-.021	.165
All Italy	Proportion married (I_m)	(.111)	(.017)	(.042)	-.482	-.481
	Infant mortality	(-.197)	.355	.611	.741	.724
	Ruralization	.115	.295	.439	.390	.358
	Industrialization	(.140)	-.298	-.435	-.366	-.314
	Male illiteracy	.033	.228	.599	.707	.697
	Urbanization	-.269	-.266	-.339	-.308	-.201

NOTE: Data in parentheses have signs contrary to expectation.

TABLE 5.5

MARITAL FERTILITY (I_g), PARTIAL AND MULTIPLE "STATIC" CORRELATIONS WITH SELECTED SOCIO-ECONOMIC VARIABLES, NORTH AND CENTER, SOUTH AND ISLANDS, AND ALL ITALY: 1881 TO 1961

Geographical area	Variable	1881	1911	1931	1951	1961
North and Center	Proportion married (I_m)	-.386[a]	-.149	-.596[a]	-.773[a]	-.361[a]
	Infant mortality	(-.087)	.523[a]	.581[a]	.527[a]	.266[a]
	Ruralization	.280[a]	.143	.248[a]	(-.166)	(-.246)[a]
	Industrialization	(.390)[a]	(.032)	(.133)	-.153	-.180
	Male illiteracy	(-.236)[b]	.177	.421[a]	.506[a]	.151
	Urbanization	-.283[a]	-.022	-.046	-.444[a]	-.368[a]
	Multiple correlation coefficient	.749	.625	.801	.882	.627
South and Islands	Proportion married (I_m)	(.470)[a]	-.530[a]	-.578[a]	-.766[a]	-.823[a]
	Infant mortality	(-.424)[a]	.330[b]	.356[a]	.307[b]	.390[a]
	Ruralization	.091	.292[b]	.140	(-.032)	(-.146)
	Industrialization	-.107	(.301)[b]	(.261)	(.179)	-.064
	Male illiteracy	.000	.336[b]	(-.108)	.349[a]	.492[a]
	Urbanization	(.439)[a]	-.187	-.427[a]	-.029	-.043
	Multiple correlation coefficient	.631	.572	.714	.792	.886
All Italy	Proportion married (I_m)	(.073)	-.323[a]	-.588[a]	-.745[a]	-.572[a]
	Infant mortality	(-.283)[a]	.454[a]	.460[a]	.341[a]	.333[a]
	Ruralization	.186[b]	.149	.162[b]	.009	(-.126)
	Industrialization	(.294)[a]	(.056)	(.012)	-.074	-.128
	Male illiteracy	.177[b]	.198[a]	.532[a]	.460[a]	.469[a]
	Urbanization	-.104	-.080	-.107	-.242[a]	-.193[a]
	Multiple correlation coefficient	.468	.567	.842	.911	.861

NOTE: Data in parentheses have signs contrary to expectation.

[a]Significant at .01 level.

[b]Significant at .05 level.

TABLE 5.6

PERCENTAGE CHANGE IN MARITAL FERTILITY (I_g), ZERO ORDER "DYNAMIC" CORRELATIONS WITH PERCENTAGE CHANGE IN SELECTED SOCIO-ECONOMIC VARIABLES, NORTH AND CENTER, SOUTH AND ISLANDS, AND ALL ITALY: 1881-1911 TO 1951-1961

Geographical area	Variable	1881-1911	1911-1931	1931-1951	1951-1961
North and Center	Proportion married (I_m)	(.085)	(.195)	-.162	-.329
	Infant mortality	(-.051)	.313	.264	.098
	Ruralization	.626	.034	(-.123)	(-.029)
	Industrialization	-.421	(.196)	(.078)	-.115
	Male illiteracy	.179	.101	.519	.421
	Urbanization	-.248	(.154)	-.013	-.032
South and Islands	Proportion married (I_m)	-.083	-.299	(.207)	-.153
	Infant mortality	.166	.196	(-.095)	(-.060)
	Ruralization	.067	.097	.210	.105
	Industrialization	(.169)	(.056)	-.349	-.400
	Male illiteracy	.105	(-.056)	.459	.259
	Urbanization	-.056	-.026	(.109)	-.090
All Italy	Proportion married (I_m)	(.055)	(.012)	-.291	-.274
	Infant mortality	(-.001)	.672	.359	.134
	Ruralization	.312	.077	.257	(-.096)
	Industrialization	-.234	-.022	-.264	-.261
	Male illiteracy	.116	.644	.605	.424
	Urbanization	-.207	(.093)	(.136)	-.028

NOTE: Data in parentheses have signs contrary to expectation.

TABLE 5.7

PERCENTAGE CHANGE IN MARITAL FERTILITY (I_g), PARTIAL AND MULTIPLE "DYNAMIC" CORRELATIONS WITH PERCENTAGE CHANGE IN SELECTED SOCIO-ECONOMIC VARIABLES, NORTH AND CENTER, SOUTH AND ISLANDS, AND ALL ITALY: 1881-1911 TO 1951-1961

Geographical area	Variable	1881-1911	1911-1931	1931-1951	1951-1961
North and Center	Proportion married (I_m)	(.078)	(.175)	-.209	-.305[a]
	Infant mortality	.131	.360[a]	.397[a]	.123
	Ruralization	.591[a]	.199	(-.286)[a]	(-.012)
	Industrialization	-.111	(.309)[a]	-.090	-.322
	Male illiteracy	(-.198)	.210	.602[a]	.524[a]
	Urbanization	(.087)	(.019)	-.109	-.055
	Multiple correlation coefficient	.692[a]	.495[a]	.665[a]	.601[a]
South and Islands	Proportion married (I_m)	-.071	-.357[a]	(.366)[b]	-.244
	Infant mortality	.100	.193	.032	.218
	Ruralization	.154	.237	(-.011)	.283
	Industrialization	(.179)	(.213)	-.236	-.491[a]
	Male illiteracy	.046	(-.011)	.511[a]	.271
	Urbanization	-.098	(.048)	(.004)	-.306
	Multiple correlation coefficient	.287	.434	.628[b]	.589
All Italy	Proportion married (I_m)	(.012)	-.039	-.101	-.186[a]
	Infant mortality	.033	.570[a]	.287[a]	.223
	Ruralization	.246[a]	.178[b]	(-.172)[b]	(-.112)
	Industrialization	(.020)	(.184)[b]	-.265[a]	-.425[a]
	Male illiteracy	(-.103)	.519[a]	.587[a]	.533[a]
	Urbanization	-.140	(.097)	(.015)	-.064
	Multiple correlation coefficient	.359	.790[a]	.689[a]	.627[a]

NOTE: Data in parentheses have signs contrary to expectation.

[a]Significant at .01 level.

[b]Significant at .05 level.

socioeconomic level and fertility disappears, giving way to relationships of different kind, often U-shaped. This process is reflected in a weaker linear association of fertility with the independent variables. On the other hand, the recovery of fertility in many areas of the North opens a new period in the history of Italian fertility in which all the traditional interpretations lose their force. Finally, certain variables, such as infant mortality and illiteracy, become negligible—the first falling to very low levels and having a low degree of territorial variability, and the second practically disappearing from the more developed provinces.

The dynamic analysis offers less satisfactory results. For instance, the multiple R between the intercensal percentage changes of I_g and the corresponding percentage changes of the six variables remains always below .700 (with the sole exception of Italy, 1911–1931), explaining from only 8 to a modest 48 percent of the variance. This generally lower level of association can be, at least in part, explained on technical grounds. Percentage changes, from one census to the other, of the independent and dependent variables are more subject than the absolute values to both random and systematic errors. For instance, the quality of censuses may change (not always for the better), and thus bias heavily the intercensal change of the variables; the bias may be milder on the rank order of the provinces according to the absolute value of the given variables (for instance, ruralization or illiteracy). Or, another case: short-term fluctuations may affect, in an opposite sense, the levels of fertility or of infant mortality at two subsequent censuses, thus greatly amplifying (or reducing) the intercensal changes.

Whatever the reasons may be, however, the dynamic association is rather weak; knowledge of the changes in the independent variables would give us a modest predictive power of the corresponding changes in legitimate fertility. The correlation is, at any time, higher for the North than for the South; for the latter region, R is significant only in 1931–1951.

5.3.3. Table 5.5 reports the "static" partial correlation coefficients for the North, the South, and Italy, 1881 to 1961. The figures within parentheses indicate that the sign of the coefficient runs in a sense contrary to our *a priori* expectations. For each variable there are 15 coefficients, in all 90 coefficients. Of these, 68 are in the expected sense and 22 in the contrary one. Urbanization is correlated in the expected sense 14 out of 15 times; proportion married and illiteracy, 13 times; infant mortality, 12 times; ruralization, 10 times; and industrialization only 6 times. Of the 22 coefficients with signs contrary to the expectations, 9 were calculated from 1881 data; 3 each from 1911, 1951, and 1961; and 4 from 1931.

If we rank the variables according to the level of partial *r* for each year and each subdivision (coefficients are, therefore, classified 15 times) and add the rank orders achieved by each variable, we get the classification reported in Table 5.8, which has a merely descriptive scope. The

TABLE 5.8

RANKING OF VARIABLES, "STATIC" PARTIAL CORRELATION, NORTH AND CENTER, SOUTH AND ISLANDS, ALL ITALY, AND ALL CASES

North and Center	South and Islands	Italy	All cases
Proportion married	Proportion married	Proportion married	Proportion married
Infant mortality	Male illiteracy	Male illiteracy	Male illiteracy, Infant mortality
Urbanization	Infant mortality	Infant mortality	--
Male illiteracy	Ruralization, Urbanization	Ruralization, Urbanization	Urbanization
Ruralization	--	--	Ruralization
Industrialization	Industrialization	Industrialization	Industrialization

: The highest "static" partial coefficient with the sign in the expected sense is assigned to rank 1.
See text for discription of table construction.

rank order has been obtained by assigning rank one to the highest partial coefficient with sign in the expected sense, and rank six to the highest partial coefficient with sign contrary to the expectations or, if all coefficients are in the expected sense, to the lowest partial *r*. Proportion married, illiteracy, and infant mortality are the three variables more closely correlated with I_g, once the effects of the other five variables are removed. These variables also have significant partial *r* in about two-thirds of the cases. Of these three variables, nuptiality in 1951 (in the three areas) and in 1961 (in the South) explains 55 percent or more of the variance of I_g. Its impact is also fairly strong in 1931 (North and South) and in 1911 (South). As for infant mortality, only in 1881 is it inversely correlated with I_g; after that date, the correlation is always as expected, positive and larger for the North than for the South. Illiteracy is, of these three variables, the one with the lowest partial association with fertility, at least in the two subdivisions of the national territory.

Of the three variables more loosely correlated with fertility (ruralization, industrialization, and urbanization), urbanization is the one with a sign almost always as expected, but its partial *r* rarely attains a significant level. The association seems to be stronger in the North than in the South. Ruralization is correlated in the expected sense with I_g until 1931; then the correlation becomes contrary to expectations. The spread of fertility control seems not to have found obstacles, after World War II, in the degree of ruralization of the economy. Finally, the role of industrialization has been, more frequently than not, contrary to the one generally assigned. The partial correlation is frequently positive and very seldom statistically significant.

5.3.4. The dynamic correlation is, as said earlier, less satisfactory (Table 5.7). For each variable there are 12 partial *r*'s (North, South, and Italy for four intercensal periods). Of these, the signs are always in the expected sense for infant mortality, 9 times out of 12 for illiteracy, 8 for nuptiality, 7 for ruralization and industrialization, and 6 for urbanization; in all, 49 coefficients out of 72 (about two-thirds) conform to the expectations. The ranking of the variables, according to the criteria set forward before, results in the classification reported in Table 5.9.

Infant mortality and illiteracy are the variables whose change is more closely correlated with changes in marital fertility. Values of partial *r*, however, are very seldom significant in the South, with the exception of proportion married in 1911–1931, illiteracy in 1931–1951, and industrialization in 1951–1961.

As in the static correlation, the dynamic analysis confirms the peculiar type of association of industrialization and ruralization with fertility. We generally find a direct correlation of industrialization with I_g in the first two periods; then in the last two periods the sign changes and the correlation conforms to expectations. The reverse is true for ruralization, whose changes are directly associated with fertility, as expected, in the first two periods; in the last two, an inverse association is most often found. Ruralization appears, therefore, to be a factor of conservation of old patterns until a certain stage of the history of fertility decline; then its role changes. The data are too weak for building a theory,

TABLE 5.9

RANKING OF VARIABLES, "DYNAMIC" PARTIAL CORRELATION, NORTH AND CENTER, SOUTH AND ISLANDS, ALL ITALY, AND ALL CASES

North and Center	South and Islands	Italy	All cases
Infant mortality	Ruralization	Infant mortality	Infant mortality
Male illiteracy	Infant mortality, Male illiteracy, Ubanization	Male illiteracy	Male illiteracy
Proportion married	--	Proportion married, Ruralization, Industrialization	Ruralization
Ruralization, Industrialization	--	--	Proportion married
--	Proportion married	--	Urbanization
Urbanization	Industrialization	Urbanization	Industrialization

: The highest "dynamic" partial coefficient with the sign in the expected sense is assigned to rank 1.
See text for discription of table construction.

but the cases of ruralization and industrialization are good examples of the changing role of a variable during the process of the decline, and of the caution required in interpreting the results.

5.3.5. Some interest lies in the comparison of zero-order with corresponding partial coefficients. The comparison may answer the following question: is the zero-order correlation between marital fertility and each of the independent variables strengthened, weakened, or reversed when the effects of the other variables are simultaneously accounted for in the partial correlation? The reader may proceed to the kind of analysis he wants by direct inspection of Tables 5.4 and 5.6 respectively with Tables 5.5 and 5.7; we will limit our analysis to whether the sense of the zero-order correlation is confirmed, or reversed, by the partial coefficients. Table 5.10 gives the answer to this question for the 162 pairs of zero-order and partial *r*'s of the static and dynamic analysis. Partial *r*'s confirm the sign of the zero-order *r*'s in 130 out of 162 instances; in 100 of the 130 cases they coincide in the expected sense. In only 32 of the 162 cases does the partial *r* reverse the sign of the

TABLE 5.10

ZERO-ORDER CORRELATIONS OF MARITAL FERTILITY (I_g) WITH SOCIO-ECONOMIC VARIABLES COMPARED WITH CORRESPONDING PARTIAL COEFFICIENTS

Variable	Signs of the zero order and of partial coefficients coincide		Signs of the partial r diff from the zero-order ones	
	In expected sense	Contrary to expected sense	Partial r in expected sense	Partial r cont to expected se
Proportion married (I_m)	17	6	4	0
Infant mortality	19	3	5	0
Ruralization	15	6	2	4
Industrialization	10	7	10	0
Male illiteracy	20	3	1	3
Urbanization	19	5	1	2
Total	100	30	23	9

zero-order *r*, and in the large majority of the cases (23 out of 32) the partial *r* sign changes in the expected sense.

In the majority of cases (four out of five), allowing for the other variables does not change the sign of the zero-order correlation; when it does change it, the chances are that the change of sign of the partial *r* is in the expected sense.

5.3.6. In general, we have given more weight to the results of the correlation analysis—static and dynamic—for the two geographic subdivisions (North and South) than to those for the whole of Italy. The reason is the following. As we have shown earlier, differences between the two areas are clear-cut, both in fertility and in socioeconomic indicators. The South has, during the twentieth century, always had a higher fertility (and a slower decline), a higher degree of ruralization, a higher infant mortality and illiteracy, and a lower degree of industrialization and urbanization. When pooling all provinces together on a scatter diagram (with I_g on the X-axis and one of the socioeconomic variables on the Y-axis), the provinces of the South form a cluster of points at a level that is significantly different than the average of the other provinces, which are generally much more dispersed around their mean. This fact often leads to the computation of significant coefficients, with signs in the expected sense, even if within each of the two subdivisions the correlation is weak or contrary to the expectations (the whole argument can obviously be reversed: the two subdivisions may have meaningful relationships that, on a national scale, disappear).

One further question could be advanced: within each of the two subdivisions (North and South) are there any provinces that because of their peculiar structure form clusters that may affect the correlation analysis? We have made the following empirical test. We have plotted the residuals of I_g, or the deviations of the actual I_g from the estimated I_g. If there were a clustering tendency within one of the areas, we might expect to find the I_g of the provinces of one given region (or of one given area) below or above the regression line. In other words, the fact that one province belongs to a given region (or to a given area) should not affect the chances of its I_g lying above (or below) the multiple regression line. Inspection of the various diagrams has convinced us that this tendency, although there are some instances of clustering in the North, cannot be consistently and clearly established. The provinces of each region of the two territorial subdivisions have actual I_g randomly distributed above and below the multiple regression line.

5.3.7. A further way of measuring the association between the socioeconomic indicators and marital fertility consists in correlating the levels assumed by the variables at a given date with the percentage changes in marital fertility during the following period. The hypothesis is that achievement of given levels (high or low) of industrialization, infant mortality, illiteracy, and so forth may generate favorable conditions for the diffusion of birth control in the following period. In other words, the decline of fertility may not be contemporary to the change of the socioeconomic variables, but subsequent to, and generated by, this change. The application of the hypothesis meets some obstacles, the main one being the difficulty of establishing an adequate time lag for the decline of fertility to take place as a consequence of the achievement of given social and economic conditions.

On the other hand, this procedure implies the assumption that changes of fertility are always the consequence of changes in the indicators, or, in other words, that there is a one-way cause and effect relationship. But which is the cause and which is the effect? A fall of infant mortality increases the number of surviving children of the average couple—if age at marriage and marital fertility remain constant—and therefore becomes a motivation for fertility control, but, on the other hand, a fall of fertility means better care for the children and generates a fall of death risks in the infant ages. The same could probably be said of illiteracy and of other variables. The word *feedback* probably describes this type of situation, but we prefer to say, more simply and clearly, that the changes in family size are only one aspect of the complex problem of social change, cause and effect at the same time. In our case, we are looking for links, associations, or relations between fertility and the other variables more than for cause-and-effect mechanisms.

There is a further point to be discussed: the nature of the "expected," *a priori*, associations. This is always a problem since the nature and the sense of the association may change through time, as we have discussed in previous pages. But in this case the situation is even more complicated. Suppose that at a given date we consider the association between industrialization and the successive fertility decline. We could formulate the following hypothesis:

(1) In areas where industrialization is high, fertility will fall more rapidly than in areas with lower industrialization. An inverse association is, therefore, expected.
(2) But in another stage it may well happen that in the more industrialized areas a high degree of fertility control has been reached by the population and that no further reduction is expected. On the other hand, the populations of the less industrialized areas will strengthen their control of fertility and therefore the expected association between the two variables will be a direct one.

We have explored this last line of investigation by correlating the levels of the various indicators at each census with the changes of the dependent variable (I_g) in the following period (1881 and 1881–1911, etc.).

The doubts we have cast upon the application of this type of analysis to the Italian situation are confirmed by inspection of Tables 5.11 and 5.12, where the zero-order, partial, and multiple coefficients are reported. The levels of multiple R are similar to those found for the dynamic correlation. The proportion of the explained variance goes from one-fourth to one-half for the North and from one-fifth to two-thirds for the South. In almost half of the cases (34 out of 72 times) the sign of the partial r is contrary to the expectations. The only variable whose partial r is mostly in the expected direction is the proportion married. For the other variables, partial r's are equally divided between the signs plus and minus.

TABLE 5.11

PERCENTAGE CHANGE IN MARITAL FERTILITY (I_g), ZERO-ORDER CORRELATIONS WITH LEVELS OF SELECTED SOCIO-ECONOMIC VARIABLES, NORTH AND CENTER, SOUTH AND ISLANDS, AND ALL ITALY: 1881 TO 1951

Geographical area	Variable	I_g, 1881-1911 Level, 1881	I_g, 1911-1931 Level, 1911	I_g, 1931-1951 Level, 1931	I_g, 1951-1961 Level, 1951
North and Center	Proportion married (I_m)	-.065	-.300	-.260	(.226)
	Infant mortality	.504	.157	.030	(-.354)
	Ruralization	(-.034)	(-.391)	(-.229)	(-.447)
	Industrialization	(.217)	-.281	(.345)	(.204)
	Male illiteracy	(-.122)	.171	(-.395)	(-.285)
	Urbanization	-.217	(.440)	-.178	(.511)
South and Islands	Proportion married (I_m)	-.227	-.036	-.276	(.022)
	Infant mortality	(-.364)	(-.272)	.184	.035
	Ruralization	(-.015)	(-.329)	(-.458)	(-.519)
	Industrialization	(.052)	(.132)	(.355)	(.148)
	Male illiteracy	(-.007)	(-.013)	.390	.418
	Urbanization	(.112)	(.198)	(.233)	(.712)
All Italy	Proportion married (I_m)	-.089	(.254)	-.027	(.197)
	Infant mortality	.290	.194	.368	(-.386)
	Ruralization	(-.026)	(-.468)	(-.066)	(-.535)
	Industrialization	(.155)	-.441	(.084)	(.334)
	Male illiteracy	(-.089)	.696	.421	(-.283)
	Urbanization	-.136	(.444)	-.110	(.547)

NOTE: Data in parentheses have signs contrary to expectation.

TABLE 5.12

PERCENTAGE CHANGE IN MARITAL FERTILITY (I_g), PARTIAL AND MULTIPLE CORRELATIONS WITH LEVELS OF SELECTED SOCIO-ECONOMIC VARIABLES, NORTH AND CENTER, SOUTH AND ISLANDS, AND ALL ITALY: 1881 TO 1951

Geographical area	Variable	I_g, 1881-1911 Level, 1881	I_g, 1911-1931 Level, 1911	I_g, 1931-1951 Level, 1931	I_g, 1951-1961 Level, 1951
North and	Proportion married (I_m)	-.102	-.452[a]	-.099	(.434)[a]
	Infant mortality	.489[a]	.349[a]	(-.216)[b]	(-.178)
	Ruralization	.063	.033	.030	(-.258)[a]
	Industrialization	(.285)[a]	-.247[b]	(.152)	-.215[b]
	Male illiteracy	(-.200)	.352[a]	(-.128)	(-.257)[a]
	Urbanization	-.182	(.498)[a]	-.152	(.119)
	Multiple correlation coefficient	.589[a]	.708[a]	.524[b]	.719[a]
South and Islands	Proportion married (I_m)	-.111	-.014	-.456[a]	-.115
	Infant mortality	(-.361)[a]	(-.033)	.356[a]	(-.099)
	Ruralization	.029	(-.350)[a]	(-.518)[a]	.005
	Industrialization	(.178)	(.299)[b]	-.409[a]	(.026)
	Male illiteracy	(-.085)	(-.095)	.487[a]	.470[a]
	Urbanization	(.039)	(.081)	-.384[a]	(.577)[a]
	Multiple correlation coefficient	.447	.487	.788[a]	.799[a]
All Italy	Proportion married (I_m)	-.194[a]	-.195[a]	-.267[a]	(.291)[a]
	Infant mortality	.278[a]	.257[a]	.010	(-.140)
	Ruralization	(-.030)	.004	(-.142)	(-.190)[a]
	Industrialization	(.161)	-.169[b]	(.026)	-.012
	Male illiteracy	(-.319)	.640[a]	.517[a]	.053
	Urbanization	-.492	(.446)[a]	-.261[a]	(.240)[a]
	Multiple correlation coefficient	.389[b]	.812[a]	.640[a]	.674[a]

NOTE: Data in parentheses have signs contrary to expectation.

[a]Significant at .01 level.

[b]Significant at .05 level.

Ranking the variables according to the criteria followed in Section 5.3.3 makes, therefore, very little sense; proportion married and illiteracy are the best of the six, with industrialization and ruralization ranking last as usual. Another distressing fact is that we cannot find any firm logic behind the changing sign of the indicators' association with fertility decline. It is true that the correlations tend to be mostly in the expected direction during the periods of strongest decline of I_g (1911–1931 for the North and 1931–1951 for the South); still they reverse their signs, in the North, during 1931–1951 when fertility decline was still very rapid. Perhaps the only exception is constituted by the last period considered, 1951–1961, when the slight recovery of fertility has taken place in the more developed areas, therefore resulting in the inversion of the secular association between the socioeconomic indicators and fertility.

5.4 *The Analysis of Covariance*

In the preceding chapter (Section 4.4.3), we studied the sources of variation in the provincial levels of legitimate fertility. The analysis of variance proved that there is an increasingly significant difference between the "within" and "between" mean square variance of fertility by region, after allowing for the number of degrees of freedom. The hypothesis that no significant difference exists between the two estimates becomes increasingly improbable with the passing of time.

In this chapter, we have shown that fertility is correlated, sometimes closely, with a few indicators of a social and economic nature. We would like now, with the help of the instruments of the analysis of covariance, to test whether, with the removal of the effects of those variables, interregional differences remain significant. Or, from another viewpoint, since we know that the six variables are associated with fertility, and territorial variation of fertility depends at least partly on the differential level of these variables, would the "adjusted" levels of regional fertility still differ significantly once the effects of the differential impact of the independent variables has been simultaneously accounted for? It is clear that in case of a 100 percent multiple correlation with fertility, allowing for the variables would result in wiping out the regional differentials.

The analysis of covariance also makes it possible to calculate "adjusted" regional means of legitimate fertility after allowing simultaneously for the differences in the independent variables. This aspect of the analysis of covariance, however, is of little interest to us.

FACTORS INVOLVED IN DECLINE

The analysis of covariance has been applied to the 90 provinces distributed in 18 (16 until 1911) regions. The same analysis has been extended to the provinces and regions of the North and of the South. Table 5.13 shows the results for North, South, and Italy. The general rule is,

TABLE 5.13

MARITAL FERTILITY (I_g), F-TEST ANALYSIS OF VARIANCE AND COVARIANCE WITH SELECTED SOCIO-ECONOMIC VARIABLES, NORTH AND CENTER, SOUTH AND ISLANDS, AND ALL ITALY: 1881 TO 1961

Date	Geographical area	Analysis of variance before allowance		Analysis of covariance after allowance	
		d.f.	F	d.f.	F
1881	North and Center	9,43	2.309	9,37	2.975
1911		9,43	7.490[a]	9,37	5.892[a]
1931		10,49	5.295[a]	10,43	8.405[a]
1951		10,47	7.634[a]	10,41	3.467[a]
1961		10,46	12.068[a]	10,40	7.798[a]
1881	South and Islands	6,27	3.829	6,21	3.385
1911		6,27	4.050	6,21	4.444
1931		6,25	7.159	6,19	3.553
1951		6,27	15.536[a]	6,21	13.247[a]
1961		6,27	8.985[a]	6,21	6.801
1881	All Italy	16,70	3.181[a]	16,64	2.908[a]
1911		16,70	6.832[a]	16,64	6.192[a]
1931		17,74	13.654[a]	17,68	6.447[a]
1951		17,74	24.770[a]	17,68	6.199[a]
1961		17,73	27.019[a]	17,67	8.087[a]

[a]Significant at .01 level.

as could be expected, that the value of *F* is higher when the six variables are not accounted for. This may sound obvious on the basis of the significant correlations found earlier.

A more detailed inspection of the results shows that in the North, interregional differentials are not significant in 1881 before allowance for the variables; after allowance, differences are still not significant, but the value of *F* has increased. Allowing for the socioeconomic variables, therefore, increases, rather than reduces, the regional differentials. This confirms that factors other than those introduced as independent variables affected the regional differentials before the beginning of the secular decline. From 1911 on, regional differentials are relevant and significant before and after allowance for the six variables. *F* is significantly reduced after allowance in 1911, 1951, and 1961, but is increased in 1931. The pattern in the South is different. Differences in the regional means are not significant, at the chosen level of 1 percent, in 1881, 1911, and 1931, and allowance for the six variables increases the value of F in 1911 and reduces it in 1881 and 1931. In 1951 and 1961, the computation of F before allowance shows significant regional differentials, but the F values decrease substantially after allowance, and regional differentials are not significant in 1961 at the chosen 1 percent level.

Summing up, in the North, after 1881, regional differentials are always significant before and after allowance for the effects of the six variables. The introduction of the variables, although it reduces regional differentials (with the notable exception of 1931), does not reduce them below significant patterns. Regional influences remain, therefore, strong and relevant. In the South, regional patterns are more homogeneous; after allowance for the variables, only in 1951 are regional differentials significant.

The analysis of covariance for the whole of Italy (92 provinces in 18 regions in 1961) shows more clear-cut results. Allowing for the six variables decreases the value of F at all dates. The value of F remains always significant, even though it is reduced by one-half to three-fourths from 1931 on.

The analysis of covariance adds further strength to the following points:

(1) When fertility is high and not too far from the so-called natural levels, traditional social and economic factors have little weight in determining territorial differentials. This is the case of the South until 1931 and of the North in 1881.

(2) Regional differences are less important in the South.

(3) The independent variables generally help to explain part of the regional differentials, but in some instances raise such differentials. In other words, the traditional variables have a changing role in explaining territorial differentials.

(4) The fact that regional differentials remain, in many instances, very relevant and statistically significant after allowance for the variables means that other factors neglected in the analysis are at work in determining such differentials. This fact is, however, scarcely surprising. We have already said several times that it would be vain to expect to find a full explanation of a very

complex phenomenon like that of procreation by the simple introduction of a few variables generally chosen because they are the only available, or, in other words, the only quantifiable data from censuses or current statistics.

5.5 *Conclusions*

Has our knowledge of the factors of Italian fertility decline improved after consideration of the results of the correlation and covariance analysis? In our opinion, and in spite of the many reservations advanced here and there, it has. Certainly, it would have been naive to expect a satisfactory explanation of territorial differentials from a limited number of variables that are, at best, indicators of aspects of life and society that may influence the behavior of the couple as far as family building is concerned. However, if we take for granted the many limitations of the empirical method employed, we have to conclude that the findings are helpful because they support some hypotheses and eliminate or modify others. This is certainly a step forward.

A first important finding is the changing degree of association between fertility and the various socioeconomic indicators simultaneously considered. It is confirmed that territorial variations around high fertility patterns cannot be adequately explained by the factors traditionally associated with the decline. This is the case of the North in 1881 and 1911 and of the South until 1931. The association tends to increase during periods of rapid fall in fertility (North in 1931 and 1951; South in 1951 and 1961), when territorial levels of fertility are very much differentiated. Multiple association, however, declines (as in the North in 1961) when a new phase of the history of fertility begins with the recovery of fertility after it has fallen to very low levels. This coincides with the substitution of a U-shaped relationship to the traditional inverse relationship between fertility and the socioeconomic level.

More evident is the changing role of each of the various indicators retained in our analysis, as can be discerned in the partial correlation analysis, especially the "static" one. We have seen, for instance, that the index of ruralization is correlated with fertility in the expected sense until 1931 and reverses its role after that date. In 1951 and 1961, the areas with a higher degree of ruralization, instead of resisting low fertility patterns, seem to favor them. We have already advanced the hypothesis that whenever modern techniques of family planning are not available, the couple, if strongly motivated, may "overdo" by over controlling their fertility with traditional techniques. The philosophy behind this behavior could be that it is better to keep on the safe side. In other words, it is better to risk remaining below the desired or envisaged family size than to risk going far beyond it.

The role of the variables may also change when the intensity of the characteristics described becomes negligible and irrelevant. Typical is the case of illiteracy in the North, where association with marital fertility is relatively strong in 1931 and 1951 but becomes very weak in 1961, when only a small fraction of the population did not know how to read or write. Some other interesting reflections are suggested by the nature of the variables more closely associated with fertility, such as the proportion married, infant mortality, and illiteracy. For the last two little commentary is needed: they are among the variables traditionally cited by demographers when dealing with fertility decline. But the fact that the proportion married (as measured by I_m) shows consistently a close and inverse correlation with legitimate fertility is worth some further consideration. The reader may recall from Table 5.5 that the partial r between I_g and I_m is particularly strong after 1931. It is in line with the expectation to find an inverse correlation between I_m and I_g when fertility is high. In this case, we may expect (1) that control of nuptiality acts as a substitute for control of marital fertility and that pressure for controlling fertility is higher when I_m is high and the family size larger; (2) that the higher the proportion ever marrying, the lower the biological selectivity of marriage; and the higher the proportion of infecund or subfecund couples, the lower the level of marital fertility; (3) that, at a given age, the higher has been the number of conceptions, abortions, and births, the lower is the probability of a pregnancy; and, (4) the longer, at a given age, the duration of marriage, the lower the frequency of sexual intercourse and, therefore, the risk of a pregnancy. All these factors contribute to an inverse relationship between nuptiality and legitimate fertility. But these factors do not seem to play a major role when fertility is under control, and, although they are still at work, their impact ought to be slight. When the average completed family size is two or three children, there is no need for a substitute for fertility control since the couples know how to plan their fertility without avoiding or postponing marriage; the influence of infecund or subfecund couples when propensity to marriage is high is less relevant since their null or weak fertility is averaged with the low or modest fertility of the other couples; finally the impact of the age at marriage is again, less relevant in determining the levels of fertility at the various ages.

Finally, two other technical factors could also have some influence in determining the inverse association between I_m and I_g. First, when I_g is low, the age composition of the population in fecund age tends to be older, therefore giving more weight, in the computation of I_m, to the older age groups where the proportion married is higher. Secondly, fertility is generally lower in areas with lower mortality and lower widowhood. But incidence of widowhood is inversely associated with I_m, and therefore I_m should be inversely associated with I_g. The effect of these two factors, however, is relatively modest, the second one being partially accounted for by the introduction of infant mortality in the multivariate analysis.

Summing up, the close relationships between I_g and I_m remain somewhat a mystery, although the sense of the relationship is not contrary to the expectations. Further analysis ought to establish which component of I_m is more closely related to marital fertility (whether the age at marriage, or the proportion ever marrying, etc.) and whether nuptiality is associated to a third factor, which, in its turn, is closely related to fertility.

Of the factors that are more loosely associated, or associated in a contradictory way, with fertility (ruralization, industrialization, and urbanization), we have already underlined the changing role of the first two indicators. We may here point out that these indicators, often indiscriminately referred to as the main determinants of fertility decline by the supporters of the so-called theory of the demographic transition, are frequently imprecise and ambiguous. The urban population is still a concept in search of application, nor is it clear which are the aspects of the urban environment affecting fertility. Industrialization is another vague concept; the housewife working at home part-time spinning wool for a textile factory should not be identified with the industrial sector in the same way as the skilled worker operating the complex machinery in a chemical plant. These rather obvious considerations suggest focusing attention, in cross-sectional analysis, on more meaningful and precise indicators.

An unexpected confirmation of our ideas came on May 12, 1974, when Italians went to the polls to decide whether to keep or to repeal the three-and-one-half-year-old divorce law. Only 40 percent of the electorate was in favor of repeal, and therefore the law was kept. The proportion of the voters against divorce is a good indicator of the attachment to the traditional concept of family and marriage prevailing in the various areas of the country. Indeed, the divorce issue cut across the boundaries of the political parties and reflected very well the predominant attitudes and feelings of the population on family matters. The proportion of voters against the divorce in the provinces correlates well with I_g of 1961 (+.743) and of 1951 (+.786). The highest correlation is with the level of fertility of 1931 (+.839), while the correlation with the 1911 I_g is lower (+.603). But in the four cases, the zero-order correlation coefficient between opponents of divorce in 1974 and I_g is well above the highest zero-order correlation coefficients between I_g and the six indicators retained in this chapter. The relation of fertility to voting behavior is especially close in the North and very weak in the South (+.831 in the North and —.007 in the South in 1961; +.876 and +.076 in 1951; +.812 and +.351 in 1931; +.699 and +.232 in 1911). In fact, the proportion voting against divorce accounts for about two-thirds to three-fourths of the variance of I_g in the provinces of the North from 1931 to 1961, as much as, or more than, the proportion accounted for by the six independent variables considered together. The close and persistent relation suggests that the vote on divorce is a good indicator of the psychological attitude of the population toward procreation, and that the differing territorial attitudes have old historical roots apt to explain rather accurately the fertility differentials of today as well as those of half a century ago.

We have thought that the introduction of the divorce variable in the multivariate analysis was not justified. Indeed, the six variables and fertility refer always to the same date, and the introduction of the divorce variable in the explanation of fertility of 20, 50, or even 100 years ago would have altered the temporal logic of the analysis.

But this example illustrates very well the limitations of multivariate analysis when indicators well suited to the purpose are not available.

CHAPTER 6: Differential Fertility as a Key to the Interpretation of Fertility Decline

6.1 *The Sources*

This chapter will deal with differential fertility as it results from the differential behavior of various sectors of the population. The same problem has already been discussed in connection with urban-rural fertility, the analysis of geographical trends, and the factors influencing fertility decline. But the definition of the sectors of the population whose fertility was measured and compared was based on geographic criteria. We have analyzed the fertility of the "mainly rural" areas; we have studied the fertility of regions, provinces, and circondari, or, in other words, the fertility of populations defined by administrative boundaries and not by their individual characteristics.

In this chapter, we will try to assemble, elaborate, and interpret a different set of information consisting of statistics on the fertility of couples having in common given social, economic, or cultural characteristics. In short, the definition of the "sectors" of the population will be based on their sharing common individual qualities and characteristics. The fertility of the educated will be compared with the fertility of the less educated; the behavior of the families drawing their livelihood from agriculture, with that of the families engaged in the industrial sector, and so on. Women, couples, or families whose behavior is measured and compared are, therefore, aggregated in groups on the basis of one or more of their individual characteristics.

The available material is very poor. Unlike many European countries, Italy is not rich in published census material on fertility. Only two census surveys have been published: that of 1931 and that of 1961. Questions on the fertility of married women were asked in 1971, but data have not yet been published. Our ambition, therefore, may run too high in comparison with the information at our disposal; however, other data on fertility, though often fragmentary and limited, may nevertheless be helpful in retracing the course of the differential procreative behavior of the Italian population. We will make extensive use of such fragmentary material in this chapter. Fertility data are not the only source of potential use to the demographer. Information on the structure of the family, as well as statistics on families according to the number of surviving children, may be of inestimable value. From the information on family structure, we may get information on the nature of the family as a social institution and a demographic unit, facts which are closely related to fertility behavior. From the number of surviving children living in the family, the level of fertility, under certain assumptions, can be estimated.

Finally, although our monograph is intended to give an account of demographic history during the nineteenth and twentieth centuries, we will also make reference to some aspects of the structure of families in the preceding centuries, since we believe that this will help to establish a better understanding of historical trends.

6.2 *Children and the Family before the Mid-nineteenth Century*

6.2.1. In the absence of a detailed nominative reconstitution of families, it is impossible to obtain direct information on differential fertility for past centuries. But when nominative censuses or counts exist, it is possible to obtain information on the number of children surviving at the census date and living in the family. If the census includes information on the characteristics of the family, such as the profession of the head of the family, or other indicators of the social and economic standing of the family, it is possible to group the families in question into homogeneous classes according to one or more qualitative characteristics (rich and poor, educated and uneducated, rural and nonrural). Furthermore, when the census lists for each family the age, marital status, and some indication of the relationship to the head of the household of the various members (wife, son, servant, etc.), it is possible to compute the average number of surviving children still living in the household per married man or married woman of a given age.

Let us consider this last and relatively favorable case. Let us suppose that for each family we know (1) the age and marital status of the members, (2) their relationship to the head of the family, and (3) some qualitative indicator of status of the family. In this case we know the number of surviving children still in the household per married man or married female of a given age-group for different segments of the population. Is this measure useful to us? It is fairly obvious that differences in the mean number of children between the various social segments may be imputed to: (1) differences in age-specific marital fertility, (2) differences in infant and child mortality, (3) differences in age at marriage, and (4) differences in the age and in the rate of departure of children from the family because of marriage, emigration, or other reasons. These four interacting factors (others could be added, but they would be of less importance) make it difficult to give an interpretation of the results. However, factor (4) may be controlled by considering only the number of children for ages or parents below, for instance, 40 years. Since the main reason for leaving the family is marriage, the differential rate of exit becomes appreciable after about age 18. Married women of 40, and with a mean age at marriage well above 20 years, probably had most of their surviving children living with them. After that age, the rate of exit rapidly increases, and factor (4) could not be accounted for. But factors (1), (2), and (3), in the absence of further data, cannot be separated and their combined effect must be considered; sometimes the direction of the differential impact of one of the factors, such as mortality, can be inferred.

Examination of some empirical data indicates that prior to the fall of mortality and fertility during the nineteenth century, the families belonging to heads of households in the higher section of the social ladder had a larger number of children at any given age than the families of less favored conditions. In other words, the burden of the family was heavier on the shoulders of the better off.

6.2.2. The Catasto of Firenze of 1427, embracing the city and a large part of the countryside, gives clear support to this statement.[1] The Catasto was an inventory of the wealth of the population of Firenze, mainly for taxation purposes; the compulsory declarations, made by every head of household, were severely and strictly controlled by the officials of Firenze. In every declaration, each member of the family was listed by name, along with his or her age, marital status, and relationship to the head of the family. There are good reasons to believe that the declarations were very complete for the times, since every member of the family who was not a slave or a servant was the basis for a deduction of taxable wealth. Citizens, therefore, had an obvious interest in listing all family members. From the Catasto, we can determine the distribution of surviving children according to the age of mother and the degree of wealth

[1] C. Klapisch, "Fiscalité et démographie en Toscane," *Annales* XXIV, no. 6 (1969); D. Herlihy, "Vieillir à Florence au Quattrocento," *Annales* XXIV, no. 6 (1969).

of the family.[2] Partial data (representing over 2,000 married women) for six of the sixteen Gonfaloni of the city of Firenze are reported in Table 6.1 and illustrated in Figure 6.1.

As expected, in each category the number of children increases until the age of 30-34, reflecting the cumulative effects of fertility. After that age, however, the cumulative effects of mortality and of the exit of children from the family offset the effects of fertility, which, of course, cease altogether after the age of 45. The interesting feature of the table is the

TABLE 6.1

MEAN NUMBER OF CHILDREN IN HOUSEHOLD, BY AGE OF MOTHER AND WEALTH OF FAMILY, SELECTED GONFALONI OF FIRENZE: 1427

Age of mother	Wealth of family		
	Low	Medium	High
15-24	1.81	1.93	2.55
25-29	3.03	3.18	3.93
30-34	2.97	3.57	4.88
35-44	3.00	3.38	4.52
45-54	2.58	2.20	3.01

SOURCE: The data have been collected and analyzed from dissertations in Economic History, (supervised by Professor F. Melis), by the following students of the Facoltà di Economia e Commercio, University of Florence, in the academic years 1970-1971 and 1971-1972: F. Barni (Gonfalone del Carro), M. Bernocchi (Bue), S. Colzi (Scala), G. Giustini (Drago), G. Novelli (Unicorno), P. Spighi (Lion Rosso).

NOTES: Data refer to surviving children still living at home. The gonfaloni are Bue, Carro, Drago, Lion Rosso, Scala, and Unicorno.

higher number of surviving children attributed in every age group to married women living in rich families, in comparison with those of moderately rich or poor families. Of the factors determining such differences—age at marriage, marital fertility, and differential mortality—we are inclined to give more weight to the third factor, although the action of the first two may have contributed to the determination of such large differentials.

[2] The data have been collected and analyzed in the dissertations in economic history supervised by Professor F. Melis, by the following students of the Facoltà di Economia e Commercio, University of Florence, in 1970-1971 and 1971-1972: F. Barni (Gonfalone del Carro), M. Bernocchi (Bue), S. Colzi (Scala), G. Giustini (Drago), G. Novelli (Unicorno), P. Spighi (Lion Rosso).

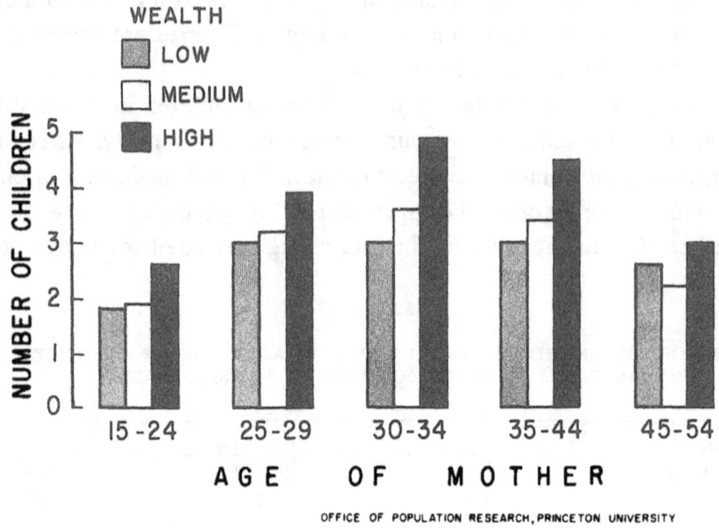

Figure 6.1 Mean Number of Children in Household, by Age of Mother and Wealth of Family, Selected Gonfaloni of Firenze: 1427

The data from Firenze confirm that:

(1) At any given age the wealthier women had a larger number of children still living in the household

(2) The differentials were presumably imputable to the lower infant mortality of the rich classes, although a lower age at marriage might have had some weight

(3) It is impossible, in the absence of an evaluation of the level of mortality and of the age at marriage, to say whether differential fertility existed between families of different wealth; if they did exist, it is likely that the wealthier families also had higher fertility.

6.2.3. Similar patterns can be found in the South of Italy in the eighteenth century.[3] De Meo has studied, in several essays, the "Catasto onciario," an enumeration of the population and of its wealth made during the second part of the eighteenth century in the *Regno delle due Sicilie.* For the city of Castellammare di Stabia, de Meo was able to distribute the surviving children still living in the household by age and

[3] P. Villani, *Mezzogiorno tra Riforme e Rivoluzione*, Bari, 1973; see particularly chapter 3, "Il catasto onciario ed il sistema tributario."

TABLE 6.2

MEAN NUMBER OF CHILDREN IN HOUSEHOLD, BY AGE AND WEALTH ("ABBIENTI" AND "NON ABBIENTI") OF FATHER, CITY OF CASTELLAMMARE DI STABIA: 18TH CENTURY

Age of father	"Non abbienti" Children per father (mean)	"Non abbienti" Fathers (number)	"Abbienti" Children per father (mean)	"Abbienti" Fathers (number)
20-29	0.94	148	1.46	58
30-39	2.19	236	2.77	124
40-49	3.25	218	3.67	174
50-59	3.24	156	3.57	128
60-69	2.78	74	3.62	69
70 and over	2.00	13	2.51	33
Total	2.74	845	3.16	586

SOURCE: G. DE MEO, Distribuzione della ricchezza e composizione demografica in alcune città dell'Italia Meridionale alla metà del secolo XVIII, in "Annali di Statistica", VI, XIX, Roma, 1931, Tables XXVII and XXVIII.

NOTES: Data refer to surviving children still living at home. "Abbienti" and "non abbienti" may be translated as "have" and "have not".

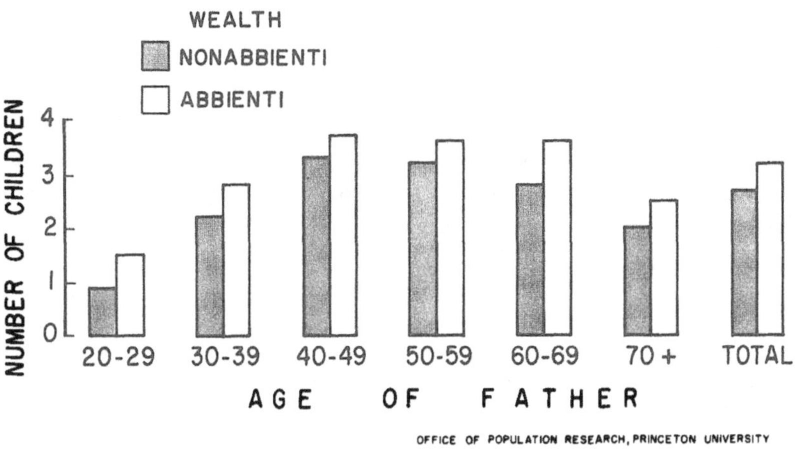

Figure 6.2 Mean Number of Children in Household, by Age and Wealth of Father, City of Castellammare di Stabia: 18th Century

TABLE 6.3

MEAN NUMBER OF CHILDREN IN HOUSEHOLD, BY AGE AND WEALTH (IN OUNCES OF GOLD) OF FATHER, CITY OF CASTELLAMMARE DI STABIA: 18TH CENTURY

Age of father	Wealth in ounces of gold Less than 10	 10 and more
20-29	.97	1.40
30-39	2.26	3.20
40-49	3.34	2.96
50-59	3.18	3.71
60-69	2.74	4.66
70-79	2.13	2.29
80-89	0.50	2.00
Total	2.52	3.24

SOURCE: G. DE MEO, Distribuzione della ricchezza e composizione demografica in alcune città dell'Italia Meridionale alla metà del secolo XVIII, in "Annali di Statistica", VI, XIX, Roma, 1931, Tables XXXVI and XXXVII.

NOTES: Data refer to children still living at home.
Both "abbienti" and "non abbienti" are included in the wealth category of less than 10 ounces of gold; only "abbienti" qualify as having 10 or more ounces of gold.

degree of wealth of the father.[4] The distinction of the heads of household among "abbienti" and "non abbienti" (broadly translated as "haves" and "have nots") gives the results reported in Table 6.2, which confirm the higher number of children in the better-off families. These data are also shown in Figure 6.2.

However, the distinction between "have" and "have not" did not satisfy de Meo as a criterion for classification of the population according to wealth. In fact, a number of proprietors of very small concerns, often extremely poor, had been included among the "haves." A further classification of the population in two extreme classes, on one side, the "have nots" together with proprietors of wealth worth not more than 10 ounces of gold and, on the other, proprietors whose wealth was worth 10 ounces or more of gold yields the results shown in Table 6.3.[5]

[4] G. de Meo, "Distribuzione della ricchezza e composizione demografica in alcune città dell'Italia Meridionale alla metà del secolo XVIII," *Annali di Statistica* VI, no. XIX, Roma, 1931.

[5] The ounce, or *oncia*, is a monetary unit of the *Regno di Napoli*, see P. Villani, *Mezzogiorno*, pp. 111ff.

Here, again, the wealthy family heads—with only the exception of those aged 40-49—had a larger number of surviving children than the poor ones. The average number of children per head of family, standardized by age, was 3.16 for the "haves" and 3.18 for those with a wealth exceeding 10 ounces, against 2.65 for the "have nots," which becomes 2.68 if those with a wealth up to 10 ounces are added.

Data from the city of Bari, also studied by de Meo, substantially confirm the findings for the city of Castellammare.[6] Here the households were subdivided according to the degree of wealth; as shown in Table 6.4, the results again demonstrate that as the level of wealth increases, the average number of living children also increases.

TABLE 6.4

MEAN NUMBER OF CHILDREN PER HEAD OF HOUSEHOLD, BY WEALTH OF FAMILY, CITY OF BARI: 1753

Wealth of family	Average number of children: Actual	Average number of children: Standardized by age
"Non abbienti"	2.02	2.02
Less than 15 ounces of gold	2.34	2.27
15 - 100 ounces of gold	2.53	2.29
100 - 300 ounces of gold	3.34	3.22
More than 300 ounces of gold	4.39	3.18

SOURCE: G. DE MEO, Caratteristiche demografiche di classi economicamente differenziate in una città italiana del secolo XVIII, in "GENUS", I, 3-4, 1935, Table VIII.

NOTES: Data refer to surviving children still living at home. "Non abbienti" may be translated as "have not".

Similar results are found for the city of Lecce in 1753, where the average number of children per head of household (standardized by age) was 1.89 for the poorest class and 2.16, 2.25, and 2.77 for the other classes with increasing degrees of wealth.[7]

[6] G. de Meo, "Caratteristiche demografiche di classi economicamente e socialmente differenziate in una città italiana del secolo XVIII," *Genus* I, nos. 3-4 (1935).

[7] G. de Meo, "Variazioni nell'assetto economico-demografico di una città dal XVII al XVIII secolo," *Genus* III, nos. 1-2 (1938).

DIFFERENTIAL FERTILITY

This sample of three cities of the South confirms that wealth was associated with a larger number of surviving children in the eighteenth century. Data for Bari exclude the possibility that this might be due to an earlier age at marriage for the rich, who, at least as far as males were concerned, seemed to have married later than the other classes. Referring to the classification adopted in Table 6.4, the proportion single at age 20-29 was 38.3 percent for the lowest class, and 39.3, 64.3, and 79.6 percent for the other classes with increasing degree of wealth.

6.2.4. At the beginning of the nineteenth century, a census of the city of Torino, elaborated by Muttini-Conti still seems to show a larger number of surviving children in the families of higher socioeconomic conditions.[8] This is shown in Table 6.5. The higher professional group had considerably more children, with an average of 1.93 against 1.18 for the lower group; the difference remains considerable if the data are calculated for only families with at least one child (2.85 against 2.25).

TABLE 6.5

DISTRIBUTION OF FAMILIES BY NUMBER OF CHILDREN IN HOUSEHOLD, BY ECONOMIC ACTIVITY OF FAMILY, TORINO: 1802

Number of children	Professional, liberal arts families		Worker families	
	Number	Percent	Number	Percent
0	180	32.3	240	47.6
1	112	20.1	100	19.8
2	92	16.3	69	13.7
3	63	11.3	46	9.1
4	51	9.2	32	6.4
5	24	4.3	13	2.6
6	11	2.0	3	0.6
7	8	1.5	1	0.2
8	10	1.8	--	--
9	2	0.4	--	--
10 and more	4	0.8	--	--
Total	557	100.0	504	100.0

SOURCE: G. MUTTINI CONTI, UN censimento torinese nel 1802, Torino, 1951, Table Xa.

NOTE: Data refer to surviving children still living at home.

[8] G. Muttini Conti, *Un Censimento torinese nel 1802*, Torino, 1951.

However, all four factors described in Section 6.2.1 are likely to be involved in determining the differences between these two groups, since we know nothing about the age distribution of husbands or wives.

These few examples—referring to different historical periods, regions, and types of enumerations—can scarcely be considered proof of a general proposition concerning a direct relationship between the number of surviving children and socioeconomic level. They do provide evidence of such a connection, however, and, lacking further statistical evidence, we may provisionally accept it as true, at least until the beginning of the nineteenth century. Italy is, moreover, exceptionally rich in nominative enumerations of all kinds in the past centuries, and it would be only a matter of patience to add further evidence on the subject.

There are interesting implications of differentials in actual family size according to socioeconomic level. In the first place, if the motivation for restricting the family size has any relationship, as we believe it has, with the pressure that a larger number of living children exerts on couples from the economic, psychological, and even physical view, then one reason to expect a reduction in fertility to first appear among couples on the higher part of the social ladder, as in fact happened, is simply the larger size of the family. In the light of these demographic considerations, the complex theory of the differential growth of the various social classes and of its consequences on social mobility and social stability could find, as it has in the past, new grounds for discussion. Here, again, Dumont's theory of social capillarity could find new material for a more modern reformulation. For our purposes it may be sufficient to retain the following points:

(1) The more favored sectors of the population had a higher number of surviving children.
(2) The fact is probably due to the effects of differential mortality and, in some instances, to differences in age at marriage.
(3) The possibility of higher marital fertility of the richer families cannot be ruled out.

6.3 *The Modern Times*

6.3.1. During the nineteenth century, the situation described in the preceding paragraph became gradually reversed. Fertility started declining in a few limited and, as far as we know, privileged sectors of the population. In Chapter 1, we analyzed and discussed the lower fertility of the aristocracy and of a religious minority (the Jews) during the nineteenth century. There is also clear evidence that the urban population practiced birth control to a larger extent, perhaps as a consequence of the heavier incidence of families with a more privileged standard of living.

Statistical evidence of an early decline of fertility among the more privileged, which starts during the nineteenth century, is very poor and scanty. We have to wait until 1931 to find the reliable and comprehensive results of the fertility survey attached to the census of that year. The survey clearly shows the inverse relationship between fertility and the social and economic level of the family that had been developing during the nineteenth century and the first decades of the twentieth.

In spite of the shortage of comprehensive information before 1931, all scholars who had been devoting attention to population problems knew very well that a strong and inverse relationship was clearly established between the level of fertility and the "standard of life" of the family. Their knowledge derived from direct and indirect evidence. Indirect evidence was linked to:

(1) The experience of other European populations where fertility declines had developed along with large class differentials.

(2) The fact that fertility had declined at a faster rate and earlier in some of the more developed areas of the country.

(3) The finding of an inverse association, in the urban areas, between the level of wealth of different sections of various cities and the level of the birth rate. Benini, Colajanni, Gini, Livi, Nitti, and others had given substantial evidence on this fact.[9]

This fairly substantial direct evidence was, moreover, consistent with the few limited and fragmentary surveys; thus further support was gained for the opinion that control of fertility was exerted with different strengths in the various segments of the population.

[9] F. S. Nitti, *La popolazione ed il sistema sociale*, Torino-Roma, 1894. R. Benini, *Principi di Demografia*, Firenze, 1901 (pp. 273ff.). N. Colajanni, *Statistica e Demografia*, Vol. II, *Demografia*, Napoli, 1909. L. Livi, "Sulla natalità differenziale in Italia," *Economia* 10, nos. 8-9 (1927). C. Gini, "Alcune richerche italiane sulla riproduttività differenziale," *Economia* 10, no. 12 (1927). For later periods, see also N. Federici, *La riproduttività differenziale*, Roma, 1939. L. Maroi, *Nuovi elementi sulla fecondità della città di Roma, Proceedings of the Fourth Meeting of the Società Italiana di Demografia e Statistica*, Firenze, 1940, II: 63-73. G. Giurovich, "Sulla natalità differenziale delle varie classi sociali a Roma nel primo trentennio del secolo XX," *Genus* X, nos. 1-4 (1953-1954).

The new trends had an interesting effect on the structure of the family. Until the beginning of the nineteenth century, the richest families apparently had the highest number of surviving children in the household; a century later the reverse was true. The increasing control of fertility in the wealthier sectors of the population more than offset the effects of lower infant mortality (which had started falling in the less privileged classes as well). The effects of higher age at marriage, which is evident for some higher professional sectors of the population in the second half of the nineteenth century, also contributed to the lower fertility of the wealthier classes.

The implications are evident. Until the beginning of the nineteenth century, the rich carried the burden of larger families; during the nineteenth century and at the beginning of the twentieth, as the more privileged classes learned how to control their fertility effectively, the burden of larger families passed to the poor, with consequences that everybody can understand. This process of change is shown in the next few pages.

6.3.2. A survey carried out by the *Ministero di Industria, Agricoltura e Commercio* on May 31, 1882, among the civil and military employees of the government provides a source for an analysis of fertility differentials.[10] The survey was intended to collect elements for the detailed study of the financial burden of pensions on the government. For every employee, information was collected on "christian and family name, the current career level, the year of birth and the year of entry into the career itself, the amount of salary . . . , marital status and the year of marriage, the year of birth of the wife (or husband) if living and of the children (if surviving), but only the minors if males and the single if females." The survey combined stepmothers with mothers, and therefore no distinction was made between the children belonging to the first or to the following marriage. The economic and financial importance of this veritable census made necessary a number of checks and corrections often unknown in surveys made for purely demographic reasons. The results have to be considered, therefore, highly reliable.

One of the tabulations is especially interesting for our purposes, since it gives the number of surviving children by age (males below 21 years and single females) and by age of the wife and qualification of the husband. This tabulation is doubly useful to us. In the first place, knowing

[10] DIRSTAT, *Statistica degli impiegati e dei pensionati dello Stato*, part 1, Annali di Statistica IV, Roma, 1884.

for each age of wife the distribution of surviving children (by age), it has been possible, with the help of an appropriate estimate of mortality (the national life table of 1881–1882), to calculate the number of children ever born.[11] But since the tabulation included only sons under 21 and single females, we have considered only the women above 30 (who were not too young, and who had completed already a substantial part of their final family size) and below 40. Women under age 40, given the prevailing high age at marriage, must have had only a negligible proportion of married daughters or emancipated sons. With regard to the national life table of 1881–1882, we may only say that it might have overestimated the mortality of our group, which, after all, was a privileged one. However, in 1881–1882 mortality had already slightly improved over the mortality levels of the preceding decade, when a large part of the children involved in our calculations were born, and this probably offsets the effects of the better sanitary conditions of our group. The results of the computations are reported in Table 6.6, where the enumerated number of surviving children and the estimated number of those ever born is shown for every category of employees.

The estimated average number of children born was 3.34 for women aged 30-34 and 3.89 for women aged 35-39. It is possible that the figure for the latter group may be slightly underestimated because of the unknown, but small, proportion of children left out because of males reaching age 21 or daughters becoming married. This bias is, at least for this age group, partly compensated by the inclusion of children born in the preceding marriage of the husband. The 3.89 children ever born at an average age of 37.5 years corresponds, at the fertility levels of the times, to 4.5-4.6 children ever born at the end of the reproductive period. The women considered, being 35-39 years of age in 1882, were born in the 1840s, before mid-century. The mean fertility level of the time (as can be deduced from the number of children ever born to women married once, husband present, born before 1871 and enumerated in 1931) was 5.84 children, with a minimum for Piedmont (5.12) and a maximum for Puglia (6.35). Therefore the estimated completed family size of government employees' wives was 23 percent below the average Italian level, 12 percent below the level of the region with the lowest fertility, and 29 percent below the region with highest fertility.

[11] C. Gini and L. Galvani, *Tavole di mortalità della popolazione italiane*, Annali di Statistica VI, Vol. VIII, Roma, 1931. The book contains the revised tables for 1881-1882.

TABLE 6.6

MEASURES OF FAMILY SIZE, CIVIL AND MILITARY GOVERNMENT EMPLOYEES: 1882

	Employees with wives aged 35-39				
	Surviving children		Estimated ever-born children		
Position	Absolute number	Average per family	Absolute number	Average per family	N
Accountants	1,309	2.57	2,098	3.97	529
Employees					
High rank	2,115	2.87	3,410	3.81	895
Low rank	3,639	2.47	5,775	3.84	1,504
Manual workers	2,294	2.47	3,630	3.94	921
Justice	1,867	2.49	1,160	4.13	452
Diplomacy	29	2.42	46	2.88	16
Education	963	2.36	1,538	3.94	390
Armed Corps	1,046	2.19	1,677	4.61	364
Army Officers 1	444	2.12	716	3.53	203
Army Officers 2	812	2.11	1,294	3.38	383
Privates	95	1.81	151	3.36	45
Total	13,906	2.44	22,202	3.89	5,702
	Employees with wives aged 30-34				
Accountants	1,179	2.52	1,827	3.22	567
Employees					
High rank	1,869	2.76	2,905	3.37	862
Low rank	3,502	2.08	5,378	3.23	1,666
Manual workers	2,116	2.22	3,248	3.31	981
Justice	1,077	2.16	1,674	3.93	426
Diplomacy	26	2.10	40	3.08	13
Education	1,011	2.17	1,563	3.44	455
Armed Corps	973	1.81	1,515	4.34	349
Army Officers 1	455	1.92	716	2.85	251
Army Officers 2	1,010	1.46	1,562	2.98	525
Privates	102	2.00	151	2.16	70
Total	13,320	2.16	20,579	3.34	6,165

SOURCE: Based on data reported in DIRSTAT, Statistica degli impiegati e dei pensionati dello Stato, Part 1, in "Annali di Statistica", IV, Roma, 1884

NOTE: Data include any of husband's children born prior to current marriage and living with the husband.

The category of government employees belonged, on the average and with some relevant exceptions at both margins, to the middle class. They were representative of the various regions of the country, probably with a certain predominance of people born in large cities. The fact that their completed fertility was almost one-fourth below the average fertility level of the Italian women of the same time reveals the existence of clear-cut class differentials in fertility.

DIFFERENTIAL FERTILITY

As for the differences in fertility between the various categories of government employees, the interpretation of the data on this point is less certain. Six out of the 11 categories have a homogeneous family size at age 35-39, estimated between 3.8 and 4.1 children. Of the other five groups, the armed forces (officers and privates) had a lower family size (3.4-3.5); this is probably due to the prevalent higher age at marriage. Wives of diplomats, as a rule belonging at that time to the aristocracy or rich bourgeoisie, had the lowest family size (2.9), but the number of cases is very small and the result probably not very significant. Armed corps (firemen, police, etc.) had the largest family size (4.6), and they occupied the lowest section of the ladder within the government employees. Therefore, fertility differentials seem to act mostly in the expected sense.

Another way of proving the lower fertility of the government employees is the following. The tabulations give, by age of mother, the number of surviving children by age (the date of birth of the surviving children was asked). We have taken the surviving children under age 1, and, through the appropriate coefficient derived from the 1881–1882 life table, we have estimated the number of children born in the 12-month period preceding the date of the survey. An analogous procedure has been followed for estimating the number of births in the preceding 24 months through the number of surviving children under age 2. With the age distribution of married women, we have computed the age-specific marital fertility rates reported in Table 6.7.

TABLE 6.7

ESTIMATED AGE-SPECIFIC MARITAL FERTILITY RATES, WIVES OF CIVIL AND MILITARY GOVERNMENT EMPLOYEES: 1882

Age of wife	Rate estimated from surviving children aged: Less than 1 year	1 to 2 years
Less than 25	305	284
26-30	285	278
31-35	208	224
36-40	144	151
41-45	54	63
46-50	8	9
Average, all ages	175	174

If we take the second estimate (which, being based on two birth-cohorts, is probably safer) as a reference for comparisons, we may observe that the general rate of marital fertility was, for the employees, 174 against 250 for the general population (in 1881–1882), or 30.3 percent less. The computation of I_g gives a value of .461 for the employees against .648 for the Italian population, or 28.9 percent less. The differences are about the same, around 30 percent below the average Italian level of the times. Finally, our data can give still further information. Using the second estimate in Table 6.7, we can calculate the hypothetical (period) number of children of a government employee's wife getting married at age 25, by summation of the age-specific marital fertility rates. This calculation gives 3.25 children per woman getting married at age 25, which can be compared with the estimated final family size of 4.5-4.6 children for government employees' wives born in the 1840s. Even assuming (but the evidence points to the contrary) that the age at marriage was one or two years below age 25, the final family size would not be larger than 3.5-3.8 children per woman. This fertility level remains well below that achieved by women born in the 1840s, and this finding informs us that the fertility of our group of women was rapidly falling. Summing up, we may conclude:

(1) That the fertility of government employees' wives was one-fourth or one-third below the fertility of Italian women of the times.
(2) That the differentials ascertained between the various categories of employees are mostly in the expected sense: higher categories seem to have had lower fertility and vice versa.
(3) That, at the beginning of the 1880s, the fertility of the group under consideration was rapidly going down.

6.3.3. Other scattered information gives some further idea as to the nature of fertility differentials at the beginning of the century. Savorgnan, for instance, studying the fertility of European aristocracies, has shown that among the Italian families in Gotha Almanach, the mean number of children was 2.14 for each marriage concluded between 1890 and 1910.[12] These marriages had been observed until 1926 and had a duration of at least 17 years. Over one-fourth of the marriages (27 percent) remained childless; only 23 percent of them had four or more children;

[12] F. Savorgnan, "La fecondità delle aristocrazie," *Metron*, IX, no. 1 (1931); see also Savorgnan's book of the same title, which includes this and other essays on the same subject (Pisa, 1942).

age at marriage was 31.7 for males and 25.9 for females, about 2.5 and 1.0 years above the average age of all Italian spouses in the same period. The very small number of marriages (only 126) and the very peculiar characteristics of the group studied limit the results to little more than a curiosity. However, it is interesting to note that the contemporary Italian marriage cohorts had a mean number of children around five.

Of a quite different nature are the data collected and published, in 1907, by the *Ufficio del Lavoro* (Bureau of Labour) concerning miners and their families.[13] The survey was carried out "with the help of a questionnaire sent to all mining concerns." The questionnaire, besides information on sex, age, marital status, salary, qualification, etc., asked information about the number of surviving children who presumably (the survey does not say so explicitly) were living with their parents at the moment of the survey (January 1906). Table 6.8 reports some basic data.

TABLE 6.8

PERCENTAGE OF MINE WORKERS SINGLE, CHILDLESS, AND HAVING LARGE FAMILIES, AND MEAN NUMBER OF CHILDREN, BY AGE: 1906

Age	Single (percent)	Childless (percent)	5 or more surviving children (percent)	Number of surviving children (mean)	N
15-20	96.6	43.2	0.5	1.19	11,116
21-29	60.6	33.5	1.1	1.13	12,582
30-39	19.3	15.5	6.8	2.20	10,375
40-49	10.0	11.6	24.7	3.23	7,514
50-59	7.4	12.7	29.8	3.42	3,765
60+	5.8	16.4	25.5	3.13	1,182
All ages	52.7	18.0	14.5	2.45	46,534

The data, for lack of elements for comparison, do not go beyond a simple description of the demographic structure of miners' families. An attempt to draw some conclusions as to the fertility level of this professional group can nevertheless be attempted.

13 Ufficio del Lavoro (Ministero di Agricoltura, Industria e Commercio), *I lavoratori delle miniere*, part 1, "Età, famiglia, occupazione, reddito," Roma, 1907.

If we take the age group 40-49, the average number of surviving children is 3.23. Making a few assumptions as to the average duration of marriage and to the age distribution of the surviving children and to the level of mortality, 3.23 surviving children correspond to 5.34 children ever born. Assuming that the average age of the miners considered was near 45 years, and that wives were three to four years younger, the mean age of wives must have been above 40: let us assume they were 41 years old. The estimated completed family size must have been, therefore, around 5.8 children per married couple. Since 84 percent of the surveyed miners came from three regions (Toscana, 12 percent; Sicilia, 49 percent; and Sardegna, 23 percent), their completed family size of 5.8 children can be compared with regional data from the 1931 census, from which we have calculated the weighted average of the number of children ever born to women married once, husband present, belonging to comparable generations (60 years and more at the 1931 survey, therefore born before 1871). The 5.8 children of the miners compare with the 5.9 children of the women of corresponding ages among the three regions: the two estimates are, therefore, almost identical.

The conclusion of this rather elaborate estimate is that the fertility of one of the less favored professional sectors—that of miners—cannot be distinguished from the fertility of the general population. On the other hand, the fertility of more privileged sectors of the population, such as the aristocracy or government employees, had clearly gone down by the end of the century. However, because of the low weight of these sectors in the total population, the general level of fertility of the entire Italian population was not affected in a visible way before the end of the nineteenth century.

In short, privileged sectors had a lower than average fertility, but the poor and disadvantaged ones did not have a tangibly higher than average one.

6.3.4. Later in the 1920s, the *Istituto Centrale di Statistica* carried out a nationwide survey on large families,[14] defined as "those families which at the end of June 1928 had had at least 7 live born children." Over 1.5 million of these families were surveyed and distributed according to the profession of the head of the family. We have reported below the

[14] C. Gini and A. Ferrarelli, "Altri risultati delle indagini sulle famiglie numerose," *Metron*, XI, no. 1 (1933): 67-109.

incidence of large families in each professional group (or among the families whose head belonged to a given professional group, the proportion having seven or more live born children):

Profession	*Percent*
Agriculture	23.3
Industrial workers	19.8
Proprietors, etc.	18.4
Servants and kindred workers	12.7
Entrepreneurs, industry, and commerce	7.1
Without profession	5.5
Army officers, clerical workers	4.5
Liberal arts, etc.	4.1

The interpretation of the proportions reported above is not simple. The proportion of famillies with seven or more children in the various professional groups depends on many factors, including the age structure of the various groups (the older the structure, the higher the proportion, other factors held constant). The differences, however, are so strong that they certainly reflect differences in the actual fertility of the various professional groups. If we exclude the category "proprietors, etc.," there is a clear inverse relationship between the social and economic level of each group and their fertility level, here very imperfectly measured by the proportion of large families.

6.3.5. The 1931 census gives the first comprehensive survey of fertility we have in Italy.[15] Unfortunately its special report on fertility gave more emphasis to various aspects of fertility by age, marital status, birth order, etc., than to fertility differentials. However, the available tabulations do not leave any doubt as to the nature, amplitude, and direction of the differentials themselves. In Table 6.9, we give the distribution, by profession of the husband and by number of children ever born,[16] of women with the following characteristics: over 45, married once, married before age 25, husband present. These women, for the most part, were born in the quarter century following the unification of the country and had

[15] ISTAT, *Indagine sulla fecondità.*

[16] L. Galvani, "Fecondità completa della donna italiana," *Notiziario Demografico*, VIII, no. 8 (1935). P. Battara, *Considerazioni sulla prolificità dei matrimoni secondo la condizione sociale dei capofamiglia, Proceedings of the Fourth Meeting of the Società Italiana di Demografia e Statistica,* Firenze, 1940, II: 58-68.

TABLE 6.9

PARITY DISTRIBUTION, WOMEN AGED 45 AND OVER, BY OCCUPATION OF HUSBAND: 1931

	Parity (percentage distribution by occupation)									Number of children	
Occupation	0	1	2	3	4	5	6	7-9	10+	Mean	Median
Agriculture:											
Self-employed	4.0	2.1	3.8	5.8	8.0	9.7	11.0	33.9	21.7	6.90	6.43
Dependent workers	4.9	2.6	4.5	6.5	8.5	9.9	11.4	22.5	18.4	6.56	6.14
Commerce, Industry, Artisans:											
Self-employed	6.5	4.2	7.0	9.1	9.8	9.7	9.7	25.8	18.3	6.08	5.38
Dependent workers	5.6	4.1	7.3	9.5	10.4	10.6	10.4	26.6	15.5	5.93	5.24
Clerical workers, etc.	8.5	8.2	14.1	14.6	12.5	9.8	8.0	16.1	8.2	4.48	3.37
Professionals, Liberal arts	9.2	8.4	14.8	14.1	12.8	10.1	7.3	15.3	8.0	4.38	3.28
Not in labor force	7.3	4.4	6.9	8.3	9.3	9.5	9.5	27.1	17.7	6.04	5.46
All occupations	5.2	3.3	5.6	7.5	9.0	9.9	10.5	30.1	18.9	6.41	5.90

NOTE: Data refer to women married before age 25.

achieved their final family size before the end of World War I; they all had spent at least 20 years of their fecund life in a continuous marital state.

The data leave little doubt as to the existence of fertility differentials. As expected, families belonging to the primary sector had the largest family size and the lowest sterility; at the other end of the social ladder, wives of people engaged in professional activities, liberal arts, etc., had a family size over one-third smaller and a level of sterility more than two times greater than the peasant. Differentials are far more evident in the median family size, which varied between 3.28 (professionals, liberal arts) and 6.43 (agriculture); the differences in the modal family size are even more striking (2 versus 7).

Unfortunately, the tabulation is available only at the national level; for studying territorial professional differentials we have to be content with a lower degree of precision and detail. Table 6.10 gives the average number of children ever born to married women of all ages according to the profession of the husband for four large geographical areas and for two classes of comuni.

It is obvious that the average number of children of women of *all ages* combined is influenced by the varying distribution of women by age and duration of marriage in each professional group. It is evident, in particular, that an older age-duration structure leads to a higher fertility because average parity increases with age and duration of marriage and becuse older women belong to generations that, in a period of currently falling fertility, had experienced the higher fertility of the past. Differences, however, are so strong that it is awkward to impute them to differences in age structure, with the sole exception of the group not belonging to the labor force because of the high incidence of retired workers. Table 6.10 and Figure 6.3 show the existence of a very marked inverse relationship between professional status and fertility in the four geographic subdivisions and the two classes of comuni. Families engaged in agriculture have, everywhere, the highest fertility, while the lowest fertility is that of the wives of clerical workers, etc., in the North and in the Center, and of the wives of professional workers, liberal arts, etc., in the South and in the Islands. It is worth noting that differentials—as might be expected—are more marked in the North and in the Center than in the South and in the Islands. In the North, the differences between the family size of the most and of the least fertile groups is 2.6 children, in the South only 1.5. Even more interesting is the fact that

TABLE 6.10

CHILDREN EVER BORN, BY OCCUPATION AND RESIDENCE OF HUSBAND: 1931

Occupation	Geographical area				Class of comune		Italy
	North	Center	South	Islands	More than 100,000	Less than 100,000	
Agriculture:							
Self-employed	4.67	4.15	4.79	4.61	4.66	4.59	4.59
Dependent workers	4.12	3.57	4.11	4.24	4.51	4.06	4.08
Commerce, Industry, Artisans:							
Self-employed	3.27	3.28	4.61	4.27	3.19	3.83	3.71
Dependent workers	2.97	3.00	4.12	4.05	2.96	3.41	3.27
Clerical workers, etc.	2.06	2.22	3.39	3.08	2.19	2.66	2.42
Professionals, Liberal arts	2.29	2.31	3.29	2.93	2.31	2.78	2.60
Not in labor force	4.46	4.15	5.30	5.07	4.19	4.85	4.66
All occupations	3.68	3.53	4.45	4.29	3.03	4.08	3.90

NOTE: Data refer to mean number of children ever born to married women of all ages with husband present.

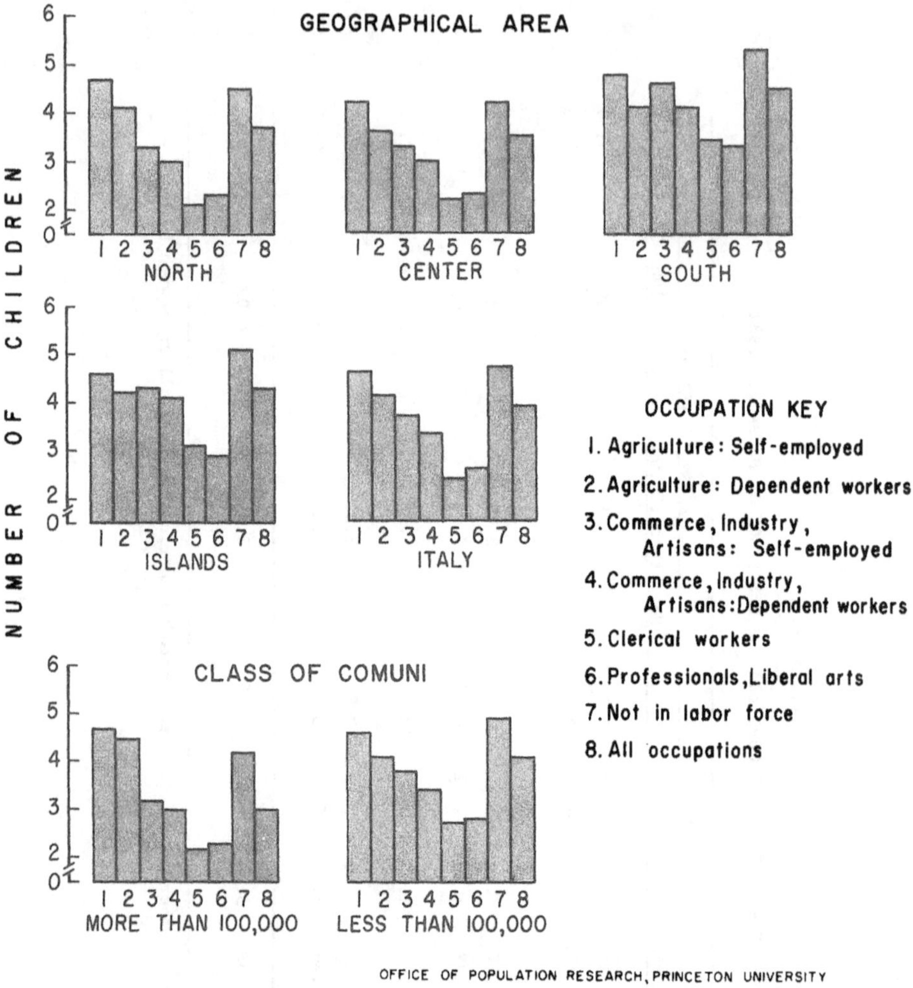

Figure 6.3 Children Ever Born, by Occupation and Residence of Husband: 1931

in the South and in the Islands, 89 percent of the married women considered had an average family size between 4.1 and 4.8 children. It is only among the "white collar" wives—slightly more than one-tenth of all women—that family size falls to about three children. In the North and in the Center, on the other hand, in addition to the "white collar" groups, the category of industrial workers, accounting for one-fourth to one-third of all women, had a family size around three, against four and over for the other categories.

It is also interesting to note that there is more difference between the family size of a white collar worker's wife in the North and in the South than there is, within the South, between a white collar worker's wife and a peasant wife, at least in relative terms. The data confirms the analysis of Chapter 4, where we found that territorial variability of fertility is, in the South and in the Islands, much lower than in the rest of the country. In this body of data it is evident that the populations of the Mezzogiorno—at the time of the survey—were much more homogeneous than in the rest of the country with respect to the fertility of different professional groups.

6.3.6. Thirty years later, the 1961 census shed new light on fertility differentials.[17] The tabulation of census results has been limited, for comparative reasons, to women married once and before the age of 45. We will present and comment on data on the mean number of children per woman, by birth cohort, according to education and main sector of activity.

Table 6.11 contains data on the fertility performance of women with different occupational and educational characteristics, by cohort. It is tempting to give a historical interpretation to the varying performance of women born in different years, but this can be done only with a certain degree of caution. Even considering only women with completed fertility (up to the cohort of 1912–1916), it is obvious that differential mortality according to age, socioeconomic status, and number of children is likely to introduce a great deal of unknown distortions. Second, while the level of education is relatively stable throughout life, the same cannot be said of occupational status; women not belonging to the labor force are more represented among older women and many women not belonging to the primary sector have, in fact, only recently abandoned the agricultural sector and may have spent part of their married life in a rural setting.

Taking in mind these precautions, an examination of Table 6.11 reveals many interesting facts. First, the decline in the mean number of children between the oldest and youngest cohort with completed fertility (those born before 1886 and in 1912–1916) is greater among women not belonging to the labor force than among women in agriculture or in

[17] ISTAT, *Indagine sulla fecondità*, "Note e Relazioni," Roma, 1974, n. 50.

TABLE 6.11

CHILDREN EVER BORN PER MARRIED WOMAN, BY OCCUPATIONAL STATUS AND EDUCATION: COHORTS OF PRE1886 TO 1942 AND LATER

		Occupational status			Degree of education				
Cohorts	Total	Agriculture	Other sectors	Not in labor force	University and high school (Class 1)	Junior high school (Class 2)	Primary school (Class 3)	Less than primary school (Class 4)	Illiterate (Class 5)
Pre1886	4.38	4.50	3.05	4.39	2.33	2.41	3.97	4.36	5.07
1887-1891	4.17	4.52	3.13	4.17	2.13	2.10	3.74	4.20	5.04
1892-1896	3.82	4.35	2.89	3.82	2.14	2.01	3.47	3.97	4.83
1897-1901	3.73	4.42	2.75	3.72	2.16	2.04	3.45	4.09	4.88
1902-1906	3.58	4.39	2.63	3.57	2.12	2.08	3.34	4.09	4.91
1907-1911	3.30	4.13	2.37	3.30	2.07	2.02	3.04	3.87	4.71
1912-1916	3.01	3.69	2.21	3.03	2.05	1.98	2.81	3.67	4.44
1917-1921	2.72	3.27	2.01	2.77	1.98	1.88	2.60	3.45	4.22
1922-1926	2.40	2.82	1.75	2.46	1.81	1.75	2.31	3.06	3.74
1927-1931	1.98	2.26	1.40	2.04	1.47	1.50	1.92	2.53	3.08
1932-1936	1.42	1.60	0.89	1.48	0.96	1.05	1.36	1.83	2.24
1937-1941	0.89	0.97	0.49	0.94	0.55	0.64	0.87	1.18	1.43
1942 and later	0.57	0.51	0.37	0.60	0.35	0.46	0.55	0.68	0.80
Total	2.64	3.06	1.70	2.71	1.67	1.61	2.43	3.31	4.26

SOURCE: Census of 1961.

NOTE: Data refer to mean number of children ever born to women married once and before age 45.

the secondary and tertiary sector. Women not belonging to agriculture, in all but the youngest cohort, have the lowest fertility (about 1.5 children less than women in the primary sector). The ratio between the fertility performance of women in agriculture and women in the other sectors remains of the same order of magnitude in the various cohorts (mostly between 1.5 and 1.8).

More interesting are the data by education of women, as indicated by Classes 1 to 5 corresponding to decreasing levels of education (Class 1, university or high school degree; Class 5, illiterate).[18] Considering only cohorts with completed fertility, differences between the oldest and youngest cohorts are almost nil for Class 1, weak in Class 2 (the youngest cohort has .4 children less, on the average, than the oldest cohort) which also has the lowest fertility; very large in Class 3 (1.2), and then decreasing again for the less educated (.7 and .6 children for Classes 4 and 5). About one-third of the total difference of 1.4 children between the oldest and youngest cohorts is attributable to the change in educational structure; indeed, had this remained the same, the mean number of children of the cohort born in 1912–1916 would have been 3.44 instead of 3.01. It is also worth noting that women born before 1886 and with a high degree of education had achieved fertility levels—given the prevailing mortality—below replacement; on the other hand, the youngest cohort with the lowest degree of education was still not too distant (10 to 20 percent below) from premodern levels of fertility.

The most striking result is the persistence of very large fertility differentials; the ratio of the fertility performance of women belonging to Class 5 to women belonging to Class 1 has remained unchanged in all cohorts. The reduction of fertility differentials in the general population, therefore, is due to the equalization of social and educational characteristics rather than to the equalization of fertility behavior of women belonging to different social strata. This is an important finding because it shows that the lack of a systematic policy in the population field—in Italy, the persistence of legislation opposing the dissemination of in-

[18] The census asked the degree achieved and not the number of years of school completed. Class 1 includes the university and high school degrees; Class 2, the equivalent of a junior high school degree; Class 3, the primary school degree (after 5 years of primary school); Class 4, women who could write and read and, therefore, had some years of school but did not achieve the primary school degree; Class 5, women who were illiterate. The census underestimated the level of education, because the years of school completed without a degree were not considered.

formation on family planning—cannot check the general fertility decline, but it does tend to maintain unchanged fertility differentials among the different social strata.

6.3.7. Tables 6.12 and 6.13 present the same data for five geographical areas (we have split the North into Northwest, including the three regions of the industrial triangle [Piemonte, Liguria, and Lombardia],

TABLE 6.12

CHILDREN EVER BORN PER MARRIED WOMAN, BY OCCUPATIONAL STATUS AND GEOGRAPHICAL AREA: COHORTS OF 1887-1891 AND 1912-1916

Cohort	Area	Agriculture	Other sectors	Not in labor force	Agriculture relative to other sectors
1887-1891	Northwest	3.31	2.31	3.35	143.3
	Northeast	4.11	3.09	4.50	133.0
	Center	4.42	2.62	3.73	168.7
	South	5.12	4.46	5.04	114.8
	Islands	4.53	3.68	4.64	123.1
	Italy	4.52	3.13	4.17	144.4
1912-1916	Northwest	2.29	1.66	2.44	138.0
	Northeast	2.67	1.99	2.68	134.2
	Center	3.05	2.04	2.63	149.5
	South	4.34	3.59	4.03	120.9
	Islands	3.71	3.15	4.00	117.8
	Italy	3.69	2.21	3.03	167.0

SOURCE: Census of 1961.

NOTE: Data refer to mean number of children ever born to women married once and before age 45.

and Northeast). The geographical analysis confirms—with the necessary variants—the conclusions drawn on the basis of the national data. Fertility differentials, particularly by educational levels, are very strong in all areas.

It is also interesting to note that, while the fertility performance of women classified by profession of husband in the 1931 fertility survey had shown a much lower variability in the South and in the Islands than in the rest of Italy, this does not happen when women are classified by educational level 30 years later. Although variability for the older cohort born in 1887–1891 is slightly lower in the South and in the Islands in relative terms, this is not true in absolute terms: educated women have

TABLE 6.13

CHILDREN EVER BORN PER MARRIED WOMAN, BY EDUCATION AND GEOGRAPHICAL AREA: COHORTS OF 1887-1891 AND 1912-1916

Cohort	Area	University and high school (Class 1)	Junior high school (Class 2)	Primary school (Class 3)	Less than primary school (Class 4)	Illiterate (Class 5)	Total	Illiterate relative to university and high school
1887-1891	Northwest	1.91	1.87	3.31	3.52	4.52	3.33	236.6
	Northeast	2.05	2.13	4.30	4.76	5.30	4.48	258.5
	Center	2.05	1.95	3.26	3.61	4.55	3.73	222.0
	South	2.67	2.83	4.66	4.88	5.33	5.04	199.6
	Islands	2.49	2.71	4.14	4.46	4.97	4.63	199.6
	Italy	2.13	2.10	3.74	4.20	5.04	4.17	236.6
1912-1916	Northwest	1.86	1.72	2.36	2.73	4.04	2.32	217.2
	Northeast	2.04	1.91	2.70	3.11	3.86	2.72	189.2
	Center	1.99	2.01	2.52	2.90	3.47	2.60	174.4
	South	2.33	2.68	3.82	4.33	4.72	4.07	202.6
	Islands	2.33	2.54	3.69	4.24	4.79	3.93	205.6
	Italy	2.05	1.98	2.81	3.67	4.44	3.01	216.7

SOURCE: Census of 1961.

NOTE: Data refer to mean number of children ever born to women married once and before age 45.

2.5 children less than illiterate ones in these two areas as in the rest of Italy. Education seems to be a more sensitive explanatory variable than profession.

On the other hand, women of the South and of the Islands have a higher fertility than women of corresponding educational level in the rest of the country. In the youngest cohort with completed fertility (1912–1916) the mean number of children per woman in the South was .5 higher than in the Northwest for Class 1, and, respectively, 1.0, 1.5, 1.6, and .7 for Classes 2 to 5. These differences are also evident in younger cohorts with incomplete fertility; for example, women in Campania born in 1927–1931 (30-34 years old in 1961) had a much higher mean number of children than women of the same age in Piemonte (.4, .8, 1.0, .8, and .4 more for Classes 1 to 5). In practice, territorial differences for the same educational level have remained constant even for women who achieved their fertility in the decade before 1961.

We have, on several occasions, discussed the peculiar behavior of the populations of the South, where fertility differentials are lower than elsewhere and where the levels of fertility have remained higher than in other areas, even controlling for several typical socioeconomic variables. What seems to be at work is the force of residual factors, which we cannot measure statistically. Attachment to traditions; a more extended and tightly knit family system; the stronger weight of social control; the lack of women's emancipation; the weight of the often very conservative teaching of the church—these are some of the manifold factors of the Southern culture. These aspects seem to affect, in a degree not appreciably different, all sectors of the population without regard to income, profession, or residence.

Territorial data show also that the inverse relationship between educational level and fertility performance is gradually changing. Table 6.13 shows that in some areas women with the highest education do not always have the lowest fertility. But some special tabulations of the census returns for the cities of Bologna and Firenze give a very clear picture of the changing relations between education and fertility in urban and socially advanced communities.[19] In Bologna (see Table 6.14) there is

[19] A. Bellettini, *Alcuni risultati di una ricerca sulla fecondità delle donne coniugate in una popolazione urbana, Proceedings of the Twenty-seventh Meeting of the Società Italiana di Statistica,* Palermo, May 1972. C. A. Corsini, *Aspetti della fecondità completa delle fiorentine secondo il Censimento demografico del 1961:*

TABLE 6.14

AGE AT MARRIAGE, NUMBER OF CHILDREN, AND PERCENTAGE CHILDLESS, MARRIED WOMEN AGED 45 AND OVER, BY EDUCATION AND BIRTH COHORT, BOLOGNA: 1961

Measure	Education (years)	-1884	1885-1894	1895-1904	1905-1914	1915+	All cohorts
Mean age at marriage	0	25.5	26.7	27.3	26.4	23.5	26.4
	1-3	26.5	26.7	26.6	25.9	24.7	26.4
	4-5	28.2	28.0	27.3	26.7	25.8	27.0
	6-8	29.8	30.2	29.4	28.3	27.1	28.6
	9-13	30.4	29.9	30.4	29.8	28.5	29.9
	Total	27.2	27.6	27.5	26.9	26.1	27.2
Mean number of children	0	3.29	2.28	1.76	1.58	1.96	2.22
	1-3	3.05	2.18	1.77	1.56	1.55	1.94
	4-5	2.45	1.84	1.54	1.45	1.34	1.57
	6-8	1.97	1.68	1.59	1.53	1.37	1.56
	9-13	1.76	1.52	1.66	1.64	1.74	1.65
	Total	2.77	2.00	1.63	1.50	1.41	1.71
Percentage childless	0	18.6	29.8	35.5	35.5	17.3	29.5
	1-3	21.0	25.6	30.9	28.8	24.4	27.6
	4-5	19.9	27.0	29.0	26.0	23.0	26.3
	6-8	23.5	33.6	34.8	26.4	26.7	28.8
	9-13	38.3	33.0	33.3	29.6	19.1	30.7
	Total	21.1	27.5	30.6	27.2	23.3	27.2

SOURCE: A. BELLETTINI, Alcuni risultati di una ricerca sulla fecondità delle donne coniugate in una popolazione urbana, XXVII meeting of the Società Italiana di Statistica, Palermo, May 1972, Tables 5, 6 and 7.

NOTE: Data refer to females born and residing in Bologna in 1961.

an evident inverse relationship between fertility and the degree of education in the cohorts born before 1895, while a U-shaped curve is evident for the following cohorts. For women born in 1905–1914 the variability of fertility was extremely low, ranging from 1.45 to 1.64; in the following cohorts, the fertility was lowest for women of intermediate levels of education, and the more educated ones had a family size perceptibly larger (1.74 against 1.34). These data are graphically shown

Riflessione sulle ricerche sulla fecondità dei centri urbani, Proceedings of the Twenty-fifth Meeting of the Società Italiana di Statistica, Bologna, 1967. On recent aspects of differential fertility, see also M. de Vergottini, *Indagine sulla fecondità della donna al Censimento del 1961*, Pisa, 1969; M. Livi-Bacci, *Recent Trends of Italian Fertility*, IUSSP General Conference, London, 1969.

in Figure 6.4. Similar conclusions can be drawn on the basis of the data for Firenze (see Table 6.15).

The cases of Bologna and Firenze are probably typical of the urban

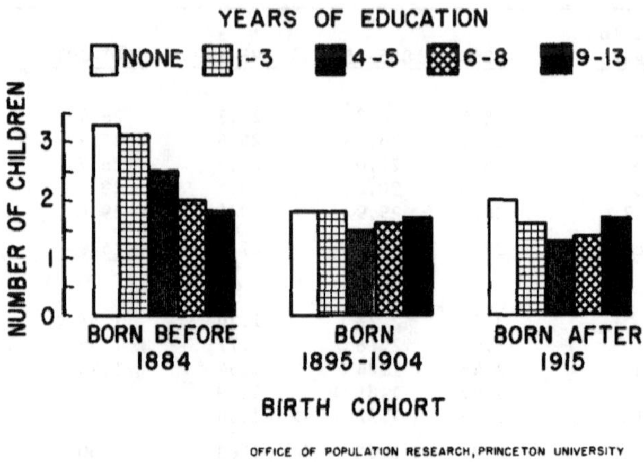

Figure 6.4 Mean Number of Children, Married Women Aged 45 and Over, by Education and Birth Cohort, Bologna: 1961

and advanced areas of the country, where family size is very low (well below replacement) and variability of the fertility performance much more reduced than in the rest of the population.

TABLE 6.15

CHILDREN EVER BORN TO MARRIED WOMEN AGED 50 AND OVER, BY EDUCATION AND BIRTH COHORT, FIRENZE: 1961

Education (years)	Birth cohort -1890	1890-1900	1900-1910
Less than 5	2.49	2.08	2.04
5 - 8	1.86	1.66	1.78
More than 8	2.00	2.07	1.91
Total	2.22	1.90	1.88

SOURCE: C. A. CORSINI, Aspetti della fecondità completa delle fiorentine secondo il censimento demografico del 1961. Riflessioni sulle ricerche sulla fecondità dei centri urbani, in Proceedings of the XXIV Meeting of the Società Italiana di Statistica, Bologna, 1967, p. 781, Table 6.

NOTE: Data refer to mean number of children born to married women living with their husbands.

6.5 *Conclusion*

A cycle is coming to an end. The relations between children and the family have undergone a number of changes since the times of the Florentine Catasto in the fifteenth century. When mortality rates were still quite high, the rich family at any given moment of its cycle had a higher number of surviving children than the poor one. The higher survival rate of children in rich families was responsible for this fact, although the influence of differential fertility cannot be ruled out. But, whatever the causal factors might have been, differentials went in the right direction since the poor had a lighter burden of family size.

During the nineteenth century, the situation gradually changed. Wealthier families started controlling—or exerted a stricter control over—their fertility, giving birth to a decreasing number of children, and gradually offsetting the influences of differential mortality. The number of surviving children for any given age of father or mother, first leveled off and then reversed the traditional relation. In the later nineteenth and in the twentieth century poor families had a larger number of both ever born and surviving children.

Changes have continued. Differential mortality has become unimportant. Fertility differentials are narrowing; the inverse relationship between fertility and the socioeconomic level of the family has disappeared, giving way to a U-shaped relation. It is not unlikely that, following the precedent set by other populations, the level of fertility may be in the future a positive function of family wealth and income. Certainly this is a new and more modern situation. But, from another point of view, it is a new logical equilibrium, one which was probably firmly established before the nineteenth century, and lost during the last one or two centuries.

CHAPTER 7: Some Fertility Determinants: Biological Factors, Family Structure, and Selected Characteristics of Italian Society

7.1 *Unanswered Questions*

"The life of the peasant can be quickly described. In the first months of his infancy, swaddled in such a way as to risk suffocation, he is abandoned to the custody of some child a few years older, until the time when, able to move about without help, he romps in the dust and mud of the farmyard with his playmates.

"Still at a tender age, he is sent to the communal school in the winter and begins to work during the summer, when, as a first task, he is required to watch after the ducks and the pigs, and, later, the cattle.

"When he reaches the age of 20, he faces the most important steps of his life: military conscription and marriage. Every country girl is certain to find a husband, as every young man is certain to find a wife, even when nature has not spared him some physical imperfection. This does not mean indifference in the choice, since in that class the art of appealing is very well known. But at the end, the girl of marriageable age does not want to condemn herself to a long wait. She brings always some dowry, usually the bed and a lot of goodwill to work and procreate many offspring.

"Subsequently the life of the peasant does not experience much change, except for an increasing number of offspring, who from early adolescence, take an active part in the economy of the family. There is much weeping for the dead and, in general, still more drinking after the funeral ceremony. . . . Much respect is kept for the memory of the loved one."[1]

This synthetic portrait of peasant society and life in Lombardia was written by Jacini in 1857; in a few lines, the main characteristics of a pre-industrial society, centered around the essential events of life, are vividly described. The question before us, however, is whether knowledge of the personal lives of individual men and women, and their values, attitudes, and interrelationships would not indeed be very helpful in the interpretation of a century and a half of demographic behavior.

[1] S. Jacini, *La proprieta' fondiaria e le popolazioni agricole in Lombardia*, Milano and Verona, 1857, pp. 102-103.

Unfortunately, this is not a question that the demographer alone can answer. At the same time, it would be naive to believe that a more detailed sociological portrait of nineteenth-century Italy would provide the key to the explanation of several obscure points of Italian demographic history. We would like, however, to escape one of the traps of empirical research: that of eluding the discussion of factors that do not lend themselves to quantitative measurement under the assumption that *quod non est in numero non est in mundo*, or of factors whose relationship with the main object of investigation—reproductive behavior in our case—is not firmly proved.

This chapter is, therefore, devoted to the discussion of topics that somehow do not find a place in classic fertility analysis but are certainly related to fertility. We shall discuss three main topics. The first concerns the nature of some of the biological factors of fertility; the second, the structure of the family; and the third, factors peculiar to the Italian situation that have delayed the process of fertility reduction and increased fertility differentials. These three topics could be easily expanded on the basis of further multidisciplinary research based on the existing, but incompletely explored, material.

7.2 *On the Biological Factors of Fertility*

7.2.1. In a population in which contraception is still rare, the role of biological factors in explaining fertility differentials is very important. Social as well as biological factors may have been the cause of variability (only a negligible fraction can be explained by the traditional social and economic indicators usually employed), but it is impossible from our present knowledge to estimate their respective share with any precision. Moreover, even if predecline variability had not been very large, it is true that the Italian population, as well as other Mediterranean ones, had a level of marital fertility below that found in other European populations. Again, the sources of these differences are partly social and partly biological, in unknown proportions.

In this section, we will try to assemble the available information concerning some biological variables of fecundity, such as the age at puberty and at menopause, the diffusion and duration of breastfeeding, and the factors possibly related to sterility. The combination of these factors and others, including the incidence of intrauterine mortality, may be responsible for part of the variation of fertility and for part of its departure from the level prevailing in other populations during the predecline period. Unfortunately, the source and quality of our information are very disparate, and it is therefore risky to give a global estimation of their possible impact. The omission of this material would, however, be more serious than its too bold presentation.

7.2.2. Onset and termination of fecundity have a certain degree of variability as a consequence of the biological characteristics of each population and of the environmental conditions at large. Demographers simplify the problem by assigning conventional age limits for the computation of indexes and rates, but the lower and upper limits of fecundity are set by the age of puberty and menopause. However, the precise knowledge of the age pattern of menarche and menopause is not enough. Ability to conceive does not appear with puberty but develops in parallel with the progressive biological transformation of the body after puberty. On the other hand, menopause indicates only the upper limit of age at which a woman becomes infecund but, in practice, infecundity takes place a few years before the termination of menstruation. Variations of the age pattern of menarche and menopause through time or among groups probably reflects variations in the age limits of fecundity, although the exact functional relationship remains unknown. The analysis of these factors may be important when fertility is not yet under the restriction of voluntary control and is, therefore, closer to the so-called "natural pattern." Age at puberty seems relatively unimportant, given the relatively high mean age at first marriage (about 23-24 years in Italy, at all times); more interesting is the age pattern of termination of reproductive capacity, which generally has a wider dispersion varying from the early 30s to the early 50s.

In 1872, the *Società Italiana di Antropologia e Etnologia* carried out a survey on some physiological characteristics of the Italian population. Although the methodology followed was far from being unbiased, some of the results are interesting since they constitute the only quantitative information available on puberty and menopause prior to the start of the decline of fertility. Territorial differences, even assuming the data to be unbiased, were not significant. As shown in Table 7.1, the mean age of menarche was around 15 years; at age 15, 63 to 74 percent of all girls had reached puberty; at age 18 practically all of them (96 percent) were menstruating. Marriages below age 18 were a small fraction of all marriages and the marriage of a girl below the age of puberty—owing to selective processes of precocious marriages—was certainly a very rare

TABLE 7.1

AGE AT MENARCHE, NORTH, CENTER, SOUTH AND ISLANDS, AND ALL ITALY: 1870s

	Percentage distribution within each area			
Age	North (N=992)	Center (N=647)	South and Islands (N=1,111)	Italy (N=2,750)
10	0.1	1.9	0.1	0.5
11	1.9	6.8	2.1	3.1
12	9.8	13.0	10.2	10.8
13	19.1	19.4	16.8	18.3
14	20.1	19.5	15.2	18.0
15	16.0	13.8	18.3	16.4
16	15.9	12.7	14.0	14.4
17	6.6	5.7	11.6	8.4
18	7.2	4.8	5.4	5.9
19	2.3	1.2	2.2	2.0
20 and over	1.0	1.2	4.1	2.2
Total	100.0	100.0	100.0	100.0
Mean age	15.19	14.65	14.44	15.16

SOURCE: E. RASERI, Materiale per l'etnologia Italiana, "Archivio per l'Antropologia e l'Etnologia", Vol. IX, Firenze, 1879, p. 280.

exception.[2] Indeed, there must be a good correlation between age at menarche and age at marriage, and territorial variations of the former ought to be taken into account in explaining variations of the latter.

More interesting, for our purposes, is knowledge of the curve of termination of female fecundity. We shall remember that menopause indicates the upper limit of age at which a woman becomes infecund; in practice, infecundity takes place several years before the termination of menstruation. In Table 7.2 are the data collected by Raseri drawn from the same survey.

Menopause seldom appeared before 35 years of age; by the age of 40, over 12 percent of women had definitely ended their fecund life, and by the age of 46 the proportion was close to 50 percent.[3] The mean age of menopause of about 46 years—assuming that the data are sound—is three to four years below the mean age observed, for instance, in contemporary American and French populations, and only slightly

[2] At the end of the nineteenth century it was reported that in Orune (Sardegna) it was not infrequent that girls were married as soon as they entered the period of puberty; examples were also quoted of marriages planned but not concluded because the wife was still in tender age. See *Atti della Giunta per l'Inchiesta agraria,* XIV, part 2, p. 326, Roma, 1884.

[3] Livi, *Le leggi naturali della popolazione,* pp. 65-66.

TABLE 7.2

AGE AT MENOPAUSE: 1870s

Age	Percentage Distribution	Age	Percentage distribution
35 and under	1.2	44	9.5
36	0.7	45	9.7
37	0.4	46	10.9
38	0.9	47	8.0
39	1.7	48	9.4
40	7.3	49	6.1
41	3.0	50	7.3
42	6.1	51 and over	11.8
43	6.0	Mean age	46.1

N=964

SOURCE: E. RASERI, Materiale per l'etnologia Italiana, "Archivio per l'Antropologia e l'Etnologia", Vol. IX, Firenze, 1879, p. 280.

above the levels observed in Punjab and in selected villages in India. Should it be proved that under different conditions of nutrition, climate, etc., termination of fecundity varies substantially, this might explain part of the premodern variability of fertility, especially in populations with a relatively high age at marriage. There are certainly grounds for further research in this area in cooperation with physiologists and anthropologists.

7.2.3. In recent times the relationship between the length of breastfeeding and fertility has been the object of much attention among demographers interested in the biology of fertility. The notion that breastfeeding contributes to extending postpartum amenorrhea and delaying the resumption of ovulation has been proved. A vast documentation has also proved that in many populations there was a conviction that during lactation the risk of becoming pregnant was considerably reduced. It has also been suggested that, in many instances, breastfeeding was coupled with sexual taboos.

The Italian population, as other Mediterranean populations, had a predecline fertility well below not only the empirical maximum (fertility of the Hutterites, etc.) but also below the levels commonly reached in many areas of Europe. It has been suggested that prolonged breastfeeding might have been one of the factors contributing to these differences. We have collected some information on diffusion and length of lactation. There is no attempt at completeness, but only an attempt to point the way for further analysis.

The fifteenth-century poet Francesco de Barberino sang "Lo suo lattar comune è dei due anni ma non si vol levar tutto ad un punto" (two years is the common duration of lactation, which cannot be all at once).[4] It is probable that the two-year period was not as common as the poet would believe. However, the existing evidence points out clearly that children were breastfed well into their second year of life. Fantini in his treatise on breastfeeding observes that it is a good rule that breastfeeding be prolonged until the milk becomes scarce, an event that might take place during the second or even during the third year.[5] He affirms that mothers and wet nurses should follow this rule and wean their children when they have 16 or 20 teeth; he adds that many hold the superstitious view that breastfeeding might be dangerous to the life of the child after his first year of life.

A good source of information is provided by the rules and policies followed by the charitable institutions for foundlings that existed in all major cities of the country and received a considerable proportion of all live births. Foundlings, generally abandoned by the mother or the parents in the first days of life, were initially nourished by wet nurses living in the hospital, and generally sent out to live with the families of wet nurses living in the countryside. Both resident and nonresident nurses were paid a monthly salary for breastfeeding; the hospital made sure also that the child was properly and continuously breastfed. During the period of breastfeeding, the monthly salary paid by the institutions was generally higher than the salary paid after the child was weaned. Accurate records were generally kept, and many have survived.[6]

In the *Spedale degli Innocenti* of Firenze, for instance, the length of breastfeeding was 18 months before the end of the seventeenth century; the duration was reduced to 15 months from 1700 to 1779, and then reduced again to 12 months "because that was the common duration

[4] Francesco da Barberino, *Reggimento e costumi di donne*, ed., G. E. Sansoni, Torino, 1957, p. 192.

[5] A. Fantini, *Discorso sopra l'allattamento dei bambini*, Venezia, 1794, p. 48.

[6] See, for instance, the sophisticated use that C. Corsini has made of these records in "La fecondité naturelle de la femme marieé: le cas des nourrices," mimeograph, Firenze, Dipartimento Statistico, 1973.

for mothers breastfeeding their own children."[7] Francesco Bruni, historian of this Florentine institution, also supplies interesting information regarding the required duration of lactation for wet nurses on the payroll of similar institutions in other cities at the beginning of the nineteenth century.[8] Nurses in Venice were requested to breastfeed children entrusted to their care for 12 months. The duration was the same in Padova, Siena, Pistoia and Lucca; it was 14 months in Roma and 24 in Perugia (Bruni, however, states that he "cannot see the advantages of such a long duration").[9]

According to Buffini, at the hospital for foundlings in Milano, breastfeeding lasted 16 months as of 1642; subsequently, in 1791, the duration was reduced to 12 months.[10] The same author reports that at the hospital for foundlings in Brescia children were breastfed for 18 months.[11]

In short, the experience of the charitable institutions tells us that the usual duration of breastfeeding was between 12 and 18 months, with some cases above the upper limit and none below. We can, of course, ask ourselves whether the regulations of these particular institutions reflected the customs of the general population. Abandoning illegitimate, and also legitimate, children to the care of the charitable institutions was a common procedure, often involving a substantial fraction (1/10 or 1/5) of all urban births. In view of the widespread dimensions of this phenomenon, we believe that the regulations of the institutions conformed to the prevailing customs. If any discrepancy can be imagined, we would be inclined to believe that breastfeeding would normally last longer in the general population, since charitable institutions had to pay a higher monthly salary to the nurse or adopting mother before the weaning of the child.

7.2.4. More extensive, although unsystematic, information was collected by the *Giunta per l'Inchiesta Agraria*, a parliamentary committee created

[7] *Ibid.*, p. 12.

[8] F. Bruni, *Storia dell'I. e R. Spedale di S. Maria degli Innocenti di Firenze e molti altri pii stabilimenti*, 2 volumes, Firenze, 1819.

[9] F. Bruni, *Storia*, Vol. II, pp. 259, 265, 288, 302, 305, 314 and 328. For Pistoia, the duration of 15 months is also given. See L. Bargiacchi, *Storia degli istituti di beneficenza, d'istruzione ed educazione in Pistoia e suo circondario dalle rispettive origini a tutto l'anno 1880*, Firenze, 1880, I: 257.

[10] A. Buffini, *Ragionamenti storici economici statistici e morali intorno all'Ospizio dei Trovatelli in Milano*, Milano, 1844-1845, Vol. I.

[11] A. Buffini, *Ragionamenti intorno alla casa dei Trovatelli di Brescia*, Brescia, 1841, pp. 64 and 136.

to inquire into the conditions of the rural classes in the 1870s, which presented the results of its investigations in volumes published between 1881 and 1885. We will refer to it as the *Inchiesta Jacini*, from the name of its chairman.[12]

Local experts were asked to compile monographs on the economic and social conditions of the rural classes in the various areas, and also to supply information on nursing habits and wet nurses. In many instances they provided very interesting material.

Duration of breastfeeding was reported to last normally only 10 months in Treviglio and Casalmaggiore (Lombardia) and over 12 months in Verolanuova (also in Lombardia). In Val d'Aosta weaning started between 15 and 20 months after birth, and, not uncommonly, after 24 months; the author (a doctor) expressly stated that "breastfeeding was deliberately prolonged in order to avoid pregnancy."[13]

In Verona (Veneto), breastfeeding lasted normally until the eighteenth month; again, the author of the monograph justifies the duration with "the hope to avoid pregnancy."[14] Eighteen months was also the reported duration for Viterbo (Lazio). In the Marche and in Umbria, breastfeeding was reported to last normally 15 to 20 months; here again it was stressed, "with the hope not to become fecund, a new way to follow Malthus's teaching."[15] From 14 to 16 months was the duration in Terlizzi and Modugno (Puglia). Moreover, the notion was widespread that infant mortality tended to be much higher among children of the same age who were not breastfed.

The use of *baliatico* was widespread in Italy, but occurred more in the Center and in the North than in the South and the Islands. Nurses breastfed foundlings entrusted to them by charitable institutions, or children of well-to-do families, particularly from the urban areas. In some instances nurses left their families and went to live with the child's family, but more frequently the children lived in the nurse's home. In general, the nurses were mothers of children who died in the first months of life. In some instances, however, their own children were weaned early; in others, their child was given to a neighbor who would nurse him for a low salary. In the latter case, the mother would then go to

[12] See *Atti della Giunta per l'Inchiesta Agraria*, 15 Volumes. Roma, 1881-1884.

[13] *Atti*, VI, part 4, p. 648 (Treviglio); *ibid.*, p. 733 (Verolanuova); VIII, part 2, p. 173 (Val d'Aosta).

[14] *Atti*, V, part 1, p. 203.

[15] *Atti*, XI, part 3, p. 218 (Viterbo); XI, part 3, p. 355 (Umbria and Marche); XII, part 2, p. 32 (Puglia).

nurse the child of a rich family in town where she would be paid a high salary, sufficient to pay for her own child's nurse and to remunerate herself with a small profit. In other cases, nurses would breastfeed children whose mothers were physiologically unable to nourish them, and part of the salary, for certain duration, was paid by the comune.

In many areas of Toscana children were generally weaned, at the beginning of this century, in the early second year of life, and the rural population was generally conscious that prolonged lactation was associated with longer birth intervals.

Late weaning was probably the common practice everywhere in Italy. The recommendations of doctors and hygienists point also in this direction. In 1881, Sormani, professor of hygiene in Pavia, gave the following recommendations: "Do not wean the child early, but only when he has his first 12 teeth—this is after his fifteenth or twentieth month of life."[16] Later, popular books on the nutrition of the child, advised weaning the child at the age of 1 year in spite of the fact that "the use of excessively long lactation prevails in many cases."[17]

7.2.5. During this century, in Italy and in much of the developed world, fewer mothers breastfeed their babies and, when they do so, the interval is shorter. It would be vain to retrace earlier habits in the current behavior, which is radically changed from that prevailing in the nineteenth century. However, a survey carried out by ISTAT in 1927–1928 on children dead during their first year of life gives an interesting picture of the situation in a period in which fertility was already under control in the Center and in the North, but in which the rest of the country had fertility levels still close to the predecline patterns.[18]

For every infant death (defined as deaths under 1 year of age) it was asked: (1) if the child was breastfed, and for how long; (2) whether lactation of the child was exclusively maternal or supplemented; and (3) if a supplemented nutrition system had been followed, the duration of breastfeeding.

This information, of course, gives only indications as to the breastfeeding habits of mothers whose children died before 1 year of age. The "sample" cannot be considered, therefore, representative of all

[16] *Atti*, VIII, part 1, p. 705.

[17] L. Colombo, *La nutrizione del bambino*, Milano, 1900, p. 101.

[18] ISTAT, *Movimento della popolazione secondo gli Atti dello Stato Civile nell'anno 1928*, Roma, 1932, pp. 157-175 and 285-324.

Italian mothers, since it is very likely that infant mortality was associated with breastfeeding habits. The association could work in two different ways:

(1) Directly, because mother's milk has to be considered healthier for the baby than other forms of nutrition; therefore in the universe of children who died in infant age, children never or only partially breastfed are to be considered overrepresented

(2) Indirectly, because we can assume that infant mortality was higher in the lower socioeconomic strata, where the habit of breastfeeding was more common. In this case, children ever breastfed are overrepresented

The two distortions work in opposite directions, but it is impossible to measure their importance.

In Table 7.3, data on infant deaths before the first year of age show the proportion who were breastfed in the 18 regions, in each region, in comuni with a center with 10,000 inhabitants or more, and in the rest of the comuni. The data show, in the first place, that an increasing proportion of children were breastfed going from North to South, the low being 41 percent in Trentino and the high 88 percent in Basilicata. In the second place, there is an evident difference between comuni including large, urban, centers and the other comuni. The proportion of children breastfed is substantially lower in the former than in the latter, in every region with the exception of Trentino.

The data of Table 7.3 not only show the existence of wide North-South and urban-rural differentials in breastfeeding habits but also give the impression that the differentials are influenced by the different stage of development of the various areas. In other words, it appears that the propensity to breastfeed children is a function less of customs related to remote traditions than of the socioeconomic status of the population. This last factor probably accounts for the lower propensity to breastfeed found in the mainly urban comuni as compared with the other mainly rural comuni.

The North-South differences in breastfeeding habits can be clearly seen in Table 7.4. Again using infant mortality data, we have reported the proportion breastfed by age at death. This proportion tends to decrease rapidly from the first to the third month, but seems to remain stable thereafter.

For children dead after the third month of life, the breastfed propor-

TABLE 7.3

INCIDENCE OF BREASTFEEDING FROM DATA ON INFANT DEATHS, BY REGION: 1927-1928

Region	Urban comuni	Other comuni	Total
Piemonte	45.0	63.4	59.5
Liguria	58.7	72.8	65.6
Lombardia	44.2	55.7	53.7
Trentino Alto Adige	43.5	41.0	41.3
Veneto	56.2	61.0	60.1
Venezia Giulia	53.1	70.6	66.0
Emilia	63.8	71.9	70.0
Toscana	67.1	75.6	73.5
Marche	69.1	80.0	78.5
Umbria	68.6	74.0	72.8
Lazio	68.8	84.8	79.2
Abruzzi	77.3	82.0	81.5
Campania	72.5	84.3	79.5
Puglia	78.6	86.2	81.5
Basilicata	87.9	88.3	88.2
Calabria	74.1	85.8	83.7
Sicilia	83.5	85.6	84.4
Sardegna	69.2	80.6	78.9
Italy	70.5	72.2	71.7

SOURCE: ISTAT, Movimento della popolazione secondo gli Atti dello Stato Civile nell'anno 1928, Roma, 1932, pp. 157-175 and 285-324.

NOTES: Data refer to percentage of infants dying under 1 year of age who were breastfed.

Urban comuni refer to those with a population center of 10,000 or more inhabitants.

tion remains slightly over 50 percent in the North and slightly below 80 percent in the South. North-South differentials remain substantially unaltered even controlling for age at death. It is interesting to note, however, that the incidence of breastfeeding is lowest among infants dead in the sixth month of life (North and Center) or in the fifth (South), with 52.7 percent and 75.2 percent; these proportions increase slightly thereafter. This peculiar trend leads to the conclusion that the proportion of breastfed children dying in the first year of life cannot be considered

TABLE 7.4

INCIDENCE OF BREASTFEEDING FROM DATA ON INFANT DEATHS, BY AGE AT DEATH OF INFANT, NORTH AND CENTER, SOUTH AND ISLANDS, AND ALL ITALY: 1927-1928

Age at death of infant	North and Center	South and Islands	Italy
0 - 1	82.8	96.3	86.6
1 - 2	70.2	85.5	77.8
2 - 3	63.4	81.8	72.1
3 - 4	58.0	79.1	67.6
4 - 5	53.7	75.2	63.4
5 - 6	52.7	76.7	63.8
6 - 7	52.9	78.1	65.2
7 - 8	52.9	78.1	65.3
8 - 9	53.7	78.4	66.0
9 - 10	52.9	78.5	65.9
10 - 11	52.8	80.7	66.7
11 - 12	54.8	80.1	67.2
Total	63.6	82.3	72.5

SOURCE: ISTAT, Movimento della popolazione secondo gli Atti dello Stato Civile nell'anno 1928, Roma, 1932, pp. 157-175 and 285-324.

NOTE: Data refer to percentage of infants dying under 1 year of age who were breastfed.

representative of the universe of breastfed children. Breastfeeding should decrease with the age of child instead of remaining stable or increasing after the fifth or sixth month of life. But because of infant mortality differentials, it is likely that after three or four months following birth, the proportion of infant deaths from low socioeconomic classes (with a higher propensity to breastfeed) increases, and therefore the proportion of breastfed babies among infant deaths (other factors remaining unchanged) also increases.

Table 7.5 again reveals substantial North-South differentials utilizing infant mortality data. (The high percentages at duration 11-12 months are due to the fact that many babies were breastfed up to the time of their deaths.)

In the Center and the North, 38 percent of babies dead in the twelfth month of life (with mixed nutrition) had been breastfed for 10 months

TABLE 7.5

DURATION OF BREASTFEEDING FROM DATA ON INFANT DEATHS, NORTH AND CENTER, SOUTH AND ISLANDS, AND ALL ITALY: 1927-1928

Duration (months)	Percentage distribution within each area North and Center	South and Islands	Italy
0 - 3	9.4	3.1	7.4
3 - 6	22.1	8.4	17.1
6 - 9	23.6	11.5	19.8
9 - 10	6.5	3.3	5.5
10 - 11	7.0	7.4	7.2
11 - 12	31.4	66.2	43.0
Total	100.0	100.0	100.0

SOURCE: ISTAT, Movimento della popolazione secondo gli Atti dello Stato Civile nell'anno 1928, Roma, 1932, pp. 157-175 and 285-324.

NOTE: Data refer to percentage breastfed among infants dying in the twelfth month of life.

or more; in the South, the proportion is 74 percent, nearly double that of the North and Center.

It is obvious that the large regional differentials in breastfeeding habits were the consequence of the different stages of development of the various regions; the correlation between the proportion of children dead in infancy who were breastfed and the proportion of women (aged 20 to 29 years) who were illiterate in 1931 is +.85. In the South, the habit of breastfeeding was very widespread, as is proved by the fact that 80 percent of the children dead toward the end of their first year of life were breastfed by their mothers.

The analysis of the unequal and scattered information on nursing habits presented in the preceding paragraphs may be summarized as follows:

(1) Breastfeeding had been a common habit until the end of the nineteenth century in all regions, and well into the twentieth century in the countryside and in the South.

(2) The normal duration of breastfeeding was probably between 12 and 18 months, with many exceptions above the upper limit.

(3) Mercenary breastfeeding was widespread, especially in the North and in the Center of the country.

(4) Women were conscious that prolonged lactation reduced fertility through a longer spacing of births.

7.2.6. The demographer wanting to provide a more complete background of the biological factors of fertility, particularly for the predecline period, would certainly try to gather material on abortion and its frequency and on diffusion of venereal diseases, especially those more likely to induce sterility. Information on sterility, if available, would also be of the utmost interest. The field is extremely wide and the result of deep investigation, particularly of hospital records, medical literature, etc., could be time-consuming and perhaps deceiving. But the interest of the subject is worth the risk.

As a mere curiosity, we have compiled Table 7.6, where we have reported the incidence of childlessness for cohorts born before 1881; the frequency of venereal diseases, and the resulting mortality; and the diffusion of these diseases among prostitutes. In the series reported in the table there is no assumption of an implicit cause and effect relationship, particularly between the diffusion of venereal diseases and sterility, which is very imperfectly measured by census data.[19] We will only note the high incidence of "registered" venereal diseases in certain regions (Liguria, Lazio, Umbria, and Campania), the high mortality of these areas due to syphilis, and the high frequency of prostitutes sent to venereal dispensaries in the South.

For the curious demographer, many questions remain unanswered. First, have venereal diseases and other infirmities had any effect on fertility and sterility? And if so, would the effect be sufficiently pronounced to depress the overall level of fertility? What was its impact on regional fertility differentials? Was the diffusion of prostitution responsible for the diffusion of venereal diseases and of contraception? In connection with the diffusion of contraception—and we are going beyond the mere discussion of the biological factors undertaken in this section—we will only remember that army doctors at the beginning of this century were very much worried by the diffusion of venereal

[19] This is the proportion of females, married once, aged 50-59 in 1931, without children ever born. This group contains women married at relatively old ages and therefore already unable to bear children, as well as women married young but with elderly husbands.

TABLE 7.6

STERILITY AND VENEREAL DISEASES, BY REGION: END OF 19TH CENTURY

Region	Percentage of wives aged 50-59 childless at 1931 Census	Venereal disease rate (average number of cases 1881-1883 per 100,000 population 1881)		Prostitutes sent to venereal disease clinics in 1885 per 100,000 females aged 15-49 in 1881	Deaths from syphilis per 100,000 population 1890-1892
		All diseases	Syphilis		
Piemonte	9.6	72.1	13.6	122.8	3.0
Liguria	11.4	122.0	22.5	280.6	4.0
Lombardia	7.9	69.6	6.3	110.8	7.0
Trentino Alto Adige	12.1	--	--	--	--
Veneto	7.5	77.2	15.4	108.0	4.0
Venezia Giulia	10.5	--	--	--	--
Emilia	9.0	104.9	20.4	150.1	5.0
Toscana	9.5	95.5	22.6	142.6	5.0
Marche	7.8	88.9	14.3	71.5	5.0
Umbria	8.1	171.4	32.5	107.7	13.0
Lazio	10.6	217.2	29.8	593.8	22.0
Abruzzi	8.2	85.3	9.3	146.2	10.0
Campania	9.7	204.5	21.7	353.4	12.0
Puglia	9.0	} 64.1	} 7.7	328.9	7.0
Basilicata	7.2			246.3	7.0
Calabria	7.8	98.7	18.4	335.9	14.0
Sicilia	9.8	141.6	19.5	537.5	7.0
Sardegna	10.6	66.5	7.9	163.9	2.0
Italy	9.1	109.4	18.3	247.3	7.0

diseases among soldiers, remarking that the men seldom used the existing "mechanical precautions" (condoms) in their contacts with prostitutes.[20] The rare use of condoms as contraceptives even with prostitutes induces one to believe that their use must have been much more rare in marriage.

In conclusion, a better knowledge of the biological determinants of fertility discussed above, and the study of the relationship of these variables among themselves and with nutritional and sanitary conditions may provide a better insight of the many questions raised in historical analysis.

7.3 *Marriage and the Family*

7.3.1. The structure of the family and the customs and traditions leading to marriage and family building, and the system of land ownership and of land transmission and its relationship to marriage and to family structure are all elements of great interest for reconstituting the socio-economic context within which reproduction took place. In this section we will present a few elements showing the possible interrelation between the marriage pattern, the structure of the family, and perhaps fertility itself during the nineteenth century.

Liberal changes during the nineteenth century, particularly after the unification of the country, eliminated many existing obstacles to marriage. In 1839, Cagnazzi, writing about the Regno delle due Sicilie, observed that "in other times, in order to preserve the wealth of the family, the practice of entailing the land to the eldest son was widespread . . . leaving to the others a very modest sum which condemned them to celibacy. . . . Nowadays, this practice has practically disappeared, except in very rich families, but the consequences are still with us, since the head of the family retains the right of entailing his wealth to the son selected for marriage."[21]

The monograph on Piemonte of the *Inchiesta Jacini* observed that since the 1848 Constitution granted by King Carlo Alberto "the laws abolishing impediments to marriage were passed in rapid succession. The custom of Maggiorascato . . . was abolished . . . ; the properties of

[20] E. Gilardoni, "Considerazioni sulla profilassi delle malattie veneree e della sifilide in specie nei militari," *Giornale di Medicina Militare*, LVIII, nos. 10-11 (1909): 861. See also F. Testi, "Sulla profilassi delle malattie veneree e della sifilide dei militari," *Giornale di Medicina Militare*, LVIII, nos. 4-5 (1910): 326.

[21] L. de Samuele Cagnazzi, *Saggio sulla popolazione del Regno di Puglia ne' passati tempi e nel presente*, part II, Napoli, 1839, p. 83.

the rich families were no longer bequeathed to the first born male child but were equally subdivided among the male children, contributing to the subdivision of land. Any check on the division of land was abolished in 1865 with the new civil code, which granted equal rights to males and females."[22]

In Susa, Piemonte, "in past times, when families had more children, only one of them got married, and others remained unmarried in order not to increase too much the size of the family living on the farm . . . but nowadays these limitations are not observed anymore."[23]

In Toscana "when both parents are dead, and the family is composed of several brothers, the unmarried one becomes head of the family; when at the death of the father all are unmarried, the elder has the choice between getting married or assuming the authority of head of the family. In the first instance, the second in age becomes head of the family, but he cannot get married."[24]

In this particular case, a specialization of functions is suggested. The farm cannot support too many people, and family limitation is practiced by the more classical observance of Malthusian teaching. Half a century before, Capponi had noted: "the population of Toscana has been increasing for some time, and it is increasing now, at the annual rate of 1 percent. It is true that this increase is lower among peasant families who, cautious and sparing, contract few improvident marriages. Confined to a limited space of land, they limit their family according to the size of the land."[25] The *Inchiesta Jacini* described the effects of land subdivision on the island of Elba, which was part of Toscana: "the peasant is not inclined to patriarchal life. His family is generally composed of few persons, and it could not be larger because of the subdivision of land, and as a consequence of his nature longing for freedom."[26]

In other instances, tradition tended to delay marriage. In Sardegna, "it is the custom to get married when the groom can take the wife in his own house, and . . . also a servant or poor peasant does not get married if, with his savings, he hasn't bought a house. It is considered a shame to take his wife to a home not belonging to the husband."[27]

[22] *Atti*, VIII, part 1, p. 454.

[23] *Atti*, VIII, part 2, p. 101.

[24] *Atti*, III, part 1, p. 456.

[25] G. Bowring, *Statistica della Toscana, di Lucca, degli Stati Pontifici e Lombardo Veneti e specialmente delle loro relazioni commerciali*, London, 1838, p. 44.

[26] *Atti*, III, part 2, p. 611.

[27] *Atti*, XIV, part 2, p. 326.

Age at marriage of Sardegna has always been significantly above the national average.

The nineteenth-century literature could certainly provide a very rich crop of information on the customs affecting marriage and the family. Writers of the time on economic and social problems made ample reference to marriage and family patterns. An extended survey on this subject would be, however, out of place in this book, since we do not have the means of testing the demographic consequences of the *Maggiorascato* or of the custom for brothers, exploiting the same farm, to reserve authority to one and marriage to the other. Only individual data and family reconstitution can provide an answer to the various hypotheses on the demographic impact of certain traditions or rules. We cannot therefore provide answers to classical questions such as: Are populations limiting growth with Malthusian means more or less prepared or receptive to contraception than those lacking Malthusian checks? Is subdivision of property an inducement to the limitation of family size?

The relationship between the size of the rural family and the size of the farm is shown in Table 7.7 for four geographical areas and all Italy. The data, taken from the agricultural census of 1930, indicate a close correlation between the two variables.

TABLE 7.7

MEAN NUMBER OF PERSONS PER FARM OWNER FAMILY BY SIZE OF FARM, GEOGRAPHICAL AREAS: 1930

Size of farm (hectares)	North	Center	South	Islands	Italy
Less than 0.5	4.1	4.1	3.8	3.4	4.0
0.5 - 1	4.3	4.1	3.9	3.4	4.0
1 - 3	4.9	4.6	4.4	3.6	4.5
3 - 5	5.7	5.7	5.1	4.0	5.3
5 - 10	6.8	7.0	5.8	4.4	6.4
10 - 20	9.0	9.0	6.6	4.8	8.3
20 - 50	9.2	9.7	6.3	4.9	8.5
All farms	5.5	5.7	4.5	3.8	5.1

SOURCE: ISTAT, Indagine rappresentativa sulle famiglie contadine imprenditrici, Rome, 1939, Table III.

NOTE: Data computed only for farms 50 hectares and less.

The results of the table must be accepted only with major qualifications, but it is evident that the size of the farm is closely correlated with the size of the family in the North and in the Center, and that this relationship is less clear in the South and especially in the Islands. In the latter area, families owning large farms could easily hire workers from the abundant and cheap labor force, but in the Center and in the North, where forms of crop-sharing between the owner and the farmer were prevalent, the family size had to be adequate for the tasks required by the size of the farm and vice versa. If the farm was large, it was generally worked by a large family: a nuclear one with many sons and daughters of working age, or an extended one with more than one nucleus living together. If the farm was small, then a small family would do. Generally, in the crop-sharing system, the farm unit was not subdivided. We can only speculate about the consequences of an increasing rural population with a fixed distribution of land; the effects can go in different directions since the responses to a similar situation might have been different, going from a more ready acceptance of family limitation to the emergence of permanent emigration. But where land was being more and more subdivided from one generation to the following, the creation of uneconomical holdings might have divergent effects: toward family limitation, toward emigration, or toward any combination of the two.[28]

On the other hand, the relative indifference of family size with respect to the size of the farm—in the South and particularly in the Islands—probably means that changes in land distribution might have exerted a very modest pressure on family size.

7.4 *Characteristics Peculiar to Italian Society*

7.4.1. It is perhaps superfluous to stress again that the battery of social and economic indicators employed for explaining the socioeconomic determinants of fertility trends and differentials is only an extremely crude and approximate tool for measuring the complex changes—of a social, economical, and cultural nature—in the attitude of individuals toward reproduction. In this section we want to stress the impact that certain particular features of the development of Italian society may have had on the rate of change of reproductive behavior and on the creation of fertility differentials.

[28] L. Livi, "Indagine sulla natalità in rapporto ai tipi di contratto agricolo dominanti ed al frazionamento della proprietà fondiaria," *Economia* VI, XII, no. 10, 1927.

In the first place, although the differential spread of social and economic development between the Northern and Southern portions of Italy increased greatly during the last decade of the nineteenth century, substantial differences already existed before the unification of the country. The indicators (reported in Table 5.2) show that the distance between the North and Center on the one side and the South and the Islands on the other in terms of industrialization, ruralization, infant mortality, and urbanization was not great. Only the level of illiteracy was significantly different in the two areas; thus, it is the only sensitive indicator that recalls in full the enormous distance in terms of social and cultural development that separated the two major areas of the country before and after unification.

Vigo has given a very complete account of the interrelationships between literacy, education, and economic development during the nineteenth century.[29] In his book, he shows the proportion of children aged 6 to 12 in school at mid-century. The differences are enormous. In the Regno di Sardegna these vary from virtually a universal education system in the provinces of Savoy (later annexed by France) to a system where hardly any children went to school in Sardegna (only 9 percent were enrolled). The maximum school attendance can be found in Lombardia, with 85 percent of children in school, and the minimum in Basilicata, with only 4 percent. These enormous differences are reflected in illiteracy. The 1848 census of the Regno di Sardegna reveals that the proportion of those who did not read and write in the total population above age 20 varied from slightly above 1/2 in the provinces of Savoy and to 95 percent in the province of Nuoro (Sardegna). In the same province, only 337 out of 61,479 women above age 20 knew how to read and write; illiteracy reached 99.5 percent. The situation of Sardegna is typical of the majority of the South.

After 1861, although the new unified state made a strong effort to increase education, regional differentials became more pronounced. The proportion in school increased from 67 percent in 1863 to 85 percent in 1901 in the North; from 28 percent to 50 percent in the Center; and from 22 percent to 44 percent in the South and Islands. Only between the two world wars did the achievement of near universal education start reducing the geographical differences.

Another factor that contributed to the isolation of the South prior to

[29] G. Vigo, *Istruzione e sviluppo economico in Italia nel secolo XIX, Archivio Economico dell'Unificazione Italiana* II, Vol. XVIII, Torino, 1971.

and after unification was the backwardness of its system of communication. In 1864, the average length of "provincial" and "national" roads per square kilometer varied between 10 and 16 km. in the regions of the Center and of the North to only 6.5 km. in the South, 9.0 in Sicilia, and 3.5 in Sardegna.[30] Before unification, no public money was spent on roads in Sicilia. The pace of railroad construction was also much slower in the South; of the 2,759 km. of tracks existing in 1864, only 334 were in the South, only 13 in Sicilia, and none in Sardegna. The disadvantage of the South and of the Islands was not eliminated until just before World War I, when the national network was practically completed.

The lack of two forms of mobility—mobility of people and circulation of ideas, via roads and schools—put the Islands and the South, in a disadvantaged position that lasted well into the twentieth century. If diffusion is an important component in the fertility decline, and, at the same time, cumulative in its nature, we may get some better understanding of the reasons behind the increasing fertility gap between North and South in the first decades of the twentieth century. Other evidence of the distance in terms of development already accumulated at the time of the unification between areas of the country ought to be brought into the picture; but this, perhaps, would not add much to the strength of our argument, which is intended to provide examples and not conclusions.

7.4.2. External migration is another factor that probably contributed to the slower fertility decline in the South. Until the 1870s, external migration originated mainly from the North and the Center. It consisted of seasonal workers, bricklayers, woodcutters, peddlers, artists, and farmers —people who emigrated both to other European countries, regions that from a geographic and cultural point of view were closer to their native areas and to the Americas. The South did not participate in this early phase of migration; mobility was extremely low not only before unification but also in the years immediately following. On the whole, the demographic impact of this early phase of migration in terms of net loss of population was relatively modest.

Mass migration started during the 1880s with the growing attraction of the labor markets in Brazil, Argentina, and, particularly, the United States. The bulk of transoceanic emigration, especially that with North

[30] Ministero dei Lavori Pubblici, *Statistica delle strade nazionali del Regno d'Italia 1.1.1864*, Torino, 1864.

American destination, came from the Southern regions. It was favored by the development of the system of communications, internal and maritime; by the elimination, with unification, of the legal and customary impediments to migration existing in the Regno delle due Sicilie; and by the economic crisis of the South during the later part of the century. Whatever the causes, the net outflow of migrants more than doubled between 1872–1881 and 1882–1891, rising from 378,000 to 845,000. These figures continued to increase, reaching 1,378,000 in the 1892–1901 period and 1,417,000 in the 1902–1911 decade. During the 1912–1921 period, in spite of the war, the net outflow was 903,000 (see Table 2.2). The number of total departures was about three times the net migration figure. In the following decades, emigration declined because of the restrictions to immigration introduced in the United States, the demographic policy of fascism, which disliked and restricted emigration, the world depression, and World War II. Later developments of emigration are less relevant to our argument. Emigrants, particularly those from the South, were essentially illiterate, poor peasants, predominately male at the beginning but soon followed, with a chain mechanism, by other family members and extended to the whole community of origin. The sociology and demography of Southern European emigration is too well known to justify a further description of its features. Moreover, we are interested in its consequences on the fertility of the population of origin.

These consequences were of a double nature. In the first place there were some direct, induced effects in the demography of the population of origin. The more the structure of the migrating population (age, sex, marital status) departed from the structure of the population of origin, the stronger the impact on the latter, given the same level of emigration. The population of the South bears the marks of mass emigration, as can be seen clearly from the censuses at the beginning of this century. These effects—at least the largest part of them—can be allowed for with the classic tools of demographic analysis: differential migration according to marital status does not affect the level of marital fertility rates; the standardization by age (I_g) takes care of the distortions in the age distribution; the elimination from the denominator of the marital fertility index of the estimated number of married women with absent husband eliminates the impact of the higher emigration of married men.

What we are interested in here are the indirect effects of migration. A classic scheme says that migration, particularly the transoceanic, mainly permanent migration we are talking about, was selective from a biological point of view. The hardships and length of the trip, the material obstacles to adaptation, and the screening of immigrants made by the host countries to prevent admission of bearers of particular diseases are all factors that worked in the same direction, discouraging or barring the departure of the unfit. With respect to fertility, this selective biological process (although the impact was probably hardly appreciable in quantitative terms) acts by depressing the level of fecundity and perhaps also of fertility in the population of origin. Quite a few proofs of this assertion exist. However, other selective mechanisms of a social and psychological nature are also put into action by emigration. It is very likely that emigration attracted those more inclined to change and innovation, those more receptive to new ways of life, those less adaptable to a static—and, of course, undeveloped—society. If this is true, there are two likely consequences that are closely interrelated. The population at the origin loses the elements more likely to be receptive to new ideas—these would include people willing to undertake innovations in their reproductive behavior. On the other hand, with emigration the society gets rid of its tensions, which are at the same time a liability—surplus manpower, for instance—and an asset—pressures likely to induce change. Emigration becomes, therefore, a factor of conservation in the population of origin; the social system, relieved of the mounting pressure of an increasing population, is deprived of an endogenous force of change. Traditional values and norms of behavior are less likely to change.

7.4.3. How true is this hypothesis formulated by sociologists and demographers? Unfortunately we cannot provide confirming evidence. It is true that most areas of Western and Mediterranean Europe with a delayed and slow decline of fertility are those with a long history of emigration. This is true for Ireland, for Northern Portugal, for Galicia and Andalusia in Spain, and for Southern Italy. Unfortunately emigration is also closely correlated with poverty, net effects on fertility are hard to measure. Another confirmatory element is represented by the migrants' ready acceptance of new fertility patterns. Italian women who immigrated into the United States, for instance, greatly reduced their fertility between 1910 and 1940, as can be seen by Table 7.8. These data, however, do not really show the great extent of fertility reduction, since a large part of fertility was completed before leaving the country of

TABLE 7.8

MEAN NUMBER OF CHILDREN EVER BORN, ITALIAN IMMIGRANT WOMEN, AGED 35-44 TO 65-74, UNITED STATES: 1910 AND 1940

Age	1910	1940	Change (percent)
35-44	5.6	3.9	-30.8
45-54	6.0	5.0	-16.7
55-64	5.8	5.6	- 3.2
65-74	6.0	5.8	- 4.2

SOURCE: Bureau of the Census, Population, Differential Fertility 1940 and 1950 - Women by Number of Children Ever Born, Washington, 1945, Tables 40 and 43.

origin. A combined use of census and vital data for the foreign-born allows the computation of general fertility rates for the Italian-born female population, 1920–1936 (Table 7.9). The fertility of Italian-born women, almost double of that of white American-born women in the

TABLE 7.9

GENERAL FERTILITY RATE, ITALIAN IMMIGRANT WOMEN AND NATIVE-BORN WHITE WOMEN, UNITED STATES: 1920 TO 1936

Date	General fertility rate		Ratio of Italian to native-born
	Italian	Native-born	
1920	206	109	1.89
1921	219	112	1.96
1922	207	104	1.99
1923	193	103	1.87
1924	186	104	1.79
1925	161	100	1.61
1926	150	96	1.56
1927	144	95	1.52
1928	137	90	1.52
1929	116	86	1.35
1930	137	86	1.59
1931	112	82	1.37
1932	100	79	1.27
1933	88	74	1.19
1934	78	76	1.03
1935	73	75	.97
1936	67	74	.90

SOURCE: M. LIVI-BACCI, L'immigrazione e l'assimilazione degli Italiani negli Stati Uniti secondo le statistiche demografiche americane, Milano, Giuffrè, 1961, p. 111.

early 1920s, dropped below the latter level in the mid-thirties during the great depression. In 1935 the standardized general fertility rate fell to 40 percent of its level in the early 1920s; during the same period, the index of overall fertility (I_f) fell by only 21 percent for the entire Italian population, and much less for the population of the South and the Islands, from which the majority of the emigrants came. One can wonder whether a decline of the proportion married might have been responsible for the rapid fall of general fertility; this is not the case, since given the large prevalence of males in the Italian-born population, the proportion remaining single has always been very low: only 2 percent and 1.3 percent for women aged respectively 35-44 and 45-54 years at the 1910 census; and 3.1 percent and 1.3 percent for the same age group at the 1940 census.

Although the use of period measures, especially if calculated for a group such as the foreign-born or for a period seriously affected by the great depression, may be a misleading way of assessing the fertility performance of a group of women, we cannot avoid inferring from the extremely rapid fall of general fertility a very ready acceptance among Italian-born women of birth control practices typical of American urban society. In a very short time span, the mainly illiterate peasant women of the South radically changed their fertility behavior. Later studies have proved that the American-born women of Italian descent had a fertility lower than that of other native Catholics. This difference of behavior could not be explained by the remoteness of the immigration of their parents or ancestors (which was, for the Italian, more recent), by socio-economic factors, or by the lesser degree of religiousness typical of the Catholic community of Italian origin.[31]

Data for Canada, although of more recent times, and therefore of less interest to us, seem to confirm the finding of a rather quick adaptability of Italian reproductive patterns, as proved by Table 7.10. The evidence, however, is not conclusive since the history and the structure of the various cohorts of the Italian-born is unknown; unknown also is the period of immigration and, therefore, the "exposure" to the new environment, and the age at marriage. However, in 1961 the Italian-born

[31] C. F. Westoff, R. G. Potter, P. C. Sagi, E. G. Mishler, *Family Growth in Metropolitan America*, Princeton, 1961, pp. 202-211. See also C. F. Westoff, R. G. Potter and P. C. Sagi, *The Third Child*, Princeton, 1963, pp. 102-107. C. F. Westoff, R. H. Potvin, *College Women and Fertility Values*, Princeton, 1967, pp. 147-148.

TABLE 7.10

MEAN NUMBER OF CHILDREN, ITALIAN IMMIGRANT WOMEN AND NATIVE-BORN WOMEN AGED 15-19 TO 65 AND OVER, CANADA: 1961

Age	Italian	Native-born	Ratio of Italian to native-born
15-19	0.4	0.7	.55
20-24	1.0	1.3	.73
25-29	1.6	2.2	.72
30-34	2.0	2.8	.72
35-39	2.5	3.1	.80
40-44	2.9	3.2	.89
45-49	3.2	3.1	1.02
50-54	3.8	3.2	1.20
55-59	3.9	3.4	1.15
60-64	4.1	3.7	1.11
65+	4.8	4.0	1.19

SOURCE: Dominion Bureau of Statistics, Census of Canada, Bull. 4.1.8, 1966.

had a lower fertility than the entire Canadian population in the ages below 40—representing the majority of women immigrating after the war. Those born in the 1920s, aged from 30 to 40 years at the 1961 census, will not have a completed family size exceeding 3.0 children, against more than 3.5 for the women who remained in the South and belonged to the same generation.

Similar suggestions can be drawn from L. H. Day's work based on a sample of the 1954 census of Australia. The median number of children of Italian-born women (children issued from the last marriage) was almost identical to the median number of children of Australian-born and British-born Catholics (Table 7.11). The geographic origin of the Italian immigrant, however, was predominantly Southern only after World War II; the women who arrived before the war had a more balanced geographic structure.[32] However, the relatively moderate level of fertility is much lower than one would expect had the immigrant women experienced the levels of fertility of their contemporaries who remained in the home country.

That the Italian-born are experiencing a rapid fertility decline is also

[32] C. A. Price, *Southern Europeans in Australia*, Melbourne, 1963, pp. 18-20.

TABLE 7.11

MEDIAN NUMBER OF CHILDREN BORN TO CATHOLIC WIVES, ITALIAN AND BRITISH IMMIGRANT WOMEN AND NATIVE-BORN WOMEN AGED 40-44 TO 60 AND OVER, AUSTRALIA: 1954 CENSUS

Age	Italian	British	Native-born	Ratio of immigrant births to native-born births: Italian	British
40-44	2.58	2.68	2.55	1.01	1.05
45-49	2.60	2.30	2.51	1.03	.91
50-54	2.52	2.97	2.68	.94	1.10
55-59	2.73	2.99	3.00	.91	.99
60+	3.93	3.49	3.75	1.04	.93

SOURCE: L. H. DAY, Fertility Differentials Among Catholics in Australia, The Milbank Memorial Fund Quarterly, XLII, 2, 1964, p. 70.

NOTE: Data refer to women married before age 26.

revealed by the following table, showing that general and marital fertility fell by 20 percent between 1961 and 1971 (Table 7.12). It is also interesting to note that the rapid reduction of fertility cannot be attributed to access to more efficient and safe contraception technology. An investigation in family planning carried out in Melbourne in 1971, found "a much wider use of withdrawal among those [wives] born in Southern Europe."[33] At the time of the survey, 74 percent of Greek-born contra-

TABLE 7.12

FERTILITY MEASURES OF ITALIAN IMMIGRANT WOMEN, AUSTRALIA: 1960-1962 TO 1970-1972

	Absolute levels			Relative levels (1960-1962 set at 100)		
Date	Birth rate	Overall fertility (I_f)	Marital fertility (I_g)	Birth rate	Overall fertility (I_f)	Marital fertility (I_g)
1960-1962	45.8	.326	.435	100	100	100
1965-1967	41.0	.298	.397	90	91	91
1970-1972	35.2	.261	.348	77	80	80

SOURCE: Bureau of Census and Statistics, Census of Population, 1961, 1966, and 1971.

[33] J. C. Caldwell and H. Ware, "The Evolution of Family Planning in Australia," *Population Studies* 27, no. 1 (1973), p. 25.

ceptors, 73 percent of Yugoslav-born contraceptors, and 54 percent of Italian-born contraceptors were using withdrawal, compared with a mere 5 percent of the Australian-born. Indeed, the Southern European, in general, made a significantly lower use of all artificial methods of contraception.

Similar conclusions were drawn by Girard and Stoetzel in their study of the assimilation of Italians who immigrated, mainly before World War II, into the Paris metropolitan area.[34] Italian women "uprooted from Italy and settled in the Paris agglomerates, although in the majority originating in the countryside, conform immediately [as far as family planning is concerned] to the new environment."

It is obvious that the ready acceptance of family limitation views in the society of immigration does not prove the existence of a mechanism of "psychological" selectivity in the migrating process. We do not know, in any case, what the reaction of the women who remained in their home villages would have been had they migrated into an advanced urban society.

Our hypothesis therefore remains suspended, awaiting further empirical demonstration. We believe that emigration has favored, in the South—perhaps also in other areas of the country (the Veneto, for instance)—the preservation of traditional modes of behavior and, therefore, of traditional fertility patterns. During the last quarter of a century, transoceanic emigration was replaced by European emigration and internal migration to the industrialized or urban areas of the North and Center. During this period, important advances were made in the South in terms of education, income, urbanization, etc.—advances, in absolute and relative terms, of unprecedented strength. Fertility has, of course, declined, but rather slowly, responding in a rather weak way to economic and social change. We believe that emigration, together with the slow modernization of the legal frame concerning fertility—which we will explain in the next section—is partly responsible for this.

7.4.4. During the Italian fascist regime, population was an important element of the government's policy.[35] Fascist policy advocated a fast

[34] A. Girard and J. Stoetzel, *Français et Immigrés*, INED, Cahier n. 19, Paris, 1953, p. 242.

[35] For a general view of the Italian population policy, see my essay "Italy," in B. Berelson, ed., *Population Policy in Developed Countries*, New York, 1974. Part of the text of pages 657-658 is reproduced here.

increase of population as a means of increasing power, in view of the many potentially declining European populations. Thus, emigration was discouraged, nuptiality and fertility stimulated, and the unity of the family sustained by an attempt to prevent the emancipation of women. People were discouraged from leaving the rural areas. From 1926 to World War II, a set of coordinated legislative and social measures were adopted in an effort to achieve a sustained growth or, at least, to check the fall of the rate of increase. It would be impossible to give a complete picture of the various aspects of this deliberate policy, which ranged from economic incentives to continuous propaganda at all levels; we will merely recall some of its main traits.

The first set of measures sought to increase nuptiality. A nuptiality allowance was introduced for those marrying before age 26. Loans were also available for young couples at a very low interest rate. The loan was partially canceled with the birth of children and completely canceled with the birth of the fourth child. These measures were coupled with several discouragements against celibacy. All unmarried males above age 26 and below the age of 65 were subject to a special tax, which increased with income. Married persons took precedence over unmarried persons in public employment, with respect to both hiring and promotion. In 1938, the state of marriage or widowhood was an essential prerequisite for being elected to an honorary or eminent public office, such as mayor (*podestà*), full professor in a university, or dean or principal in a public school.

Another important set of measures sought to stimulate fertility and the unity of the family. These were inspired by a commission, nominated in 1926, one of whose objectives was to ensure that "the order of the family system could be maintained against the many menaces of neo-Malthusianism, scientific and empirical." The ban against the spreading of contraceptives and birth-control information was instituted in 1926 and reinforced in the new penal code of 1931, together with severe penalties for induced abortion.

There were many fiscal inducements for large families, both in the case of personal income tax and inheritance tax. In 1934, a family allowance system was introduced; allowances increased with every additional child. A bonus was given at the birth of a child, and the sum increased with every additional birth. The number of children was a preferential factor in hiring and promotion for public employment. A few limitations to the employment of women were also introduced in an effort to protect the role of the woman in the family. Special public honors were granted to mothers of large numbers of children.[36]

Fascist policy discouraged emigration, which was also made difficult, if not impossible, by both the depression and the restrictions on immigration introduced in the United States. Schemes were, however, produced for emigration and settlement in the Italian colonies, particularly in Libya. These included the eradication of malaria and the subsequent effort to populate the areas. The regime followed a policy of slowing internal migration and the exodus from the rural areas. Citizens were prohibited from taking residences in comuni with 25,000 inhabitants or more or in comuni of special administrative or industrial importance, unless they could demonstrate that they had found permanent employment there.

In Table 7.13 we have assembled a few indicators of the financial inducements used during the 1930s. The effort was intensified in the late 1930s: the amount of exemptions for large families increased threefold for income taxes and twofold for local taxes; taxation of the unmarried more than doubled; and nuptiality and natality premiums, established in 1932, skyrocketed, as did marriage loans. On the whole the policy was well coordinated; it involved a considerable amount of financial resources and heavy pro-natalist propaganda at all levels.

The effectiveness of these policies is difficult to evaluate. Italy was in a period of very rapid fertility decline; in many areas of the North and the Center fertility was already below replacement; in the South and in the Islands the diffusion of birth control had started to produce its first visible effects. Complex pro-natalist policies such as the Italian one cannot offset long-term tendencies, especially if they are not pursued for a long time. World War II and the fall of fascism interrupted the pro-natalist policy only a few years after its full enforcement. Table 7.14 shows a few demographic indicators for the 1930s and for the marriage cohorts of the same period. The period measures of fertility show a remarkable stability during the years 1932–1940. However, the fertility of the marriage cohorts continued its steady fall throughout the period. This may be, to a certain extent, the effect of the World War I years, which negatively affected all cohorts in this series. But even

[36] A comprehensive review of the population policy of fascism is contained in the well-documented volume of ISTAT, "L'Azione promossa dal governo nazionale a favore dell'incremento demografico," Annali di Statistica VII, Roma, 1943.

TABLE 7.13

FASCIST DEMOGRAPHIC POLICY, SELECTED ECONOMIC INDICATORS: 1928-1931 TO 1939

	Provisions encouraging large families						Provisions encouraging marriage					
	Income tax exemptions		Local tax exemptions		Natality bonuses		Marriage bonuses		Marriage loans		Bachelor tax	
Date	Families (number)	Value in thousands of lira	Families (number)	Value in thousands of lira	Number	Value in thousands of lira	Number	Value in thousands of lira	Number	Value in thousands of lira	Bachelors (number)	Value in thousands of lira
1928-1931	27,586	7,882	--	--	--	--	--	--	--	--	--	--
1932	30,196	8,105	24,233	3,955	9,946	2,746	2,080	764	--	--	974	101,722
1933	30,583	8,338	31,394	4,895	15,721	4,405	6,885	2,195	--	--	1,027	104,841
1934	30,705	8,274	34,219	5,104	21,156	4,934	10,952	3,033	--	--	1,076	132,505
1935	30,401	8,138	38,338	5,296	72,065	36,673	38,553	27,073	--	--	1,115	165,975
1936	30,146	7,853	41,511	5,485	129,663	64,644	53,553	27,460	--	--	1,131	199,657
1937	29,945	7,605	45,247	5,830	160,223	74.914	59,717	42,926	7,554[a]	12,945[a]	1,139	209,349
1938	30,418	7,853	50,225	6,467	179,422	80,997	58,588	41,216	54,034	89,259	1,185	219,679
1939	--	23,251	55,961	7,053	191,635	86,304	65,172	55,718	55,078	89,497	1,287	230,426

SOURCE: ISTAT, L'azione promossa dal governo nazionale a favore dell'incremento demografico, "Annali di Statistica", VII, VII, Roma, 1943.

[a]Second half of year.

TABLE 7.14

FERTILITY MEASURES: 1930 TO 1940

	Period measures		Cohort measures			
Year	Total fertility (per 1000)	Mean number of children per marriage	Mean number of children (married 25 years)	Percentage childless	Number of children after 1-2 years of marriage	Percentage ever married by age 50
1930	3,507	3.61	3.28	14.1	.94	88.4
1931	3,329	3.38	3.23	13.5	.94	88.9
1932	3,169	3.29	3.22	12.6	.94	88.8
1933	3,150	3.33	3.14	12.8	.94	88.3
1934	3,104	3.30	3.07	12.9	.92	90.5
1935	3,085	3.29	3.01	14.1	.91	89.5
1936	2,966	3.19	2.93	12.6	.91	90.1
1937	3,030	3.23	2.83	13.0	.91	89.1
1938	3,162	3.28	2.75	12.6	.91	92.1
1939	3,166	3.31	2.71	14.2	.86	91.3
1940	3,172	3.31	2.70	12.7	.83	92.1

if we take the fertility in the first two years of marriage for these cohorts (thus, it would be unaffected by the war and probably much more sensitive to the effects of natality provisions and marriage loans), there is a considerable fall. The proportion childless, on the other hand, remained very nearly constant. The proportion married by age 50 also remained almost unchanged.

On the whole, the direct long-range effects of the fascist demographic policy seem to have been very modest, if any existed at all. We are convinced, however, that a strict statistical consideration of the problem understates the real impact of the policy, which has been more far reaching than suspected.

Twenty years of propaganda for a pro-natalist mystique have created a persistent reluctance, particularly at the public level, to take positive steps for recognizing and implementing the right to space and plan the number of children. The ban on birth control information remained in full effect until 1971. Even after this date, the extensive public health system ignored family planning. Contraceptives have always been widely available, but access to them has always been extremely uneven in the various social strata. The medical class has always maintained an extremely conservative attitude in this field, impeding, rather than facilitating, dissemination of knowledge and techniques. Catholic hierarchy has provided the ideological cement for the complex institutional frame opposing the modernization of reproduction. The few private organizations concerned with family planning have played only a minor and insufficient role in the dissemination of contraceptive knowledge.

The indirect effects of the pro-natalist fascist policy, then, have been to reinforce the conservative elements in Italian society that impeded the spread of controlled fertility. It is likely that this reinforcement was most pronounced in the less developed areas of the country, where it slowed the natural development of rationalized reproductive behavior, but was ineffectual in the more developed areas where the limitation of families was far advanced when the fascist policies were initiated.

7.5 *Conclusion*

We have raised more problems in this chapter than we have solved. Three sets of problems have been discussed: (1) the impact of certain biological factors on fertility, particularly before the onset of the decline; (2) the complex interrelations between the economic functions of the family, the norms regulating its formation and growth, and the effects on fertility; and (3) the factors that delayed changes in fertility patterns, particularly in the South and in the Islands.

As for the biological factors, it is possible to establish with a certain degree of confidence, that breastfeeding was generally well prolonged into the second year of life and that women were generally aware of the relationship between prolonged lactation and duration of intervals between births. Indeed, prolonged lactation may be one of the factors that produced the relatively low level of fertility before the decline. It is impossible to establish, however, whether or not it was responsible for regional or class fertility differentials. Two other aspects of fertility have also been considered: age at menarche and at menopause, and the role of morbidity. Age at menarche, given the relatively high age at marriage of Italian women, has little importance; on the other hand, the relatively low age at menopause indicated in nineteenth-century data may have had some effect on fertility at the older ages. Finally, we have suggested that more research into the consequences of morbidity, particularly that of venereal diseases, on sterility and subfecundity could be helpful in completing a basic picture of the biological factors of fertility.

FERTILITY DETERMINANTS

A second set of problems concerns the interrelations between the social and economic functions of the family, and the norms determining its structure and functions. An area in which quantitative insight may be gained is that of the system of land ownership and land use in its relations with the mechanisms controlling the process of family formation. The hypothesis that the increasing subdivision of land through inheritance strongly affects nuptiality patterns and may provide a strong motivation for limiting fertility is not a new one, but it has rarely been tested. It is likely that clear-cut relationships between land ownership and land use and fertility will not be found, unless the investigation is very detailed.

A third set of factors, concerns the forces that have concurred with the slow social and economic development of the South and of the Islands in holding back fertility changes. These forces include education and communications, the role of emigration, and the impact of the fascist demographic policy. At the time of unification, the South and the Islands were already far behind the rest of the country in terms of literacy, education, and system of communications. If diffusion is the vehicle of behavioral changes in fertility, then the hard-core illiteracy of the population and the lack of adequate communications constituted two of the many obstacles to the spreading of new forms of behavior.

As for emigration, its effects are certainly not limited to Southern Italy, since many other areas of the country historically contributed to a permanent outflow of people. But it is from the South and Sicilia that an almost continuous stream of emigrants departed, with the only interruption being the interwar period. It is possible that migration constantly carried away the young members of the society who were potentially most receptive to change, and that migration therefore helped perpetuate traditional patterns of behavior. Those who emigrated did demonstrate their responsiveness by the rapid decline in their fertility, and those who remained did lag behind the rest of Italy in practicing control of fertility. But of course we cannot be sure that the emigrants would have modified their fertility if they had stayed at home.

We have shown that the demographic pro-natalist policy of fascism had only a modest influence on the performance of the cohorts directly affected by this policy, an influence hardly detectable in the aggregate data; but there is ample reason to believe that other effects of a more subtle nature survived the fall of the fascist regime and delayed the demographic change in the socially disadvantaged sectors of the population. These effects can be seen in the survival of antiliberal legislation concerning birth control until very recent years; in the survival of an antisecular mentality in the public administration in matters concerning the family and fertility; in the persistence of a very conservative mentality of the medical class; in the long-lasting influence of the less-enlightened sectors of the clergy; and in the timidity of private action in the field of family planning. Twenty years of pro-natalist propaganda have had a pervasive, long-lasting, and subtle influence, not easily measurable, but nonetheless quite evident in the historical analysis of Italian society.

Conclusion

The broad picture of the decline of fertility in Italy that took place during the last century conforms well to the classic pattern in which birth rates fall when modernization occurs. The decline represented primarily a change in marital fertility. Once started, it proved irreversible. The movement to lower fertility was led by the well-to-do, the better educated, and the residents of the cities; the poor, the illiterate, and the rural population trailed in the reduction of childbearing. In our conclusion, we shall review predecline fertility in Italy, possible deviations from a more general model, aspects of the decline that are generally not included in such a model, and problems of interpretation that still remain.

Of some interest to the demographer and to the historian are certain characteristics of fertility before the end of the nineteenth century when the decline started. One is the relatively moderate level of legitimate fertility, which was about two-thirds of the Hutterite fertility and well below the levels of many populations of Central or Eastern Europe. Indeed, it has been proved that predecline levels of fertility had wide variations; these do not fit the concept of the existence of natural fertility levels determined mainly, if not exclusively, by biological factors. Predecline fertility levels of Spain and Portugal, for instance, were very close to the Italian levels prevailing after the mid-nineteenth century. That populations with high mortality and morbidity, generally poor levels of nutrition, and a very low standard of living had a fertility level one-third below that of a well nourished, healthy, rich, small, and selected population giving religious emphasis to large families hardly comes as a surprise. What is surprising is that other nineteenth-century populations had matched the Hutterite levels, under living conditions in many ways comparable to those of the Mediterranean populations with lower fertility. Therefore, even in populations with comparable degrees of development, very large fertility differentials existed before the beginning of the secular decline.

While the factors underlying the moderate performance of the Italian population cannot be easily explained with available evidence, a few facts give some interesting clues and suggestions for further research. First, there is ample evidence of the existence of fertility differentials during the nineteenth century. Populations living in the urban areas of the North and Center; minorities such as the Jews or the aristocracy of Lombardia, Veneto, or Toscana; and the well-educated middle class were showing unmistakable evidence of controlled fertility before the decline became apparent for the entire population. These low fertility minority groups, however, were too small in number to account for the relatively moderate level of the entire population. Excluding them would not appreciably raise the overall fertility of the national, or even of the provincial, population.

A second fact that may have some weight in explaining the reasons for the moderate predecline fertility is the widespread habit of breastfeeding children well into their second year of life. Closely related to this is the fact that couples seem to have been aware of the logical link between the duration of breastfeeding and birth intervals. In some cases, people disapproved of couples having many children and short intervals between births and considered their behavior as deviant. It appears, therefore, that concern for the dimensions of the family was not alien to the psychology of the Italian couple prior to the beginning of the decline, and that their natural fertility was influenced by a conscious effort to prolong interbirth intervals.

The existence of groups that controlled fertility, in some cases before the nineteenth century, does, however, prove two important facts. First, it proves that groups sufficiently motivated had the knowledge and the necessary will to lower fertility. That the decline did not spread to other segments of the population until the end of the century may be the consequence of both the relative rigidity of class and group structure within the society and the lack of mobility between classes and groups. On the other hand, it is also possible that a certain degree of fertility control existed in other groups of the population, but we were unable to detect it owing to the lack of statistical evidence. Second, differential fertility prior to the general decline proves that the roots of behavior modification often come into being far before a particular change becomes apparent in any way. This is hardly a novelty for the historian, but demographers tend to overlook this fact when only a limited period of the demographic history of a population is well known.

There is ample ground for research in the field of premodern demography. Family reconstitution and ad hoc surveys for selected social groups may add further evidence of fertility differentials. Investigation of the folklore and of medical evidence may deepen our knowledge on the diffusion of breastfeeding. More data on customs and culture, particularly with reference to marriage and the family, may broaden our knowledge of the attitudes and preferences regarding procreation held by the nineteenth-century population. Greater understanding of the impact of biological factors and morbidity on fertility might be obtained through better use of medical and hospital records.

The Italian data suggest an interesting cycle in the average number of living children in well-to-do, as compared to poor, families. The decline of fertility radically changed a situation that, as far as we know, may have lasted for centuries; the end of the decline may restore the previous pattern once again. Historical evidence clearly shows that, before the nineteenth century, rich families had, at any given point of their life, a higher number of surviving children than poor families. This difference is probably due to a lower age at marriage among the rich, the lower mortality of their children, and, possibly, their higher fertility. The result was that those who had the greater means had also a larger number of mouths to feed. During the nineteenth century and the first half of the twentieth, in Italy as in other western countries, this logical pattern was broken; the rich started to limit offspring, while the poor continued their traditional behavior. The classical inverse relationship thus developed between the wealth of a family and the number of children requiring support: the poor, at all ages, had the largest family burdens. The higher mortality of the poor classes was not sufficient to balance the lower fertility of the rich. In general, nuptiality differentials seemed to accentuate, rather than dampen, the differences between the poor (who tended to marry at younger ages) and the rich. In any society it is probably possible to identify the period in which the differential burden of raising a family between the poor and the rich attained its maximum. In Italy this point was reached between the two world wars; many large areas of the country had fallen below replacement, while in other areas entire regional populations still maintained premodern levels of fertility.

Then the course of events brought about the reappearance of the traditional balance; fertility fell rapidly among the poor and rose among the rich. Data for urban areas in 1961 show that fertility differentials had been greatly reduced and that a U-shaped relationship between economic and social levels and fertility had replaced the inverse relationship; it is probable that this foreshadows a direct relationship. When this direct relationship will be achieved, a historical equilibrium, broken by the rapid fall of fertility beginning in the nineteenth century, will be restored.

Seen in this broad historical perspective, the development of an inverse relationship between economic level and fertility is revealed as a transient and unnatural situation: it is a deviation from a natural historical pattern that is bound to be eliminated. The rapidity of the decline of fertility may be viewed therefore as a function of the differences in family size created between privileged groups and the rest of the population, and as a function of the competition between these two segments of the population. Innovation, imitation, or diffusion are the technical means through which the behavior of the privileged groups is accepted by the rest of the population.

This scheme seems to fit the Italian experience well. In the North and the Center, where ample group differentials in fertility were evident before World War I, the decline was relatively rapid and, for the largest part, accomplished between 1911 and 1931. In the South, group differentials have always been very minor, and there was only a very gradual erosion of the levels of fertility. Not even the unprecedented development after World War II could accelerate the decline. The reasons for the lack of large group fertility differentials are hard to explain. Differences in social and economic level were perhaps more marked in the South than elsewhere in Italy. Feudalism survived until very recently in fact if not in a legal sense. The elites, however, derived their wealth from the land; they were more the guardians of tradition than the innovators; they drew part of their strength from the support of the church and from the system of values that a not too enlightened clergy was happy to impose on the masses. The middle class, the professionals, and the urban industrial workers were few in number, and very much integrated into the value system of the agrarian South. The census of 1931 showed that there was less difference between the fertility of the professionals and the fertility of the rural workers in the South than between the fertility of the professionals in the South and that of the professionals in the North. The lack of fertility differentials (and, therefore, of the stimulus for the response from the less-privileged sectors of the population) and the lack of competition between groups have probably deprived the South of two powerful factors bringing about a fertility decline.

The attempt to explain the decline of fertility with the help of several social and economic indicators met with moderate success. In Chapter 5 we discussed at length the limitations of the multivariate analysis for evaluating the association between fertility levels and changes in different periods and the characteristics of the provincial populations. Of the six indicators employed in the analysis—proportion married, infant mortality, illiteracy, industrialization, ruralization, and urbanization—the first three show the highest partial association. Multiple correlation is relatively high when fertility differentials are high but multiple regression is a poor predictor of provincial fertility either before the onset of the decline or when fertility has reached moderate levels.

The analysis of covariance, on the other hand, clearly shows that in the North and the Center, when allowance is made for the effects of the various socioeconomic variables, fertility differences among regions remain significant. In other words, if we make the hypothesis that regions had the same socioeconomic level, we still would find significant, although reduced, fertility differentials. This means that other factors, not accounted for by the variable retained, were at work in determining regional differentials. The nature of the finding is negative: the indicators employed that we believe to have some action in determining fertility levels, especially during the decline, reduce, but only to a minor extent, the differences in the fertility performances of the regions.

In the South and the Islands, fertility differentials are generally not significant before allowing for the different impact of the socioeconomic indicators; when allowance is made for the effects of the six variables, regional differences are diminished.

In less technical words, if we want a full explanation of the regional fertility differentials in the North and the Center, we have to look for factors not included in the six retained in the multivariate analysis. The difference among regions is a residual that depends on factors not included in the available statistics. The situation in the South and the Islands is different; the regional populations have a very homogeneous behavior as far as fertility is concerned. The lack of geographical differentials in the South is consistent with the lack of group differentials that we have discussed before, and that we hold in part responsible for the slow fertility decline of the South.

The success of multivariate analysis depends very much on the choice of independent variables. The quality of census data, the limited number of social and economic characteristics measured by early censuses or by other statistical sources, and the loose relationship tying these characteristics to the causal determinants of fertility are all serious limitations to this type of analysis. The proportion of the Italians voting in favor of, or against, the divorce law in 1974 is the best single predictor of the provincial fertility levels not only in 1961 and in 1951 but also in 1931 and 1911. This fact clearly shows that when the independent variables are not well suited for the purpose, the results of the multivariate analysis have to be accepted with a great deal of circumspection.

Other factors, often unmeasurable, have certainly been at work in determining fertility trends during the last century. In the last chapter we discussed some of the factors that were responsible for the slow decline of fertility in the South and contributed to the differential development of Italy during the last century. Education, closely correlated with the diffusion of ideas and innovation, and a system of communications, closely tied with the mobility of people, have developed at a much slower pace in the South than in the rest of the country. The continuous emigration from the South during the last century has also had a negative effect by depriving the population both of tensions that might have led to innovation and of people who probably were more receptive to new ideas and new modes of behavior. Emigration had had selective effects, and the extremely rapid adaptation of the Italian emigrants to the fertility levels of the receiving country is one element in favor of the theory. Finally, the pro-natalist policy of fascism has had long-range effects by retarding the recognition of personal rights in the field of procreation and creating an institutional frame in which the public administration, the medical class, and the educational system have consistently hindered access to the knowledge and the technical means of family planning. This attitude, still in part surviving, has particularly affected the less-developed sectors of the population and particularly the South.

It is our opinion that further research at the aggregate level is not likely to add to the general picture of fertility decline given in this book. However, two different approaches do merit attention.

With the first approach, at the micro-level, the characteristics of fertility decline could be followed for selected groups of the population. For instance, the comparative evolution of fertility and nuptiality in the agricultural classes, according to the type of land-ownership system and in connection with the analysis of the structure of the family and of the response to changing economic conditions, could prove extremely productive. This type of approach, however, could be followed only on a small scale, and on the basis of data collection from nominative records.

On the other hand, a satisfactory interpretation of the factors of fertility decline cannot be done without a careful reconstitution of the *histoire des mentalités.* The gradual acceptance of fertility control has to be explained in the light of the general evolution of the attitudes of the population. Modifications of religious feelings and of the prevailing morale, changes in the relations between men and women and parents and children, and the development of a political conscience and the formation of a class conscience among the rural, urban, industrial, and middle classes are some of the many important elements necessary for the reconstitution of the general cultural climate generating the changes of attitudes on procreation.

The first approach is the demographer's task. But he cannot ignore the second, unless he is resigned to accepting a purely deterministic interpretation of demographic trends.

Appendix A

Notes on the Quality of Data

1. We have already pointed out the main reasons for believing birth registration to be relatively accurate.[1] In short, registration of baptism had an old tradition, going back in its primitive form to the fourteenth century. The thick network of parishes covered the entire territory, and the watchful eye of the priest, together with the common feeling of performing a necessary religious act, made baptism of children almost universal. In many instances, the health of the child was jeopardized by taking him to the church in spite of adverse season and distance. Before the unification of the country, registration of vital events was certainly not faultless, but it was sufficiently complete for our purposes. Serious biases affected the classification of births as live or as stillbirths, the latter being systematically underregistered, as well as the distinction between legitimate and illegitimate. These inconveniences lasted for several decades after the unification of the country and the centralization of the statistical services. It is likely that the major sources of errors, particularly in pre-unification times, derived from the very imperfect criteria followed in the collection of parish data and in their presentation at the aggregate level (diocese, province, region, etc.).

2. Unlike in other Mediterranean countries, such as Spain or Portugal, there is in Italy no evidence of differential completeness of registration by sex. In Appendix Table A.1 we have reported the sex ratio ($M/F \cdot 100$) for 16 regions in 1862–1970. The ratio ranges between a minimum of 1.052 and a maximum of 1.076. In the following decades, the sex ratio continues to remain within the normal range.

3. A good way of testing the completeness and consistency of registration is through the matching male cohorts at birth, early infancy, and at the time of the compulsory military draft.[2] At the age of 20, every male was drafted and underwent a medical examination. Escaping the draft was a rare event, and in many occasions proof of compliance with mili-

[1] For a historical evaluation of the sources, see the first volume of the Gruppo di Demografia Storica, *Atti del Seminario*, Roma, 1973, particularly the essay by C. Corsini.

[2] R. Benini, *La demografia italiana nell'ultimo cinquantennio*, Roma, 1911, p. 15.

APPENDIX A

APPENDIX TABLE A.1

SEX RATIO OF LIVE BIRTHS, BY REGION: 1862-1870

Region	Ratio	Region	Ratio	Region	Ratio
Piemonte	1.064	Marche	1.062	Calabria	1.064
Liguria	1.057	Umbria	1.072	Basilicata	1.056
Lombardia	1.057	Lazio	1.064[b]	Sicilia	1.056
Veneto	1.076[a]	Campania	1.058	Sardegna	1.070
Emilia	1.061	Abruzzi	1.054		
Toscana	1.064	Puglia	1.052	Italy	1.064

NOTE: Data refer to ratio of males to females, multiplied by 100.

[a]1867-1875

[b]1862-1870

tary obligations was required. Every year the cohort born 20 years before was drafted; the draft call was based partly on the same birth records, but partly also on census records and on any other direct or indirect information. The two sources are, therefore, partially independent, and their good matching is a good index of their consistency and of their quality.

In Appendix Table A.2 we have reported, for each cohort born from 1866 to 1894, the number of male live births; the number of males surviving at age 5 (calculated on the basis of death records), and the number of draftees belonging to the same generation at a mean age of 20.

The difference between the number of survivors at age 5 and the number of draftees of the same cohort is the result of mortality, emigration, and various errors in the data.

Appendix Table A.2 offers two checks of the consistency and quality of data. The first can be made by observing the percentage of change between each cohort and the successive one in the number of survivors at age 5 and of draftees aged 20. The coincidence of variations is almost perfect; the coefficient of correlation is +.980, explaining 96 percent of the variance. The close similarity of variation of survivors at age 5 and draftees, from one cohort to the following, demonstrates that the sources, although partially independent, are consistent in their fluctuations. This is not, however, a proof of their quality since one of the two (i.e. birth statistics) could be biased by a constant amount and still fluctuate in close agreement with the other.

APPENDIX TABLE A.2

MALE BIRTHS, SURVIVORS AT AGE 5 AND DRAFTEES AT AGE 20 :
BIRTH COHORTS 1877 TO 1894

Cohort	Live male births	Male survivors at age 5	Draftees mean age 20	Percentage change between preceding cohort and		Ratio of draftees to survivors at age 5
				Survivors at age 5	Draftees	
1877	529,867	329,723	287,816	--	--	.8729
1878	521,495	324,691	283,464	-1.53	-1.51	.8730
1879	548,959	338,867	294,277	+4.37	+3.81	.8684
1880	493,591	306,887	267,723	-9.44	-9.02	.8723
1881	557,029	351,923	311,423	+14.68	+16.32	.8849
1882	545,714	345,916	311,059	-1.71	-0.12	.8992
1883	551,402	353,053	315,220	+2.06	+1.34	.8928
1884	581.413	374,520	329,994	+6.08	+4.69	.8809
1885	580,079	375,279	323,440	+0.20	-1.82	.8618
1886	559,441	363,932	313,814	-3.02	-2.98	.8624
1887	592,936	387,414	338,525	+6.45	+7.87	.8738
1888	575,081	378,798	336,351	-2.22	-0.62	.8879
1889	591,480	392,132	354,163	+3.52	+5.30	.9031
1890	556,378	368,725	333,644	-5.97	-5.79	.9048
1891	581,818	392,567	353,488	+6.47	+5.95	.9004
1892	570,782	388,341	352,807	-1.08	-0.19	.9084
1893	579,076	396,213	356,786	+2.03	+1.13	.9004
1894	566,412	386,582	348,235	-2.44	-2.37	.9008

SOURCES: Male survivors at age 5: L. GALVANI, Calcolo delle probabilità di morte in generale ed applicazione alla misura della mortalità infantile nella popolazione italiana dal 1873 in poi, "Annali di Statistica", VI, Vol. XVII, 1931 pp.36 and ff.
Draftees: A. COSTANZO, La statura degli italiani ventenni nati dal 1854 al 1920, in "Annali di Statistica", VIII, Vol. II 1948, and Annuario Statistico Italiano, various issues.

However, the second check shows that there was also a considerable consistency in the estimate of the numerical size of each cohort as provided by the two sources. The ratio of draftees to survivors at age 5 oscillates between 86 percent and 91 percent and tends to increase from 87 percent in 1877–1878 to 90 percent in 1893–1894. During the same period, expectation of life at birth for males grew from about 35 years (life table of 1881–1882) to 40 years (life table of 1900–1902); this means that the first cohorts must have experienced a mortality, between 5 and

20 years of age, of about 9 percent, against 7 percent for the more recent cohorts. The residual loss of 3 to 4 percent can be easily explained by emigration, which reached its peak during the last decade of the nineteenth century and the first fifteen years of the twentieth century (net migration amounted to —1,378,000 in 1892–1901 and —1,417,000 in 1902–1911, or 4.2 percent and 4.1 percent of the 1891 and 1901 populations).

4. Other minor biases of vital registration are of a lesser interest in our case. We have discussed at length illegitimacy; we will not take time to discuss in detail the nature and reasons of the bias in the stillbirth statistics, whose increasing completeness is revealed by the rising trend from the 1860s to the beginning of this century. Another curious bias, of little relevance for us, was the tendency, until the 1920s, to postpone the registration of live births, particularly of boys, from December to January of the following year.[3] This was done to delay the military service for one year and also, it is believed, to render girls one solar year younger. Whichever the motivation, the bias affected 8 percent of all December male births from 1885 to 1914, against 3 percent for females; it rose to 14 percent in 1915–1919 and 19 percent in 1920–1924 for males, and to 7 percent in the latter period for females.[4]

At the regional level, this bias was much stronger in the South than in the rest of the country; in 1924–1925 it was estimated that the unlawful postponement of births affected approximately 40 percent of the December male births of Campania and Puglia, and 50 percent of those of Puglia and Sicilia.[5]

5. We must stress again here the better quality of vital records as compared to the quality of censuses, particularly of the first ones. The inexperience in census taking and the high degree of illiteracy of the population are the main causes of the imperfections of the first census operations. In practice, only the Regno di Sardegna had an established experience in census taking, with the three enumerations in 1838, 1848, and 1858. In other states experience was totally lacking (Veneto and Regno delle due Sicilie) or was limited to primitive forms of census

[3] L. Livi, "Sulle false dichiarazioni della data di nascita per i nati alla fine dell'anno, e rettifica della distribuzione mensile delle nascite nel triennio 1923-25," Annali di Statistica VI, Vol. III, 129.

[4] Livi, "Sulle false," p. 49.

[5] *Ibid.*, pp. 63-73.

taking (Toscana and Stato Pontificio), or was very recent in a modern form (Lombardia, Parma, and Modena: censuses of 1857–1858).

Misreporting of age was one of the main biases. Only with the census of 1901 was the exact date of birth requested; in preceding censuses, only the age (in completed years) was asked.[6] This resulted in a very strong underestimate of children under 2 years of age and, in general, in a very marked heaping at "round" ages.

Galvani devised a formula for the estimate of age-heaping in age groups terminating in zero (in case of age distribution in 5-year age groups).[7] The index of regularity is:

$$\frac{S_p}{S_d} : \frac{S'_d}{S'_p}$$

where designing with $y_1, y_2, \ldots y_{11}$ the 5-year age groups from 25-29 to 75-79,

$$\begin{aligned} Sp &= y_2 + y_4 + y_6 + y_8 + y_{10} \\ Sd &= 1/2(y_1 + y_{11}) + y_3 + y_5 + y_7 + y_9 \\ S'd &= y_3 + y_5 + y_7 + y_9 \\ S'p &= 1/2(y_2 + y_{10}) + y_4 + y_6 + y_8 \end{aligned}$$

In case of a relatively unperturbed age structure, the index approaches 1 when ages are stated correctly, but, supposing that no other biases are at work but age rounding, Sp/Sd tends to be above 1 if there is a tendency to rounding at ages terminating in 0 stronger than for ages terminating in 5, while, on the contrary, $S'd/S'p$ tends to be below 1.

For the entire Italian population, the index of regularity is reported, for males and females, in Appendix Table A.3. The regularity of the age distribution is rapidly increasing, and a radical progress is made with the 1901 census (exact date of birth was asked for the first time). The age distribution is more regular for males than for females. There is also ample evidence that age-heaping was much stronger in the less literate regions. One example is sufficient: in 1881, the index of regularity for the population of Piemonte was 1.11 for males and 1.15 for females, against 2.04 and 2.35 for the male and female population of Sicilia.

[6] Benini, *La demografia*, pp. 21-23, ISTAT, *VII Censimento Generale della popolazione*, Vol. IV, part I, Roma, 1935, p. 45.

[7] L. Galvani, "Alcune osservazioni sul VI Censimento generale della popolazione Italiana," Annali di Statistica VI, Vol. XVIII, 1931, pp. 78-83.

APPENDIX TABLE A.3

INDEX OF REGULARITY OF THE AGE STRUCTURE (20-80), BY SEX: 1861 TO 1931

Census	Males	Females
1861	1.53	1.76
1871	1.31	1.36
1881	1.31	1.38
1901	1.02	1.06
1911	1.04	1.06
1921	1.02	1.04
1931	1.01	1.01

6. Given their better quality, vital statistics have always been used as a yardstick for measuring the accuracy of census taking. This has been done in particular for the infant age groups, almost always under-enumerated. In the Appendix Table A.4, the census population under age 5 is compared with the estimate of the same age group based on births

APPENDIX TABLE A.4

ENUMERATED AND ESTIMATED POPULATION UNDER AGE 5: 1881 TO 1921

Date	Census population, 0-4	Estimated population, 0-4	Difference, Census-Estimate Absolute	Percentage
		MALES		
12.31.1881	1,751,493	1,878,530	-127,037	-6.76
1. 1.1901	2,099,721	2,146,787	- 47,066	-2.19
6.30.1911	2,204,269	2,262 213	- 54,944	-2.42
12.31.1921	1,799,933	1,842,487	- 42,554	-2.30
		FEMALES		
12.31.1881	1,588,556	1,805,314	-116,758	-6.45
1. 1.1901	2,016 972	2,067 554	- 50,582	-2.44
6.30.1911	2,123,064	2,191,952	- 68,888	-3.14
12.31.1921	1,728 439	1,766,731	- 38,292	-2.20

SOURCE: L. GALVANI, Alcune osservazioni sul VI Censimento generale della popolazione Italiana, "Annali di Statistica", Serie VI, Vol. XVII, 1931, pp.142-144.

and deaths of the five years preceding the census. The underenumeration of this group is 6 to 7 percent for the 1881 census, and falls to 2 to 3 percent for the 1901, 1911, and 1921 censuses. Since we have to admit that emigration also took place among infants, these later census enumerations match rather closely the estimates based on vital statistics. Similar comparison is impossible for the 1861 census (vital statistics for 1857–1861 are not available), and for the 1871 census, vital statistics were not available for Lazio, and the age distribution of deaths was inadequate).

7. The 1921 census reported a clearly overenumerated population in the regions of the South. Many comuni inflated their populations both not to show a declining or slowly increasing population (as a result of emigration and of war deaths) and not to lose the administrative, financial, and political prerogatives by falling in a lower class dimension. ISTAT was aware of the fraud, and in 1931 gave a correction—without stating what criteria were followed—of the total population of these regions. If the ISTAT correction is true, the population of Campania had been inflated by 5.6 percent, that of Abruzzi and Molise by 2.0 percent; Puglia, 5.0 percent; Basilicata, 2.5 percent; Calabria, 4.2 percent; Sicilia, 11.2 percent; and Sardegna, 0.5 percent.[8]

The computation of the fertility indexes for 1921 has been made on the basis of the corrected population, using the same correcting factor for the various age and marital status groups. The closer control of ISTAT has avoided similar macroscopic distortions in later censuses, although many comuni are reluctant, even now, to admit that many emigrants have departed for good and try to keep them in their records.

[8] O. Vitali, *Aspetti dello sviluppo economico italiano alla luce della ricostruzione della popolazione attiva*, Roma, 1970, p. 282.

Appendix B

The Computation of the Mean Number of Children per Marriage, F

In the absence of census data, it may be possible to estimate the level of fertility, without recourse to family reconstitution, on the basis of the series of legitimate births and marriages. When births are recorded according to the duration of marriage, fertility rates by duration of marriage can be computed for any year in which the distribution of married women by duration of marriage is known or can be estimated. If M_i is the number of women in the ith year of marriage, and n_i is the number of births occurring to them, then f_i is the duration-specific fertility rate for the ith *year*, and $F = \underset{i=0}{\overset{k}{S}} f_i$

(where k is largest duration yielding children) is the mean number of children per marriage according to the fertility of the year in question. F is a period measure of the aggregate production of children by married couples, analogous to the total fertility rate.

F can be approximated in the absence of the rarely found tabulation of births by duration of marriage provided the number of married women at duration i does not differ excessively from the number of marriages i years earlier—in other words if the effects of migration and marital dissolution are moderate. Under these circumstances M_i can be approximated by the number of marriages i years before the year in question, and F can be approximated by a procedure analogous to indirect standardization.

Specifically, a standard distribution of duration-specific fertility rates $\bar{f}_i$, adjusted in scale so that $\Sigma \bar{f}_i = \bar{F}$ is 1.0, is used to calculate the number of births that would occur, given these rates and the observed number of marriages, M_i, in the preceding years. The ratio of the observed births to this calculated number is the estimated mean size of family—ignoring the effects of migration and marital dissolution, and assuming that the *structure* of fertility by duration was the same as in the standard duration-specific schedule. This simple method was applied, for the first time, by Gini for estimating Italian fertility on the basis of a special tabulation of births by duration of marriage in 1927.[1]

[1] C. Gini, *Di un procedimento per la determinazione del numero medio dei figli legittimi per matrimonio*, Atti del Congresso Internazionale per gli Studi sulla Popolazione, Vol. x, Roma, 1934, pp. 41-68. See also a critical discussion of Gini's procedure in G. Mortara, "Sui metodi di studio della fecondità dei matrimoni," *Giornale degli Economisti*, XLVIII (Dec. 1933), pp. 890-897.

For the computation of F for the nineteenth century, we have applied the percentage distribution (graphically smoothed) of birth by duration of marriage for 216 families of Fiesole (Firenze), marriages 1630–1680. This distribution, typical of a population with little fertility control has been used for the estimate of F for the Italian regions prior to the end of World War I. For the period between the two wars (1919–1940), we have used another standard distribution based on the 1927 national schedule. For the last quarter of a century (1941–1965), we have employed the national schedule of 1931 for the regions of the South, which still had a relatively high level of fertility, and the 1953 national schedule for the regions of the North and Center, where fertility was very low. Appendix Table B.1 clearly shows the increasing concentration of fertility at the low durations of marriage as F decreases; it would be a useful and not too difficult job to provide a series of "model" distributions of f_i according to the general level of fertility and to the age at marriage.

APPENDIX TABLE B.1

DISTRIBUTION OF BIRTHS ACCORDING TO MARRIAGE DURATION: FIESOLE, 1630-1680, AND ITALY, 1927 AND 1953

Duration of marriage	Fiesole, 1630-1680 (F = 6.0)	Italy, 1927 (F = 3.6)	Italy, 1953 (F = 2.5)
0 - 4	38.5	46.9	52.5
5 - 9	18.2	24.9	24.2
10 - 14	19.2	15.6	13.7
15 - 19	10.3	8.9	6.9
20 - 24	3.4	3.2	2.5
25 and over	0.4	0.5	0.2

The standard schedule employed has a relatively mild effect on the level of the estimated F when the series of marriages is relatively stable, as it happens to be in the majority of cases. To test this assumption, we have computed F for the regions in 1880 and 1914 using both the Fiesole (1630–1680) and the Italian schedules (1927). In 1880, the differences between the two sets of estimates are very small, going from a maximum of 2.2 percent (Marche) to a minimum of zero (Veneto, Liguria, and Campania). In 1914, differences are between a high of 1.2 percent (Puglia) and a low of zero (Emilia and Basilicata).

APPENDIX B

We have done the same test for 1925 and 1938, using the national 1927 and 1953 schedules. The differences between the two sets of estimates are all below the maximum of 3 percent in 1925 (Veneto) and 2.8 percent (Lazio) in 1938.

Appendix C

Provincial Series

The administrative subdivision of the country into provinces has changed considerably throughout the last century: the number of provinces has increased from 59 in 1861 to 94 in 1961.

The variation in the number of provinces resulted from:

(1) Annexation of new territories (Veneto in 1866, Lazio in 1870, Trentino and Venezia Giulia in 1918), adding a total (1961 boundaries) of 16 provinces
(2) Loss of part of Venezia Giulia to Jugoslavia after World War II, entailing the loss of two provinces
(3) Creation of new provinces with the territory of one or more provinces

This process was particularly intense during the 1920s. The new provinces, by year in which they were set up, and, within parentheses, by provinces with whose territory they have been formed, are:

1923: Taranto (Lecce)
1927: Vercelli (Novara); Aosta (Torino); Savona and La Spezia (Genova); Varese (Como, Milano); Pistoia (Firenze, Lucca); Terni (Perugia); Rieti (Perugia, L'Aquila); Frosinone (Roma, Caserta); Viterbo (Roma); Pescara (Chieti, Teramo); Brindisi (Lecce); Matera (Potenza); Enna (Caltanissetta, Catania); Ragusa (Siracusa); Nuoro (Cagliari, Sassari)
1934: Latina (Roma)
1935: Asti (Alessandria)

These extensive changes make it impossible to compare provincial series throughout the century. As far as the series of fertility and nuptiality measures are concerned, provincial indexes have been computed for all provinces at all censuses, with the exclusion of the 1901 and 1921 censuses because the combined distribution of the sex, age, and marital status population was not published at the provincial level.

We have therefore attempted the reconstitution of the populations of the provinces in 1881 and 1911 in their 1961 boundaries. This has been possible because the necessary tabulations had been published, in 1881 and 1911, for the circondari, the smaller administrative unit within each province. In many cases, the subdivision of a province to create a new province had been done following the boundaries of one or more circondari. In these instances it was sufficient to take the population of the circondario forming the new province, or to add together the populations of the two or more circondari forming the new province, and subtract it from the old one. In some instances, however, a circondario was subdivided, one part remaining to the old province, the other going to the new province. In these cases we had to go to the smallest administrative unit, the comune, to apportion the population of the circondario between the old and the new province. In these instances, however, since the population of the comune was not available at the two censuses in question by sex, age, and marital status, we had to make the hypothesis that the two parts of the circondario (the one remaining in the old province and the other going to the new one) were identical as far as these characteristics were concerned. By so doing, we were able to compute a comparable series of provincial fertility and nuptiality measures and socioeconomic indicators for 1881, 1901, 1931, 1936, 1951 and 1961. Provincial fertility and nuptiality measures for 1861 and 1871 are comparable only when no territorial change has taken place.

The identification of the provinces in the maps has been made with numbers (see Map 4.1). Numbers without primes refer to the original provinces in 1861 or at the moment of the territorial annexation. A number with one or more primes refers to a province created with the territory of the province having the same number but no prime.

Official Statistical Sources

1. *Census Statistics*

[1861] DIRSTAT, vv. I, II, III: *Popolazione, Relazione; Popolazione di diritto; Popolazione delle provincie, circondari e comuni*, Firenze, 1863-1867.

[1871] DIRSTAT, v. I: *Popolazione presente ed assente per comuni, centri e frazioni di comuni*; v. II: *Analfabeti distinti per età – Popolazione per sesso, stato civile ed istruzione*; v. III: *Popolazione classificata per professioni; Classificazione dei comuni secondo la popolazione; Censimento degli italiani all'estero; Stranieri in Italia*, Roma, 1874-1876.

[1881] DIRSTAT, v. I, parte I: *Popolazione dei comuni e dei mandamenti*; parte II: *Popolazione secondo la qualità della dimora degli abitanti, nei Comuni – Assenti – Famiglie o convivenze sociali – Abitazioni – Nati all'estero e cittadini stranieri – Numero dei ciechi, dei sordomuti e degli idioti e dei cretini*; v. II: *Popolazione per età, sesso, stato civile ed istruzione elementare*; v. III: *Popolazione classificata per professioni o condizioni; Relazione generale; Tabella della popolazione presente e residente; Circoscrizioni giudiziarie e circoscrizioni ecclesiastiche in relazione alle circoscrizioni amministrative*; 2 volumes; *Censimento degli italiani all'estero*, Roma, 1882-1885.

[1901] DIRSTAT, v. I: *Popolazione dei comuni e delle frazioni divisa in agglomerata e sparsa*; v. II: *Numero delle famiglie e degli abitanti secondo la qualità della dimora, luogo di nascita, sesso, età, stato civile e istruzione – Ciechi – Sordomuti – Stranieri – Lingue parlate*; v. III: *Popolazione presente classificata per professioni o condizioni*; v. IV: *Popolazione presente classificata per sesso, età e professione – Convivenze in alberghi, collegi, ospedali, ecc. – Temporaneamente disoccupati – Proprietari di beni immobili – Religione*; v. V: *Relazione; Tabella della popolazione residente o legale e della popolazione presente o di fatto*, Roma, 1901-1904.

[1911] DIRSTAT, v. I: *Popolazione presente (di fatto), popolazione temporaneamente assente e popolazione residente (legale)*; v. II: *Popolazione presente classificata per sesso, età, stato civile e istruzione*; v. III: *L'alfabetismo della popolazione presente*; v. IV: *Popolazione presente, di età superiore ai 10 anni, classificata per sesso e per professione o condizione*; v. V: *Popolazione presente, di età superiore ai 10 anni, classificata per sesso, età e professione o condizione*; v. VI: *Popolazione presente classificata secondo la religione – Popolazione presente classificata secondo il luogo di nascita – Proprietari di beni immobili – Ciechi – Sordomuti – Popolazione presente di età superiore a 90 anni – Stranieri – Famiglie – Convivenze non familiari*; v. VII: *Relazione; Popolazione di fatto dei comuni*, Roma, 1912-1916.

[1921] ISTAT, *Risultati sommari*; 18 volumes with the regional results; *Relazione generale; Tabella della popolazione residente o legale censita nei singoli comuni del Regno; Censimento della popolazione delle colonie italiane al* 1-12-1921 *e rilevazione degli abitanti del Possedimento delle isole Egee al* 20-8-1922, Roma, 1924-1930.

[1931] ISTAT, v. I: *Relazione preliminare e appendici*; v. II: *Popolazione dei comuni e della frazioni di censimento*, parti I, II, III; v. III: 92 provincial volumes; v. IV: *Relazione generale*; v. V: *Colonie e Possedimenti*; v. VI: *Indagine sulla fecondità della donna*; v. VII: *Centri abitati; Diagrammi di distribuzione della popolazione per età, sesso, stato civile; Indagine sulle abitazioni; Elenco dei comuni e frazioni*, Roma, 1933-1936.

[1936] ISTAT, v. I: *Atti del censimento*; v. II: 94 provincial volumes; v. III: *Popolazione – Territorio –Famiglie – Convivenze – Sesso – Stato civile – Età – Stranieri.* Parte I: *Relazione*, parte II: *Tavole*; v. IV: *Professioni*, parte I: *Relazione*, parte II: *Tavole*; v. V: *Libia – Isole italiane dell'Egeo – Tientsin; Popolazione residente e popolazione presente secondo le categorie di attività economica, in ciascun comune del Regno; Caratteri economici, agrari dei compartimenti; Elenco dei comuni e loro popolazione residente*, Roma, 1937-1939.

[1951] ISTAT, v. I: *Dati sommari per comune* (92 provincial volumes and one Appendix with summary data); v. II: *Famiglie e convivenze*; v. III: *Sesso, Età Stato civile, Luogo di nascita*; v. IV: *Professioni*; v. V: *Istruzione*; v. VI: *Abitazioni*; v. VII: *Dati generali riassuntivi*; v. VIII: *Atti del censimento*, Roma, 1952-1958.

[1961] ISTAT, v. I: *Dati riassuntivi comunali e provinciali sulla popolazione e sulle abitazioni*; v. II: *Dati riassuntivi comunali e provinciali su alcune principali caratteristiche strutturali della popolazione*; v. III: *Dati sommari per comune* (92 provincial volumes); v. IV: *Famiglie e convivenze*; v. V: *Sesso, età, stato civile, luogo di nascita*; v. VI: *Professioni*; v. VII: *Istruzione*; v. VIII: *Abitazioni*; v. IX: *Dati generali riassuntivi*; v. X: *Atti del censimento; Popolazione legale dei comuni*, Roma, 1962-1970.

2. *Vital Statistics*

DIRSTAT, *Movimento della popolazione secondo gli atti dello stato civile.* Annual series from 1862 to 1923.
ISTAT, *Movimento della popolazione secondo gli atti dello stato civile.* Annual series from 1924 to 1937.
ISTAT, *Movimento naturale della popolazione presente nei singoli comuni del Regno.* Annual series from 1932 to 1940.
ISTAT, *Movimento della popolazione e cause di morte.* Annual series from 1938 to 1942.
ISTAT, *Movimento della popolazione secondo gli atti dello stato civile negli anni* 1943-48, 1 v., p. 214; *negli anni* 1949-50, 1 v. p. 83.
ISTAT, *Annuario di statistiche demografiche.* Annual series from 1951 to date.

NOTE: DIRSTAT refers to the *Direzione Generale di Statistica*, the public body charged of the collection and publication of official statistics until 1926. After 1926, ISTAT stands for *Istituto Centrale di Statistica*, or Central Statistical Office, created in 1926.

Index

Library of Congress Cataloging in Publication Data

Livi Bacci, Massimo.
A history of Italian fertility during the last two centuries.

Includes index.
1. Fertility, Human--Italy--History. 2. Italy--Population--History. I. Title.
HB1009.L59 301.32'1'0945 76-3271
ISBN 0-691-09369-5

GPSR Authorized Representative: Easy Access System Europe - Mustamäe tee 50, 10621 Tallinn, Estonia, gpsr.requests@easproject.com

www.ingramcontent.com/pod-product-compliance
Lightning Source LLC
LaVergne TN
LVHW011113300926
849160LV00008B/365

* 9 7 8 0 6 9 1 6 0 4 4 6 6 *